Case Reports in Cardiology

From the earliest days of medicine to the present, case reports have been a critical aspect of clinical education and knowledge development. In this comprehensive volume, Dr. William C. Roberts, a renowned expert in the field, explores the rich history and ongoing importance of case reports in cardiology.

Through engaging and insightful analysis, the book demonstrates how case reports have provided physicians with crucial insights into rare diseases, complex conditions, and ground-breaking treatments. Drawing on a vast range of sources, from seminal manuscripts to cutting-edge journals, it offers a unique perspective on the role of case reports in medical education and management of cardiovascular diseases with a special emphasis on diseases and complications related to aorta such as aortic valve stenosis, aortic aneurysm, and others. It underscores how case reports can be used to enhance diagnostic accuracy, identify new treatment options, and promote innovation in the field. In addition, the book provides valuable insights into the process of writing and publishing case reports, including tips for young physicians looking to break into the field.

The book will be an indispensable guide to the history, practice, and ongoing significance of case reports for medical students, physicians, and researchers alike.

KEY FEATURES

- Provides a rich repository of diverse case reports in cardiology published by the editor and his colleagues over 61 years

- Features 46 clinical case studies related to broad Cardiovascular Diseases with a focus on aortic diseases useful for medical students and practicing cardiologists

- It is a valuable resource for young physicians seeking to establish a foothold in medical research and academics

Case Reports in Cardiology

Series Editor

William C. Roberts, MD

Baylor Heart and Vascular Institute, Baylor University Medical Center, Dallas

Case Reports in Cardiology: Congenital Heart Disease
Edited by Dr. William C. Roberts, MD

Case Reports in Cardiology: Valvular Heart Disease
Edited by Dr. William C. Roberts, MD

Case Reports in Cardiology: Coronary Heart Disease and Hyperlipidemia
Edited by Dr. William C. Roberts, MD

Case Reports in Cardiology: Cardiomyopathy
Edited by Dr. William C. Roberts, MD

Case Reports in Cardiology: Cardiac Neoplasm
Edited by Dr. William C. Roberts, MD

Case Reports in Cardiology: Cardiovascular Diseases with a Focus on Aorta
Edited by Dr. William C. Roberts, MD

For more information on this series, please visit https://www.routledge.com/Case-Reports-in-Cardiology/book-series/CRIC

Case Reports in Cardiology
Cardiovascular Diseases with a Focus on Aorta

Edited by

William C. Roberts, MD

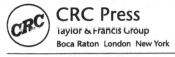

CRC Press
Taylor & Francis Group
Boca Raton London New York

CRC Press is an imprint of the
Taylor & Francis Group, an **informa** business

Designed cover image: Shutterstock

First edition published 2024
by CRC Press
6000 Broken Sound Parkway NW, Suite 300, Boca Raton, FL 33487–2742

and by CRC Press
4 Park Square, Milton Park, Abingdon, Oxon, OX14 4RN

CRC Press is an imprint of Taylor & Francis Group, LLC

ISBN: 978-1-032-52770-3 (hbk)
ISBN: 978-1-032-52768-0 (pbk)
ISBN: 978-1-003-40832-1 (ebk)

DOI: 10.1201/9781003408321

Typeset in Palatino LT Std
by Apex CoVantage, LLC

William Clifford Roberts, MD [1932–2023]
A Remembrance

As a cardiac surgical associate at the NIH in Bethesda for 2 years, I attended my father's Monday conference regularly. There was a case of a healed traumatic aortic rupture. The fellow discovered that the patient was in a motor vehicle accident "several years before death." To this fellow, WCR said, "Write this case up and have it on my desk by Friday." He added, "It takes about as long to write a brief report as it does to write up the chart. Know the case precisely before going to the library to search the literature." He told the fellow to put the aorta in his pocket to remind him what it looked like. "This is a single task, a single mission." What to search for in the library? "Are there any cases of healed traumatic aneurysm of the descending thoracic aorta?" In 30 years, WCR had seen only 1 other, who died 7 days later, not 7 years. This was 1989, of course, before the ubiquitous use of CT scans.

The material for his case reports was this weekly conference in cardiovascular pathology over 6 decades. During these conferences, WCR would personally examine each surgical and autopsy cardiovascular specimen that was submitted—a heart or valve or aorta—and a chart would be created for each patient. He would typically examine each specimen as "an unknown." To him it was a provocative way to conduct the conference. He urged his students and residents and fellows to "remember one thing about each case." To him that was >600 "new things" a year. He believed that studying the case at hand was better than general reading.

In a personal review of his own publications, William Clifford Roberts, MD (WCR) listed 269 case reports out of a total of 1784 publications over a 60-year period, 1961–2022. This sheer number of case reports by one physician in cardiovascular disease is perhaps a record in the field.

As an editor in chief of 2 medical journals, he carefully considered the value of case reports:

> Usually, case reports have only 1 point, and information not pertinent to that point is unnecessary. Indeed, unnecessary words and nonessential details actually prevent clear focus on the patient. Thus, these "Brief Reports" must be brief—no more than 2 or 3 double-spaced typed pages with few references. Reports only 1 page long will be favored over those 3 pages long. Pertinent illustrations may be the dominant element in conveying the message...Brief Reports require clear thinking. Each word must count.

In nearly every case report of WCR, there is an illustration or photograph. WCR preferred "drawings not words." He would say, "There is nothing more important than absolutely perfect photographs." In his first 20 years at NIH, he spent every Tuesday and Thursday morning from 9am to noon with a photographer. He believed the subject should occupy "85% of the frame."

WCR graduated from Southern Methodist University (1954) and Emory University School of Medicine (1958), then had 6 years of residency training. For the next 60 years (1964-2023), he focused exclusively on cardiovascular pathology. The first 30 years were spent at NIH in Bethesda and the second 30 years at Baylor University Medical Center in Dallas. He held his weekly conference past 90 years of age.

My younger brother, John David Roberts, observed that WCR was "an intense scholar, but also a loving person. He had both qualities. He was loved for the person, not the accomplishments. One would never know he was a physician in daily interactions. He was satisfied to be unknown. Though in the Public Health Service for 30 years, he never wore the Navy uniform, even when it was recommended at NIH. As a father he required respect, which included "Yes Sir" and "No Sir." Manners were important to him, especially at the table for the evening meal, where each of his children was asked to express what he or she learned that day.

He will be remembered by his family not only for his contribution to the field of medicine, but for his hungry intellect, his indominable work ethic, his high standards, and his loyalty to loved ones.

Charles Stewart Roberts, MD
October 1, 2023

Contents

Preface..xi

About the Editor..xiii

Introduction..xv

Miscellaneous Cardiovascular Disease

Case 55.   Roberts WC, Fredrickson DS. Gaucher's Disease of the Lung
            Causing Severe Pulmonary Hypertension with Associated Acute
            Recurrent Pericarditis. *Circulation*. 1967;35(4):783–789 3

Case 57.   Glancy DL, Yarnell P, Roberts WC. Traumatic Left Ventricular
            Aneurysm. Cardiac Thrombosis Following Aneurysmectomy.
            Am J Cardiol. 1967;20(3):428–433 11

Case 63.   Glancy DL, Bohjalian O, Roberts WC. An Unusual Nephritis in
            Malignant Hypertension. *Arch Intern Med*. 1967;120(5):625–630......19

Case 283.   Lachman AS, Spray TL, Kerwin DM, Shugoll GI, Roberts WC.
            Medial Calcinosis of Mönckeberg. A Review of the Problem
            and a Description of a Patient with Involvement of Peripheral,
            Visceral and Coronary Arteries. *Am J Med*. 1977;63(4):615–622 26

Case 342.   Roberts WC, Brownlee WJ, Jones AA, Luke JL. Sucking Action of
            the Left Ventricle: Demonstration of a Physiologic Principle by
            A Gunshot Wound Penetrating Only the Right Side of the Heart.
            Am J Cardiol. 1979;43(6):1234–1237 37

Case 384.   Waller BF, Brownlee WJ, Roberts WC. Self-Induced Pulmonary
            Granulomatosis. A Consequence of Intravenous Injection of
            Drugs Intended for Oral Use. *Chest*. 1980;78(1):90–94. 42

Case 412.   Waller BF, Dean PJ, Mann O, Rosen JH, Roberts WC. Right
            Ventricular Outflow Obstruction from Thrombus with Small
            Peripheral Pulmonary Emboli. *Chest*. 1981;79(2):224–225 49

Case 431.   Siegel RJ, Cabeen WR Jr, Roberts WC. Prolonged QT Interval—
            Ventricular Tachycardia Syndrome from Massive Rapid Weight
            Loss Utilizing the Liquid-Protein-Modified-Fast Diet: Sudden
            Death with Sinus Node Ganglionitis and Neuritis. *Am Heart J*.
            1981;102(1):121–122 52

Case 438.   Waller BF, Roberts WC. Systolic Clicks Caused by Rocks in the
            Right Heart Chambers. *Am Heart J*. 1981;102(3 Pt 1):459–460 55

Case 462.   Lindgren KM, McShane K, Roberts WC. Acute Rupture of the
            Pulmonic Valve by a Balloon-tipped Catheter Producing a
            Musical Diastolic Murmur. *Chest*. 1982;81(2):251–253 58

Case 653.   Ross EM, Macher AM, Roberts WC. *Aspergillus Fumigatus*
            Thrombi Causing Total Occlusion of Both Coronary Arterial
            Ostia, All Four Major Epicardial Coronary Arteries and
            Coronary Sinus and Associated with Purulent Pericarditis. *Am J
            Cardiol*. 1985;56(7):499–500 63

---

* **Note:** *Cases are numbered based on their number in WCR's CV.*

Case 703.   Barbour DJ, Inglesby TV, Roth JA, Roberts WC. Pulmonary
              Arterial and Venous Hypertension and Left Ventricular
              Calcification of Undetermined Etiology. *Am J Cardiol.*
              1986;58(7):661–663 66

Case 728.   Levine S, McManus BM, Blackbourne BD, Roberts WC. Fatal
              Water Intoxication, Schizophrenia, and Diuretic Therapy for
              Systemic Hypertension. *Am J Med.* 1987;82(1):153–155 70

Case 834.   Mann JM, Pierre-Louis M, Kragel PJ, Kragel AH, Roberts WC.
              Cardiac Consequences of Massive Acetaminophen Overdose.
              Am J Cardiol. 1989;63(13):1018–1021 75

Case 867.   Van Buren PC, Roberts WC. Cholesterol Pericarditis and Cardiac
              Tamponade with Congenital Hypothyroidism in Adulthood. *Am
              Heart J.* 1990;119(3 Pt 1):697–700 80

Case 1021.   Harvey LAC, DeMaio SJ, Roberts WC. Radiation-Induced
              Cardiovascular Disease Including Stenosis of Coronary Ostium,
              Coronary and Carotid Arteries, and Aortic Valves. *Proc Bayl
              Univ Med Cent.* 1994;7(3):33–36 85

Case 1030.   Shirani J, Zafari AM, Hill VE, Roberts WC. Long Asymptomatic
              Survival with a Bullet Adjacent to the Left Main Coronary
              Artery, the Only Site of Atherosclerotic Plaque in the Coronary
              Tree. *Am Heart J.* 1994;128(5):1043–1044 91

Case 1207.   Roberts WC, Phillips SD, Escobar JM, Capehart JE. Cardiac
              Transplantation 40 Years After a Stab Wound to the Heart. *Proc
              Bayl Univ Med Cent.* 2001;14(3):241–242 93

Case 1222.   Bang LS, Black RD, Hall SA, Roberts WC. Dyspnea with
              Hemoglobin SC Disease. *Proc Bayl Univ Med Cent.* 2002;15(1):86–90 96

Case 1251.   Mason DT, Roberts WC. Isolated Ventricular Septal Defect
              Caused by Nonpenetrating Trauma to the Chest. *Proc Bayl Univ
              Med Cent.* 2002;15(4):388–390 106

Case 1590.   Fazel P, Vallabhan RC, Roberts WC. Massive Bloody Pericardial
              Effusion as an Initial Manifestation of Chronic Kidney Disease.
              Proc Bayl Univ Med Cent. 2013;26(1):33–34 111

Case 1618.   Roberts WC, Rosenblatt RL, Ko JM, Grayburn PA, Kuiper JJ,
              Guileyardo JM. Cardiac Restriction Secondary to Massive
              Calcific Deposits in the Left Ventricular Cavity. *Am J Cardiol.*
              2014;113(8):1442–1446 114

Case 1746.   Zhang J, Baugh L, Guileyardo J, Roberts WC. Thrombotic
              Thrombocytopenic Purpura with Graves' Disease During
              Pregnancy. *Proc (Bayl Univ Med Cent).* 2020;33(2):270–272 121

Diseases of the Aorta

Case 44.   Roberts WC, Wibin EA. Idiopathic Panaortitis, Supra-Aortic
              Arteritis, Granulomatous Myocarditis and Pericarditis. A Case
              of Pulseless Disease and Possibly Left Ventricular Aneurysm in
              the African. *Am J Med.* 1966;41(3):453–461 127

Case 87.   Roberts WC, MacGregor RR, DeBlanc HJ Jr, Beiser GD, Wolff
              SM. The Prepulseless Phase of Pulseless Disease, or Pulseless
              Disease with Pulses. A Newly Recognized Cause of Cardiac
              Disease, Monoclonal Gammopathy and "Fever of Unknown
              Origin". *Am J Med.* 1969;46(2):313–324 140

Case 127. Fortuin NJ, Morrow AG, Roberts WC. Late Vascular Manifestations of the Rubella Syndrome. A Roentgenographic-Pathologic Study. *Am J Med.* 1971;51(1):134–140 154

Case 135. Buja LM, Ali N, Fletcher RD, Roberts WC. Stenosis of the Right Pulmonary Artery: A Complication of Acute Dissecting Aneurysm of the Ascending Aorta. *Am Heart J.* 1972;83(1):89–92 . . . 163

Case 386. Brosius FC III, Blackbourne BD, Roberts WC. Death in the Disco. *Chest.* 1980;78(2):321–323 168

Case 679. Barth CW III, Bray M, Roberts WC. Rupture of the Ascending Aorta During Cocaine Intoxication. *Am J Cardiol.* 1986;57(6):496 171

Case 837. Roberts WC, Satler LF, Wallace RB. Hemodynamic Confirmation of Peripheral Pulmonary Stenosis Caused by Aortic Dissection. *Am J Cardiol.* 1989;63(18):1418–1420 173

Case 971. Mautner SL, Mautner GC, Curry CL, Roberts WC. Massive Perigraft Aortic Aneurysm Late After Composite Graft Replacement of the Ascending Aorta and Aortic Valve in the Marfan Syndrome. *Am J Cardiol.* 1993;71(7):624–627 177

Case 1063. Comfort SR, Curry RC Jr, Roberts WC. Sudden Death While Playing Tennis Due to a Tear in Ascending Aorta (Without Dissection) and Probable Transient Compression of the Left Main Coronary Artery. *Am J Cardiol.* 1996;78(4):493–495 183

Case 1178. Lander SR, Roberts WC. Aneurysm of the False Channel of Descending Thoracic Aorta Years After Operative Excision of the Initiating Aortic Dissection Tear in Ascending Aorta. *Am J Geriatr Cardiol.* 2000;9(2):91–93 185

Case 1381. Roberts WC, Ko JM, Pearl GJ. Abdominal Aortic Aneurysm in Nonagenarians. *Am J Geriatr Cardiol.* 2006;15(5):319–321 189

Case 1390. Roberts WC, Ko JM, Matter GJ. Isolated Aortic Valve Replacement without Coronary Bypass for Aortic Valve Stenosis Involving a Congenitally Bicuspid Aortic Valve in a Nonagenarian. *Am J Geriatr Cardiol.* 2006;15(6):389–391 192

Case 1501. Roberts WC, Lensing FD, Kourlis H Jr, et al. Full Blown Cardiovascular Syphilis with Aneurysm of the Innominate Artery. *Am J Cardiol.* 2009;104(11):1595–1600 195

Case 1568. Benjamin MM, Roberts WC. Fatal Aortic Rupture from Nonpenetrating Chest Trauma. *Proc Bayl Univ Med Cent.* 2012;25(2):121–123 202

Case 1667. Roberts WC, Won VS, Weissenborn MR, Khalid A, Lima B. Massive Diffuse Calcification of the Ascending Aorta and Minimal Focal Calcification of the Abdominal Aorta in Heterozygous Familial Hypercholesterolemia. *Am J Cardiol.* 2016;117(8):1381–1385 207

Case 1674. Zhang J, Guileyardo JM, Roberts WC. Origin of the Left Subclavian Artery as the First Branch and Origin of the Right Subclavian Artery as the Fourth Branch of the Aortic Arch with Crisscrossing Posterior to the Common Carotid Arteries. *Proc Bayl Univ Med Cent.* 2016;29(4):423 214

Case 1675. Zhang J, Guileyardo JM, Roberts WC. Frequency and Potential Consequences of Origin of the Left Vertebral Artery (Or The

Arteria Thryoidea Ima) Directly from the Aortic Arch. *Proc Bayl Univ Med Cent.* 2016;29(4):424–425 216

Case 1705.   Velasco CE, Hashemi H, Roullard CP, Machannaford J, Roberts WC. Asymptomatic Ascending Aorta Aneurysm with Severe Aortic Regurgitation Caused by Multiple Intimal-Medial Tears Unassociated with Aortic Dissection. *Am J Cardiol.* 2018;121(5):668–669 219

Case 1739.   Roberts CS, Salam YM, Moore AJ, Roberts WC. Pseudoaneurysm of the Ascending Aorta at the Cannulation Site Diagnosed More Than Four Decades After Repair of Ventricular Septal Defect. *Am J Cardiol.* 2019;124(12):1962–1965 223

Case 1773.   Roberts WC, Roberts CS. Combined Cardiovascular Syphilis and Type A Acute Aortic Dissection. *Am J Cardiol.* 2022;168:159–162 229

Index 235

Preface

When these case reports (numbering 272) were sent to the publisher my intention was that all would be published in one or two volumes. The publisher, however, convinced me that the collection of case reports would be too large if they were all published together, and that decision resulted into dividing the collection into six smaller books arranged by subject. I find case reports useful and often they are the first publication of many authors. William Osler published many case reports in the later decades of the 19th century. Today, the JACC has a journal devoted solely to case reports. The doctor-patient relationship is one on one. Most journals today publish case reports, but their name is usually disguised as something else.

William C. Roberts, MD

About the Editor

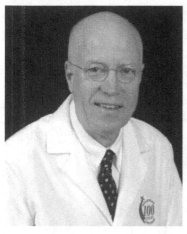

William C. Roberts, MD, was born in Atlanta, Georgia, on September 11, 1932. He graduated from Southern Methodist University (1954) and Emory University School of Medicine (1958). He did his training in internal medicine at the Boston City Hospital and at The Johns Hopkins Hospital. He had a 1-year fellowship in cardiology at the National Heart, Lung and Blood Institute. He did his training in anatomic pathology at the National Institutes of Health (1959–1962). From July 1964 to March 1993, he was Chief of Pathology in the National Heart, Lung, and Blood Institute, National Institutes of Health, Bethesda, Maryland. He has written 1784 articles. Additionally, he has edited 31 books and lectured in more than 2200 cities around the world.

From December 1992 through December 2018, Dr. Roberts was program director of the Williamsburg Conference on Heart Disease held every December in Williamsburg, Virginia. The American College of Cardiology Foundation sponsored this conference for 30 years. Since March 1993, Dr. Roberts had been the executive director of the Baylor Heart and Vascular Institute at Baylor University Medical Center in Dallas, Texas. He served as the editor in chief of the *Baylor University Medical Center Proceedings* from 1994 to 2022 (29 years) and the editor in chief of *The American Journal of Cardiology* from June 1982 until July 2022 (40 years).

He received many honors, including: the 1978 Gifted Teacher Award from The American College of Cardiology; the 1983 College Medalist Award of the American College of Chest Physicians; the Public Health Service Commendation Medal in 1979; the 1984 Richard and Hilda Rosenthal Foundation Award from the Council of Cardiology of the American Heart Association; an honorary Doctor of Science degree from Far Eastern University, Manila, Philippines in 1995; the designation of *Master* from The American College of Cardiology in 2004; the Lifetime Achievement Award of The American College of Cardiology in 2016; and the Lifetime Achievement Award for D's CEO's Excellence in Healthcare Awards in 2021.

Sadly, Dr. William C. Roberts passed away in June 2023 at the age of 90, just as this book series went into production.

Introduction

Case reports have had a long history. Many diseases have been reported initially as a case report. The first publication of many authors, including the present author, was a case report. William Osler's curriculum vitae (CV) is loaded with individual case studies on a variety of conditions. Paul Dudley White's CV, particularly his early publications, is loaded with individual case reports. Indeed, he indicated that he tried to write a case report on a variety of cardiovascular conditions to familiarize himself quickly with them.

The physician-patient relationship is a one-on-one encounter. Although randomized clinical trials are favored today, often it is difficult to fit a single patient into these types of studies due to the heterogeneous nature of the populations. Some patients or circumstances cannot be described except in the case-report format. An example might be case #342 included in this volume, which described a man who was shot; the bullet coursed through the right atrium and then through the right ventricular outflow tract, preventing flow to the left side of the heart. Autopsy disclosed the left atrial appendage to have protruded through the mitral orifice, suggesting that the left ventricle had a negative pressure during ventricular diastole, something confirmed physiologically in a subsequent publication. We recently received a manuscript describing a young boy who was thrown from his vehicle and landed on a rattlesnake who bit him on his leg that was the site of a compound fracture suffered during the accident. The case-report format is the only mechanism to report such events.

Many disease entities have been described initially as case reports: Ochronosis by Rudolph Virchow (1821–1920), sickle cell anemia by James B. Herrick (1861–1954), and the Pickwickian syndrome (obesity-hyperventilation syndrome) by Charles Sydney Burwell (1893–1967) are just a few examples. Multiple first operations were described initially in the case report format, as well as the first effective anesthetic drug.

Another benefit of case reports is that they provide the opportunity for young physicians to break into the medical publishing arena. They can be used to describe a new facet of a disease or provide a fuller description of an entity described previously. New journals often begin by publishing case reports. (See the early issues of the *Mayo Clinic Proceedings* or the *Cleveland Clinic Medical Quarterly* or the *Baylor University Medical Center Proceedings*.)

Some authors, editors, and readers minimize the usefulness of case reports to medical education. We recently received a case report from an important and established investigator who indicated that he was really not in favor of publishing case reports but that his was "special" and deserved rapid acceptance and publication. This type of comment is fairly frequent.

In more modern times, several collections of case reports have been published. *The New England Journal of Medicine* calls them "Images in Clinical Medicine" or "Case Records of the Massachusetts General Hospital"; *The Lancet* calls them "Clinical Picture"; *Circulation* calls them "Cardiovascular Images" or "Cases and Traces" or "ECG Challenge"; *JAMA Cardiology* calls them "JAMA Cardiology Clinical Challenge"; and *The American Journal of Medicine* calls them "Diagnostic Dilemma" or "Images in Dermatology" or "Images in Radiology" or "ECG Image of the Month," to name a few examples. *The Journal of the American College of Cardiology* has an entire journal devoted to case reports (*JACC Case Reports*).

The present collection of case reports, of course, is not the first. An early collection of case studies was by Ambroise Pare called *Oeuvres* in 1628 (in French) and compiled and edited by Wallace B. Hamby and titled *The Case Reports and Autopsy Records of Ambroise Pare* (in English) in 1960. These short descriptions of patients are fascinating and enjoyable reading. Richard C. Cabot, who started the clinicopathologic conferences at the Massachusetts General Hospital, published *Case Teaching in Medicine—A Series of Graduated Exercises in the Differential Diagnosis, Prognosis and Treatment of Actual Cases of Disease* in 1906. Cabot described 78 patients, most of whom went to autopsy and some to surgery. The collection included patients with a variety of conditions. Cabot's 1906 book led to "The Case History Series": *Case Histories in Pediatrics* by John Lovett Morse; *Surgical Problems* by James G. Mumford in 1911 (100 cases); and *Case Histories in Neurology* by E. W. Taylor in 1911.

In more modern times, several collections of case reports have been published. The most popular are under the general heading of *Clinicopathologic Conferences of The Massachusetts General Hospital:* the collection of cases, published individual books, are variously titled *Selected Medical Cases; Surgical; Bone and Joint; Neurologic;* and *Cardiac.* The latter by Benjamin Castleman and Roman W. De Sanctis presents 50 cases of various cardiovascular diseases studied both clinically and at necropsy. (The gross photos of the hearts cannot be recommended.)

Finally, case reports are fun reading (particularly Ambroise Pare's *Selections*). They are a "break" from the data-heavy multicenter placebo-controlled trials and metaanalyses.

When these 272 case reports were sent to the publisher, my intention was that all would be published in one or two volumes. The publisher, however, convinced me that the collection of case reports would be too large if they were all published together, and that decision resulted into dividing the collection into six smaller books arranged by subject:

1. Congenital Heart Disease
2. Valvular Heart Disease
3. Coronary Heart Disease and Hyperlipidemia
4. Cardiomyopathy
5. Cardiac Neoplasm
6. Cardiovascular Diseases with a Focus on Aorta

The case reports were written by me and colleagues over a 61-year period (1961 to 2022). All 272 describe a single patient with a cardiovascular disease, nearly all of whom were studied both clinically and morphologically, i.e., at autopsy or after cardiac transplantation or after another cardiovascular operation. Thus, the collection is unique. Each report is numbered as it appears in my CV, which includes as of August 15, 2022, a total of 1784 publications (Table 1). Some were book chapters, published interviews of prominent physicians, or published symposia in which I participated, but most (952) were patient-centered studies.

William C. Roberts, MD
May 5, 2022

Disclaimer:

All case reports are reprinted exactly as first published.

Table 1: Number and types of articles published by William C. Roberts, MD, 1961–2022

Article Type		N
1. Patient-centered studies		952
a. Single patient	269	
b. Multipatient	666	
c. Nonpatient	17	
2. From-the-editor columns		342
a. AJC (1982–2022)	234	
b. BUMC (1994–2021)	108	
3. Other editorials, mini reviews, forewords, historical pieces (all journals)		67
4. Chapters in books		143
5. Interviews		197
a. AJC	77	
b. BUMC	96	
c. Visiting professors	24	
6. Published symposia ("AJC editor's roundtable")		43
7. AJC in month (25 years earlier) (May 1983–August 1988)		40
Total		**1784**

AJC indicates *American Journal of Cardiology;*
BUMC, *Baylor University Medical Center Proceedings.*
Note: Additional publications were added after this table was compiled, including additional case studies, with a new total of 272.

MISCELLANEOUS CARDIOVASCULAR DISEASE

Case 55 Gaucher's Disease of the Lung Causing Severe Pulmonary Hypertension with Associated Acute Recurrent Pericarditis

William C. Roberts, M.D., and Donald S. Fredrickson, M.D.

SUMMARY The clinical and pathological features of a 30-year-old man with Gaucher's disease are described. He had severe pulmonary hypertension resulting from obstruction of pulmonary capillaries by Gaucher cells. Acute recurrent pericarditis of unknown etiology terminally led to hemopericardium and cardiac tamponade.

Additional Indexing Words
Cerebral involvement
Cor pulmonale
Anemia
Elastic fibers
Bronchial constriction
Ruptured pericardial vessels

GAUCHER'S DISEASE is a familial disorder characterized by accumulation in reticuloendothelial cells of glucocerebrosides, compounds containing sphingosine, fatty acid, and glucose in equimolar amounts. The storage cells, called Gaucher cells, have a characteristic appearance, and their increasing numbers in the liver, spleen, lymph nodes, and bone marrow are responsible for most of the clinical manifestations of the disorder.[1] Although nearly all patients have hepatosplenomegaly, Gaucher cells in marrow aspirates, and an abnormally high concentration of non-tartrate-inhibitable serum acid phosphatase, at least two forms of Gaucher's disease exist clinically. They probably represent expression of different mutations. In the *infantile* or *acute* form, the children have a characteristic stereotyped appearance (strabismus, opisthotonus, retracted lips and often spastic and flexed extremities), and death generally occurs before 2 years of age. The *adult* or *chronic* form comprises the majority of cases of Gaucher's disease. It may be detected at any age, usually because of hepatosplenomegaly. Neurological signs rarely if ever occur, osseous lesions are often pronounced, and hematological abnormalities associated with hypersplenism, skin pigmentation, and pingueculae usually develop. It is relatively common among Ashkenazi Jews, in contrast to the infantile form, which is very rarely seen in a Jewish child. Death in the infantile form is usually related to the cerebral involvement and cachexia, and, in the adult form, to anemia or superimposed infection. The present report describes an adult patient with Gaucher's disease followed for 25 years, who developed severe pulmonary hypertension, recurrent acute pericarditis, and finally hemorrhagic cardiac tamponade. Pulmonary hypertension, which has not been documented previously in a patient with Gaucher's disease, resulted from the plugging of alveolar capillaries by Gaucher cells.

From the Laboratory of Pathology, Clinic of Surgery and Laboratory of Molecular Diseases, National Heart Institute, National Institutes of Health, Bethesda, Maryland.

DOI: 10.1201/9781003408321-2

REPORT OF PATIENT

A.K. (02–62–62), a 30-year-old lawyer, died at the National Heart Institute on January 3, 1962. He had been followed from age 5 to age 16 years (1936–1947) by Dr. Siegfried J. Thannhauser, who described this patient's course during this interval in detail in his monograph on the lipidoses (patient 48).[2] This patient was the younger of two male children of parents who were both Ashkenazi Jews. A single bone marrow aspiration in the mother, who came from Palestine, showed no abnormality. The father, who came from Lithuania, died at age 32 of an acute myocardial infarct. The patient's oldest sibling is normal. Between the ages of 9 and 12 months, the patient was taken to physicians with a question of retarded growth and abdominal enlargement. At age 4 years hepatosplenomegaly was established and Gaucher cells were discovered in the sternal marrow. By age 7 years the spleen had become so large (7 pounds; patient weighed 35 pounds) that abdominal discomfort and dyspnea resulted, and it was therefore removed. For the next 20 years he led an outwardly normal life. He was an excellent student, and was admitted to the bar. Throughout his school life, however, he had repeated episodes of bone pain and fractures, some spontaneous and others associated with minor trauma, eventually leading to permanent deformities of the left hip and leg.

The patient was first seen by one of us (D.S.F.) in August 1959. His only complaints during the previous 5 years were easy fatigability and rare bone pain. Five days earlier he had fainted while lifting a heavy table. On examination, the liver was enormous, extending to the iliac crest. The skin had a sallow yellow color with duskiness over the tibias, and each eye had small pingueculae. The pulmonic second sound was markedly accentuated, but there was no precordial murmur or rub. The blood pressure was 120/80 mm Hg. The axillary, cervical, supraclavicular and inguinal lymph nodes were not enlarged. No abnormalities were detected on neurological examination.

The electrocardiogram (figure 1) showed right axis deviation, right atrial and right ventricular hypertrophy, and the chest roentgenogram (figure 2) showed a large right ventricle and pulmonary trunk. The blood hematocrit was 46%, white blood cell count, 18,000 mm^3 with 48 neutrophils, 49 lymphocytes and 3% monocytes; serum acid phosphatase, 3.08 Bessey-Lowry units (upper limit of normal = 0.6), 0.15 being tartrate-inhibitable, Bromsulphalein retention in 45 minutes, 11%; total serum bilirubin, 0.7 mg per 100 ml; total cholesterol, 135 mg per 100 ml with free cholesterol 46; phospholipids 176; and triglycerides, 192 mg per 100 ml (upper limit of normal for triglycerides = 150 mg per 100 ml).

Fifteen months later (November 1960) he had the first episode of acute lower substernal and precordial pain, which worsened with inspiration and movement and lasted 18 hours. Several days later the pain reappeared and a loud precordial friction rub was heard as well as a ventricular gallop. Six similar episodes of anterior chest pain occurred during the next 13 months. A pericardial friction rub was audible on each occasion, sometimes accompanied by a pleural friction rub. Atrial flutter occurred during four of these episodes. He was afebrile and had normal erythrocyte sedimentation rates during each episode. On one occasion the antistreptolysin-O titer was 500 units. His last acute illness began 7 days before death with the onset of a severe, nonproductive, hacking cough. He was brought to the hospital 2 hours before death, and at this time was severely dyspneic, cyanotic, and had tachycardia, distended neck veins, pulsus paradoxus (20 mm Hg), and a white blood cell count of 31,000 mm.^{3} Chest roentgenogram showed an enormous cardiac silhouette, a massive increase in size as compared to his previous x-rays (figure 2). Pericardiocentesis yielded 150 ml of blood. Shortly thereafter asystole occurred.

At autopsy (A62–4), 600 ml of blood was found in the pericardial sac; the pericardial surfaces were "shaggy" and contained numerous acute and chronic

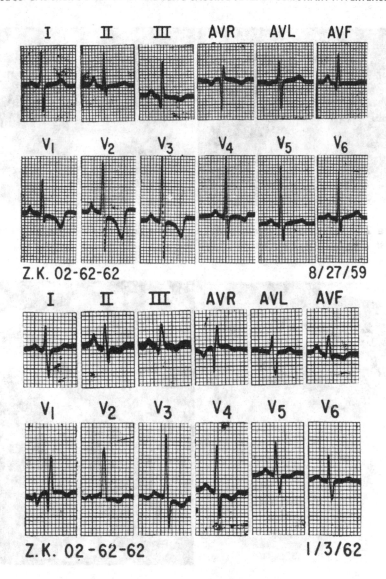

Figure 1 *Electrocardiograms.* Upper. *Recorded 29 months before death.* Lower. *Recorded 1 hour before death at the time of massive hemopericardium.*

inflammatory cells and vascular channels, but no Gaucher cells. The left pleural space contained 600 ml of serosanguineous fluid, but the pleural surfaces were normal. The heart weighed 500 g; the right ventricle and atrium were markedly hypertrophied (figure 3) and contained focal fibrous scars. The cardiac valves were normal and coronary arteries were within the range of normal for this age. The lungs together weighed 850 g, and showed evidence of pulmonary edema. The walls of both small and large pulmonary arteries were thickened and contained atheromata. The histological sections of lung disclosed the presence of numerous Gaucher cells plugging the lumina of alveolar capillaries throughout the lung (figure 4). In addition, Gaucher cells were seen occasionally in the alveolar spaces.

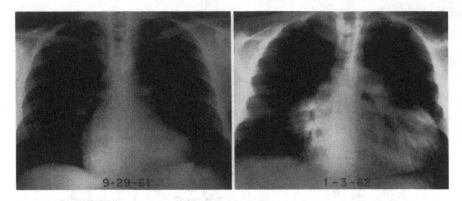

Figure 2 *Chest roentgenograms.* Left. *Two months before death.* Right. *Day of death, demonstrating massive pericardial effusion.*

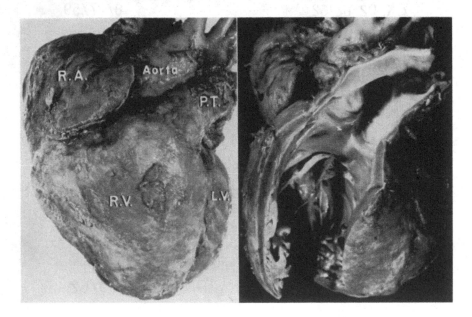

Figure 3 *Exterior of heart* (left) *and opened right ventricle and pulmonary trunk* (right). *The right ventricle (R.V.) is markedly hypertrophied; the left ventricle (L.V.) is small. Atheromata are present in the pulmonary trunk (P.T.). R.A. = right atrium.*

The pulmonary arterioles, muscular arteries, and elastic arteries showed changes characteristic of severe (grade V/VI) hypertensive pulmonary vascular disease (classification of Heath and Edwards[3]) (figure 5). Plexiform lesions were present throughout all lobes of both lungs (figure 5). The liver, bone marrow, and lymph nodes contained massive numbers of Gaucher cells. The liver weighed 8.1 kg, and its architecture was disrupted by infiltrates of Gaucher cells, hemopoietic elements, and fibrous tissue. Analysis of the liver revealed 77 mg of chloroform-soluble glycolipids per gm of dry weight (normal <10 mg per g). The abdominal lymph nodes were

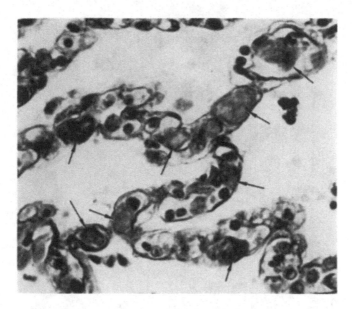

Figure 4 *Pulmonary alveolar capillaries occluded by Gaucher cells* (arrows). *Periodic acid-Schiff stain; × 780.*

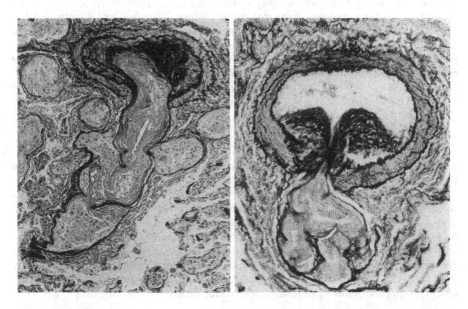

Figure 5 *Muscular pulmonary arteries, each demonstrating changes indicative of severe pulmonary hypertension. Left. The muscular artery and its branching arteriole shows extensive intimal proliferation. Numerous large thin-walled dilated vessels surround the obstructed arteriole. Right. Classical plexiform lesion arising from a muscular artery, which has hypertrophied media and intimal fibrous proliferation at the site of origin of the plexiform lesion. Elastic-van Gieson stains; × 150 (left), × 195 (right).*

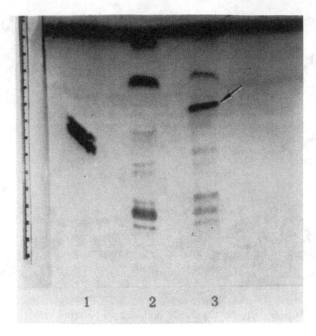

Figure 6 *Thin-layer chromatography of the chloroform-soluble glycolipids prepared from lung according to the technique of Mårtensson et al.[4] Extracts representing equal amounts of wet lung tissue are chromatographed in lanes 2 (control) and 3 (patient A.K.). Chromatographed in lane 1 is a mixture of galactocerebrosides obtained from beef spinal cord. The arrow designates a dense band of material in the lung of A.K. having an Rf comparable to glucocerebrosides. Note the absence of significant amounts of this material in the control extract. Chromatographs were developed in one dimension in chloroform/methanol/ H_2O (65/25/4) and the spots identified by spraying with an acid solution of anisaldehyde and heating 20 minutes for 120°.*

enlarged (up to 3 cm in diameter) and were virtually replaced by Gaucher cells. The thoracic lymph nodes were not enlarged.

The glycolipids from a sample of frozen lung from patient A. K. and from a control were extracted and partially purified according to the technique of Mårtensson and associates.[4] The control patient (I. D., A56–217) was a 12-year-old boy who had idiopathic left ventricular hypertrophy. His pulmonary arterial pressure was 16/9 mm Hg, and his left ventricular pressure was 130/10 mm Hg. The cerebroside contents of the lungs were compared qualitatively by thin-layer chromatography (figure 6). The lung from A. K. contained massive amounts of material having the chromatographic behavior of glucocerebrosides relative to the control.

COMMENTS

In 1933 Merklen and associates reported the finding of Gaucher cells in the sputum of a 51-year-old man with this disease.[5] In 1937 Myers described Gaucher cells in the alveolar walls and sacs and in the hilar and mediastinal lymph nodes of an 8-year-old girl who died of Gaucher's disease.[6] In addition to pleurisy this child had signs of bronchial constriction, which were attributed to compression on these structures by the enlarged hilar lymph nodes. In 1948 Groen and Garrer described an "especially accentuated" pulmonic second sound, diffuse crepitant pulmonary rales, bilateral pleural effusions, cardiomegaly, and dilatation of the pulmonary trunk in a 48-year-old woman who died of Gaucher's disease after repeated attacks of severe dyspnea with extreme cyanosis.[7] An autopsy was not performed but these authors speculated that the clinical picture of cor pulmonale and pulmonary hypertension resulted from "obstruction in the smaller circulation . . . due to an accumulation of Gaucher cells in the lungs." In 1950 Kaiser described a miliary pattern on chest roentgenogram in a patient with Gaucher's disease.[8] Subsequently, this miliary-type appearance had been described in other patients with this disease.[1,9–12] The 3-year-old child (case VII) reported by Levin died from "massive hemoptysis" and necropsy disclosed "numerous Gaucher cells in the lungs."[9] The patient reported by Jackson and Simon was also a 3-year-old girl who died of severe respiratory distress.[12] The lungs of this child on chest roentgenogram also demonstrated a miliary pattern, and at autopsy "enormous numbers of Gaucher cells" were present in the alveolar septa and spaces.

Although Gaucher cells have been described in alveolar septa, their location within the alveolar capillaries has not been previously described. In the present patient, obstruction to these capillaries by Gaucher cells appears to have been the cause of his severe pulmonary hypertension. The configuration of the elastic fibers in the pulmonary trunk were of the adult type, indicating that the pulmonary hypertension was acquired and not present at birth.[13] There is no mention of the cardiovascular or pulmonary systems in the description of this patient during childhood by Thannhauser.[2] When first seen at this clinic 29 months before his death, he demonstrated signs of severe pulmonary hypertension.

The cause of the acute recurrent pericarditis was never determined. Although a wide variety of inflammatory cells were present, no Gaucher cells were identified in the pericardium. Since this patient's pericardium was exceedingly vascular and since he experienced uncontrollable coughing during his last several days, the terminal hemopericardium and cardiac tamponade may have resulted from rupture of one or several of the pericardial vessels during the coughing episodes. Hemopericardium with cardiac tamponade has been described previously in a patient with Gaucher's disease.[14] This 59-year-old woman, however, also had an adenocarcinoma, probably primary in the lung, and malignant cells were found in the aspirated pericardial and pleural fluids. Zlotnick and Groen in 1961 described massive pericardial calcification in a 46-year-old woman who died of Gaucher's disease.[15] The cause of the pericardial calcification was not determined although "hemorrhagic diathesis . . . secondary to unrecognized hemorrhage into the pericardial cavity, with organization and deposition of calcium" was suggested. No Gaucher cells were described in her pericardium at necropsy, but interestingly these cells were found in her lungs. This patient had had an accentuated pulmonic second sound, but electrocardiogram did not indicate ventricular hypertrophy.

ACKNOWLEDGMENT

The authors wish to acknowledge the invaluable participation of Dr. Eugene Braunwald and other members of the Cardiology Branch of the National Heart Institute in the clinical management of patient A. K.

REFERENCES

1. FREDRICKSON, D. S.: *Cerebroside Lipidosis: Gaucher's Disease in the Metabolic Basis of Inherited Disease*, ed. 2. New York, The Blakiston Division-McGraw-Hill Book Co., 1966, p. 565.
2. THANNHAUSER, S. J.: *Lipidoses: Diseases of the Intracellular Lipid Metabolism*, ed. 3. New York, Grune & Stratton, 1958, 600 pp.

3. HEATH, D., AND EDWARDS, J. E.: The pathology of hypertensive pulmonary vascular disease: A description of six grades of structural changes in the pulmonary arteries with special reference to congenital cardiac septal defects. *Circulation* 18: 533, 1958.
4. MÅRTENSSON, E., PERCY, A., AND SVENNERHOLM, L.: Kidney glycolipids in late infantile metachromatic leucodystrophy. *Acta Pediat Scand* 55: 1, 1966.
5. MERKLEN, P., WAITZ, R., AND WARTER, J.: Un cas de maladie de Gaucher ã dèterminations osseuses, avec cellules de Gaucher dans les crachats. *Bull Soc Med Hop Paris* 49: 36, 1933.
6. MYERS, B.: Gaucher's disease of the lungs. *Brit Med J* 2: 8, 1937.
7. GROEN, J., AND GARRER, A. H.: Adult Gaucher's disease, with special reference to the variations in its clinical course and the value of sternal puncture as an aid to its diagnosis. *Blood* 3: 1221, 1948.
8. KAISER, A.: Morbus Gaucher-specifìsche lungeninfiltration unter dem bilde einer miliar-Tb. *Mschr Kinderheilk* 98: 252, 1950.
9. LEVIN, B.: Gaucher's disease: Clinical and roentgenologic manifestations. *Amer J Roentgen* 85: 685, 1961.
10. MACCIONI, L., AND CAPPELLI, B.: Le alterazioni polmonari nel morbo di Gaucher ad evoluzione cronica. *Policlinico* 69: 157, 1962.
11. PRATESI, V.: Un casodi malattia di Gaucher a prevalente localizzazione polmonare. *Riv Clin Pediat* 72: 396, 1963.
12. JACKSON, D. C., AND SIMON, G.: Unusual bone and lung changes in a case of Gaucher's disease. *Brit J Radiol* 38: 698, 1965.
13. ROBERTS, W. C.: The histologic structure of the pulmonary trunk in patients with "primary" pulmonary hypertension. *Amer Heart J* 65: 230, 1963.
14. ROSENFELD, S., AND EPSTEIN, S.: Gaucher's disease complicated by metastatic carcinoma presenting symptoms of recurrent pericardial tamponade with secondary acute renal failure. *New York J Med* 61: 4080, 1961.
15. ZLOTNICK, A., AND GROEN, J. J.: Observations on a patient with Gaucher's disease. *Amer J Med* 30: 637, 1961.

Case 57 Traumatic Left Ventricular Aneurysm

*Cardiac Thrombosis Following Aneurysmectomy**

D. Luke Glancy, M.D., Philip Yarnell, M.D. and William C. Roberts, M.D., F.A.C.C.
Bethesda, Maryland

The usual cause of left ventricular aneurysm is coronary atherosclerosis with transmural myocardial infarction, and one of the rare causes is blunt trauma to the chest. Seven patients with well documented traumatic left ventricular aneurysm have been reported[1-6]; in 5 the aneurysm ruptured between 2 and 90 days after the injury,[1-3,6] and in the other 2 the left ventricular aneurysm persisted.[4,5] The present report describes a young man with a left ventricular aneurysm that developed following blunt injury to the chest. Multiple systemic emboli occurred, and the aneurysm was resected. Although no thrombus was found in the resected aneurysm, fatal multiple systemic emboli occurred many months postoperatively, and at necropsy a large thrombus was found attached to the left ventricular suture line. The authors know of no previous reports describing left ventricular thrombosis following resection of a cardiac aneurysm under cardiopulmonary bypass.

REPORT OF PATIENT

The patient was well until November 1962, when at age 20 he was struck in the chest while playing football. Ten minutes later severe subslernal and interscapular pain, dyspnea and diaphoresis developed. The pain lasted for two days. A month later, intermittent claudication of the left calf and coldness of the left foot developed. In January 1963 numbness, paralysis and pain in both legs suddenly developed, and the popliteal, posterior tibial and dorsalis pedis arterial pulses were found to be absent bilaterally. Warfarin sodium was administered. Several superficial areas of necrosis on the left foot subsequently healed, and the pain at rest and the sensory and motor deficits diminished. An electrocardiogram taken in February 1963 showed an anterolateral myocardial infarct of indeterminate age.

When first seen at the Clinical Center in August 1963, the patient was asymptomatic except for claudication of the left leg on walking five blocks. The left pedal pulses were absent. The blood pressure was 130/70 mm. Hg. Examination of the precordium disclosed no abnormalities. The chest roentgenogram and electrocardiogram are shown in Figures 1 and 2, respectively. The serum cholesterol was normal (190 mg./100 ml.), as were the serum phospholipids and triglycerides.

By October 1964 he was able to play touch football without discomfort, and he stopped taking warfarin sodium. Three weeks later he noted transient pain in the right flank, numbness of both legs and coldness of both feet; the arterial pulses in each foot were diminished.

Operative Findings and Treatment: In June 1965 he underwent cardiac catheterization and cineangiocardiography at another institution. The pressures were normal, and the left ventriculogram showed an apical aneurysm with paradoxic

* From the Laboratory of Pathology, Clinic of Surgery, National Heart Institute, and the Surgical Neurology Branch, National Institute of Neurological Diseases and Blindness, National Institutes of Health, Bethesda, Md. 20014.

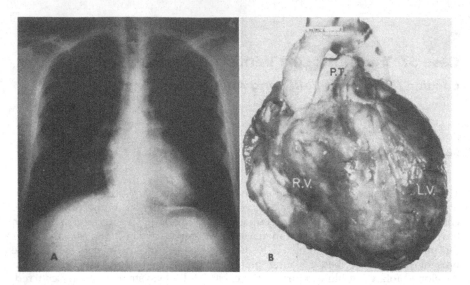

Figure 1 A. *chest roentgenogram*, 15 months after injury, is normal. B, *anterior surface of the heart at necropsy*. L.V. = left ventricle; R.V. = right ventricle; P.T. = pulmonary trunk.

pulsations and irregular filling defects suggesting the possibility of mural thrombi (Figure 3). Coronary cinearteriography showed normal left circumflex and right coronary arteries but variations in the diameters of the lumens of the distal anterior descending and diagonal branches of the left coronary artery. In July 1965 a cardiac operation under cardiopulmonary bypass was performed. The left ventricular apical wall, measuring approximately 3 by 3 cm., was found to be densely fibrotic and slightly thinned, but only minimal paradoxic motion was observed in it. The central 2 by 2 cm. of this area was excised, and no intra-aneurysmal thrombus was found. The patient's early postoperative course was uneventful, and he was discharged on no medication. One and a half months following the procedure, however, he had a transient episode of numbness of the right side of his tongue and face and clumsiness of the right arm and leg.

Subsequent Course: Thereafter, he was well until Jan. 26, 1966, when he was readmitted to the Clinical Center because of the sudden appearance of signs and symptoms diagnostic of brain-stem infarction. A right vertebral arteriogram performed two weeks later showed occlusion of the basilar artery. A variety of complications arose during this final illness: inability to handle secretions necessitating tracheostomy; thrombosis at the site of the right brachial arteriotomy requiring thrombectomy; right femoral arterial embolization leading to embolectomy, recurrent cerebral emboli; and gastrointestinal hemorrhage requiring nine transfusions and cessation of heparin therapy. Electrocardiograms during the first three weeks of hospitalization were unchanged from those in 1963 (Figure 2). However, concomitant with the femoral arterial embolization and gastrointestinal bleeding, changes of acute inferior infarction appeared (Figure 2). On May 11, 1966, the clinical picture of mesenteric arterial occlusion developed, and the next day he died. Numerous tests were done during this admission to determine if this patient had blood constituents which would increase his propensity to form clots, but none were found.

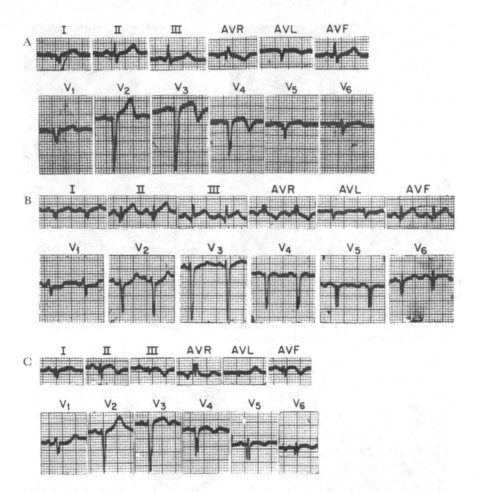

Figure 2 *Electrocardiograms.* A, *Aug. 21, 1963, nine months after injury* an anterolateral myocardial infarction of indeterminate age is indicated. Electrocardiograms shortly after operation and until four months before death were similar. B, *Feb. 17, 1966, three months before death,* additional changes of acute posteroinferior injury. C, *Mar. 7, 1966, nine weeks before death,* further evolution of the posteroinferior myocardial infarct. *At necropsy* there was, in addition to the dense anteroapical scar shown in Figure 4, extensive, patchy, cellular and acellular fibrosis of the posterior left ventricular wall from apex to base. The generalized circulatory problems experienced by the patient at the time of the acute electrocardiographic changes probably contributed greatly to the posterior wall infarction, since the coronary arteries supplying this area were widely patent.

Autopsy: The left ventricular apex of the heart (wt. 330 gm.) was extensively scarred, and a thrombus was attached to it (Figure 1 and 4). In addition, there was patchy but extensive scarring of the posterior left ventricular wall. The anterior descending coronary artery was severely narrowed 9 cm. from its origin by an organizing and fresh thrombus (Figure 5). The proximal anterior descending and the other major coronary arteries were free of thrombi and atheromata. The midline

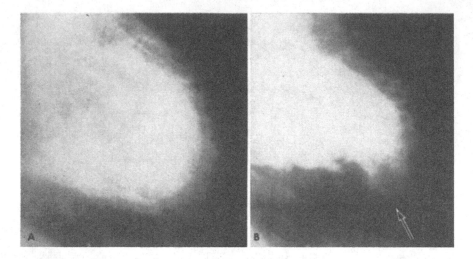

Figure 3 Left cineventriculograms, right anterior oblique projection. A, *ventricular diastole*. The apical aneurysm is not apparent. B, *ventricular systole*. The arrow points to the apical aneurysm, which bulges paradoxically as the ventricle contracts. The radiolucent filling defect within the aneurysm suggests a possible mural thrombus, but none was found at cardiac operation.

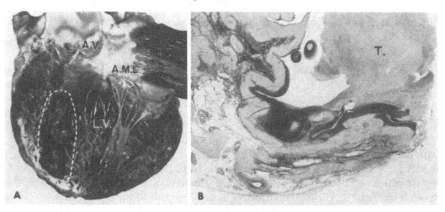

Figure 4 *Left ventricular thrombus. A, opened left ventricle.* At its apex is a dense fibrous scar, which extends half way up the anterior wall. Attached to the apex is a large mural thrombus, enclosed in dashes. A.M.L. = anterior mitral leaflet; A.V. = aortic valve; L.V. = left ventricle. B, *section through the left ventricular apex* shows scarring of the free wall and interventricular septum and the attachment of the mural thrombus (T.) to the free wall. There is a large amount of elastic tissue, which stains black, in the scar. (Elastic tissue stain, × 5.5 reduced by 31%.)

basilar portion of the pons was necrotic, and the basilar artery was focally occluded by thrombotic material, as were several of the midline perforating branches. There was a fresh thrombus in the superior sagittal sinus and in the superior mesenteric artery 5 cm. from its origin. The small intestine was distended and focally infarcted. Infarcts also were found in the kidneys and spleen, and the right femoral artery was occluded by a recent thrombus.

COMMENTS

Nonpenetrating chest trauma is frequently followed by transient clinical, electrocardiographic, or roentgenographic evidence of myocardial or pericardial injury,[7,8] and when fatal, often by cardiac laceration or rupture,[2,8-11] even without overt signs of a chest injury.[2,3,8,12] However, clinically detectable cardiac damage in late survivors of blunt trauma to the chest is unusual, although ventricular septal defect,[8] aortic regurgitation,[13] ruptured papillary muscle,[8] and constrictive pericarditis[14] all have been reported. Myocardial contusion, the most frequent cardiac injury following blunt chest trauma, rarely leaves clinically detectable evidence of cardiac abnormality in those patients surviving the injury by several months.[7,8,15] Animal experiments and observations on patients who survived blunt chest trauma, but subsequently died of unrelated diseases, indicate that the myocardial injury heals with little and sometimes no detectable scar.[8,9,11]

The coronary arteries are relatively resistant to injury by blunt chest trauma. Laceration of these vessels is uncommon, and thrombosis is rare. Of 546 patients with fatal nonpenetrating cardiac trauma reported by Parmley and associates,[8] only 10 had lacerations, and none had thrombosis of a coronary artery, despite the frequency of myocardial contusion adjacent to extramural coronary arteries. Hawkes[2] likewise recorded no coronary arterial injuries in 70 autopsy subjects who died of blunt trauma involving the heart. Furthermore, Moritz[12] found that the coronary arteries of dogs were much more resistant to injury by direct trauma than the adjacent myocardium, thrombosis of the coronary vessels in these animals was especially difficult to produce, and when it did occur, the vessels were only partially occluded.

Coronary Thrombosis Due to Blunt Chest Trauma: It is usually exceedingly difficult to establish blunt chest trauma as the cause of coronary arterial thrombosis. Before coronary thrombosis is attributed to trauma alone, ideally three criteria should be satisfied: (1) a history of chest trauma which shortly antedates the onset of cardiac signs and symptoms; (2) evidence of damage to the myocardium adjacent to the thrombosed coronary vessel; and (3) absence or near absence of intrinsic disease in the coronary arteries. Utilizing these strict criteria, we have found no reports of patients in whom coronary thrombosis could be unequivocally attributed to blunt chest trauma. In the patient described by Joachim and Mays[4] and in 1 patient (No. 4) described by DeMuth and Zinsser[11] chest trauma may have been the sole cause of coronary thrombosis, but insufficient description of the coronary arteries was given to be certain. At least 4 additional patients have been reported in whom blunt chest trauma probably played a contributory role in causing coronary thrombosis.[12,16-18] Each of these patients, however, had considerable coronary atherosclerosis. Very often patients who receive blunt chest trauma also incur other injuries which cause hypovolemia and shock, and it is possible that these consequences of the injury play a more important role in producing coronary thrombosis than direct injury to these vessels themselves. In the present patient the initial episode of myocardial necrosis, which led to formation of the aneurysm, could have been the direct result of myocardial contusion, the indirect result of traumatic coronary thrombosis, or a combination of these factors.

Mural Thrombosis in Myocardial Contusion and Aneurysm: Small mural thrombi frequently develop when the endocardium is contused,[8] and systemic embolization occasionally follows. Two of the 546 patients with fatal, nonpenetrating, cardiac trauma described by Parmley and associates[8] died of thromboembolic complications. Hildebrandt's patient (Warburg[5]) suffered blunt chest trauma at age 9 and became hemiplegic shortly before his death at 27; at necropsy a mural thrombus was found within an old left ventricular aneurysm. Randerath's[6] 34 year old patient died two days after extensive myocardial contusion, and at necropsy a left ventricular aneurysm containing a mural thrombus and occlusions by emboli of one femoral and of two coronary arteries were found. Parsons-Smith and Williams[19] described

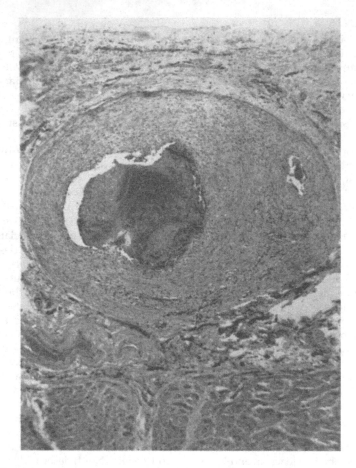

Figure 5 *Cross section of the anterior descending coronary artery 9 cm. from its origin. It* is almost completely occluded by an organizing and fresh thrombus. Recanalization of the organizing thrombus can be seen in the right half of the photomicrograph. The organized thrombus presumably dates from the time of injury. The fresh thrombus may have arisen *in situ,* perhaps coincident to hypovolemia, or may represent embolic material. (Hematoxylin and eosin stain, × 39 reduced by 8%.)

a 15 year old boy who recovered from myocardial contusion and left hemiparesis, which had developed the day after the contusion.

Postoperative Embolization: Systemic emboli are common, however, in patients with chronic left ventricular aneurysms due to coronary atherosclerosis,[20] and they constitute one of the indications for operative intervention. Before cardiopulmonary bypass was available, a left ventricular aneurysm was resected by applying a clamp across its mouth and excising the tissue distal to the clamp. As a consequence of this closed procedure, a port on of the mural thrombus frequently was dislodged into the circulation or was not removed, a problem that often led to operative or postoperative systemic embolization,[21, 22] With cardiopulmonary bypass, complete removal of the aneurysm and intra-aneurysmal thrombus became possible. In 51 reported patients who have undergone left ventricular aneurysmectomy under cardiopulmonary bypass, operative and postoperative emboli have not been recorded.[23–26]

In retrospect, it would appear that the present patient should have been placed on anticoagulants postoperatively on a long term basis. Anticoagulation following left ventricular aneurysmectomy is not a common practice of any clinic of which we are aware, but this procedure needs further consideration.

SUMMARY

The clinical and pathologic features of a 23 year old man with a left ventricular aneurysm that developed following blunt trauma to the chest are described. Systemic emboli occurred both before left ventricular aneurysmectomy under cardiopulmonary bypass was performed and several months following the operation. This complication proved to be fatal. A large mural thrombus in the left ventricle was the apparent source of the emboli.

ACKNOWLEDGMENT

We wish to thank Dr. Ayub Oinmaya, under whose supervision this patient was admitted, for his permission to publish this case. Also, we would like to thank Drs. Earl K. Shirey and William L. Proudfit of the Cleveland Clinic Foundation, who performed the cineangiocardiographic studies and permitted us to reproduce the frames shown in Figure 3.

REFERENCES

1. FRENCH, H. A case of traumatic aneurysm of the heart. *Guy's Hosp. Rep.*, 66: 349, 1912.
2. HAWKES, S. Z. Traumatic rupture of the heart and intrapericardial structures. *Am. J. Surg.*, 27: 503, 1935.
3. PITTS, H. H. and PURVIS, G. S. Ruptured traumatic aneurysm in a child. *Canad. M. A. J.*, 57: 165, 1947.
4. JOACHIM, H. and MAYS, A. T. Case of cardiac aneurysm probably of traumatic origin. *Am. Heart J.*, 2: 682, 1927.
5. WARBURG, E. *Subacute and Chronic Pericardial and Myocardial Lesions Due to Nonpenetrating Traumatic Injuries*, p. 24. Translated by ANDERSEN, H. and SEIDELIN, G. London, 1938. Oxford University Press.
6. RANDERATH, E. Fruhveranderungen des Herzens nach Commotio Cordis. *Verhandl. deutsch, Path, Gesellsch.*, 30: 163, 1937.
7. BARBER, H. The effects of trauma, direct and indirect, on the heart. *Quart. J. Med.*, 13; 137, 1944.
8. PARMLEY, L. F., MANION, W. C. and MATTINGLY, T. W. Nonpenetrating traumatic injury of the heart. *Circulation*, 18: 371, 1958.
9. BRIGHT, E. F. and BECK, C. S. Nonpenetrating wounds of the heart. *Am. Heart J.*, 10: 293, 1935.
10. KISSANE, R. W. Traumatic heart disease: Nonpenetrating injuries. *Circulation*, 6: 421, 1952.
11. DEMUTH, W. E. and Zinsser, H. F. Myocardial contusion. *Arch. Int. Med.*, 115: 434, 1965.
12. Moritz, A. R. Injuries of the heart and pericardium by physical violence. In: *Pathology of the Heart*, ed. 2, p. 849. Edited by GOULD, S. E. Springfield, IL, 1960. Charles C. Thomas.
13. LEVINE, R. J., ROBERTS, W. C. and MORROW, A. G. Traumatic aortic regurgitation. *Am. J. Cardiol.*, 10: 752, 1962.
14. GOLDSTEIN, S. and YU, P. N. Constrictive pericarditis after blunt chest trauma. *Am. Heart J.*, 69: 544, 1965.
15. ROSE, K. D., STONE, F. and FUENNING, S. I. Cardiac contusion resulting from "spearing" in football. *Arch. Int. Med.*, 118: 129, 1966.

16. JOKL, E. and GRUNSTEIN, J. Fatal coronary sclerosis in a boy of ten years. *Lancet*, 2: 659, 1944.
17. LEVY, H. Traumatic coronary thrombosis with myocardial infarction. *Arch. Int. Med.*, 84: 261, 1949.
18. LEHMUS, H. J., SUNDQUIST, A. B. and GIDDINGS, L. W. Coronary thrombosis with myocardial infarction secondary to nonpenetrating injury of the chest wall. *Am. Heart J.*, 47: 470, 1954.
19. PARSONS-SMITH, G. and WILLIAMS, D. Cerebral embolism following contusion of the heart. *Brit M. J.*, 1: 10, 1949.
20. SCHLICHTER, J., HELLERSTEIN, H. K. and KATZ, L. N. Aneurysm of the heart: A correlative study of one hundred and two proved cases. *Medicine*, 33: 43, 1954.
21. BAILEY, C. P., BOLTON, H. E., NICHOLS, H. and GILMAN, R. Ventriculoplasty for cardiac aneurysm. *J. Thoracic Surg.*, 35: 37, 1956.
22. SULLIVAN, J. J., MANGIARDI, J. L. and JANELLI, D. E. Successful resection of ventricular aneurysm. *Ann. Surq.*, 131: 22, 1960.
23. KAY, J. H., ANDERSON, R. M., BERNSTFIN, S. and TOLENTINO, P. Removal of left ventricular aneurysm with heart exposed and circulation maintained by heart-lung machine. *California Med.*, 92: 434.1960.
24. GLENN, W. W. L., TOOLE, A, L., LONCO, E., Hume, M. and GENTSCH, T. O. Induced fibrillatory arrest in open-heart surgery *New England J. Med.*, 262: 852, 1960.
25. NEPTUNE, W. B., BOUGAS, J. A. and PANICO, F. G. Open-heart surgery without the need for donor-blood priming in the pump oxygenator. *New England J. Med.*, 263: 111, 1960.
26. TELLING, M. and WOOLER, G. H. Excision of cardiac aneurysm. *Lancet*, 2: 181, 1961.
27. CHAPMAN, D. W., AMAD, K. and COOLEY, D. A. Ventricular aneurysm: Fourteen cases subjected to cardiac bypass repair using the pump oxygenator. *Am. J. Cardiol.*, 8: 633, 1901.
28. EFFLER, D. B., WESCOTT, R. N., GROVES, L. K. and SCULLY, N. M. Surgical treatment of ventricular aneurysm. *Arch. Surg.*, 87: 249, 1963.
29. LAM, C. R., GALE, H. and DRAKE, E. Surgical treatment of left ventricular aneurysms. *J. A. M. A.*, 187: 1, 1964.
30. LILLIHEI, C. W., LEVY, M. J., DEWALL., R. A. and WARDEN, H. E. Resection of myocardial aneurysms after infarction during temporary cardiopulmonary bypass. *Circulation*, 26: 206, 1962.
31. CATHCART, R. T., FRAIMOW, W. and TEMPLETON, J. W. III. Postinfarction ventricular aneurysm: Four year follow-up of surgically treated cases. *Dis. Chest*, 44: 449, 1903.

Case 63 An Unusual Nephritis in Malignant Hypertension

D. Luke Glancy, MD; Oshin Bohjalian, MD; and William C. Roberts, MD
Bethesda, Md, and Washington, DC

IN 1932 Rich[1] described a peculiar and morphologically unique nephritis with two distinctive histologic features: (1) focal spherical nodules of interstitial, chronic, inflammatory cells which invaginated the walls of tubules into their lumina, and (2) the presence in the tubular lumina of cholesterol crystals associated with degenerating epithelial cells, polymorphonuclear leukocytes, and lipid-laden macrophages. Since Rich's report, only one subsequent paper[2] describing this form of nephritis has appeared, although similar lesions were illustrated in the monographs of Allen[3] and Heptinstall.[4] In 25 other texts and monographs on renal disease published during the past 30 years either no mention is made of this focal, interstitial nephritis or Rich's observations are simply summarized. Recently, we encountered this lesion in a patient who died of malignant hypertension, and the clinicopathologic findings in him are summarized in the report which follows.

REPORT OF A CASE

A 26-year-old Negro man (DCGH 24–05–59), was known to have systemic hypertension since 1960 but was asymptomatic until November 1966, seven weeks before death, when he developed exertional and nocturnal dyspnea. A week later he was hospitalized because of pulmonary edema. He received antihypertensive agents, and two weeks later (four weeks before death) he was discharged and given methyldopa and furosemide. Three weeks before death he began vomiting and four days later had the first of several generalized seizures and was admitted to the District of Columbia General Hospital. He had no history or signs or symptoms at any time of venereal disease. A serum Wassermann in April 1962 had been negative. He had never received penicillin. The patient had no previous history of renal disease and no symptoms of urinary tract infection. An urinalysis in 1962 had been normal.

The blood pressure was 225/180 mm Hg. Retinal exudates, narrowed arterioles, and signs of papilledema were seen on funduscopic examination. A forceful left ventricular precordial impulse and a loud ventricular gallop were present. The remainder of the physical examination was unremarkable.

The blood urea nitrogen (BUN) on admission was 100 mg/100 ml, and the serum creatinine, 14.4 mg/100 ml. The urine contained both red and white blood cells in small numbers and 4 gm protein per liter. Two urine cultures, obtained before the administration of ampicillin and cephalothin sodium, yielded no growth.

The patient's 18 days in the hospital were characterized by progressive renal failure. His urine volume was initially 640 to 1,350 ml/24 hr, but after the third

Received for publication May 8, 1967; accepted June 26.

From the Section of Pathology, Clinic of Surgery, National Heart Institute, National Institutes of Health, Bethesda, Md, and the Department of Pathology, District of Columbia General Hospital, Washington, DC.

Reprint requests to Section of Pathology, Clinic of Surgery, National Institutes of Health, Bethesda, Md 20014 (Dr. Glancy).

DOI: 10.1201/9781003408321-4

19

hospital day it ranged from 150 to 500 ml/24 hr. Despite transient reductions by each of two peritoneal dialyses, the BUN rose to 180 and was 143 mg/100 ml the day before death. Hyperkalemia never developed.

A pericardial friction rub was first heard 14 days before death. Two days before death the rub disappeared, and diminished heart sounds, distended neck veins, an increased area of precordial dullness to percussion, and enlargement of the cardiac silhouette on chest roentgenogram were noted. On Dec 29, 1966, the patient became hypotensive, and several hours later his heart stopped. During unsuccessful resuscitative efforts, 60 ml of sanguineous fluid were aspirated from the pericardial cavity.

NECROPSY FINDINGS

The pericardial cavity contained 100 ml of hemorrhagic fluid, and there was diffuse fibrinous pericarditis. The heart weighed 500 gm, all chambers were dilated, and the left ventricle was hypertrophied. There were numerous fibrotic and calcified plaques in the descending and abdominal portions of the aorta, but they were rare in the ascending aorta. The right kidney weighed 140 gm, the left, 120 gm, and each contained punctate, subcapsular hemorrhages (Figure 1).

A proliferative endarteritis of small muscular arteries (Figure 1) and arterioles, characteristic of malignant nephrosclerosis, scattered hyalinized glomeruli, and occasional dilated tubules containing hyaline casts were found on histologic examination of the kidneys. An unexpected finding was bilateral interstitial nephritis (Figure 1 and 2) with the following characteristics:

1. There were dense, focal, interstitial collections of mononuclear cells, predominantly small lymphocytes, which were confined to the cortex.
2. Spherical masses of these cells invaginated renal cortical tubules, most of which appeared to be distal tubules or upper collecting ducts. Occasionally capillaries were seen entering these masses.
3. These projections of mononuclear cells were always covered by renal tubular epithelium, even when they herniated far enough for their attachment to the interstitium to be out of the plane of section so that they appeared to lie free within the tubule. The basement membrane of the portion of the tubule overlying the projecting mass, however, was frequently thinned or fragmented.
4. The tubules were often dilated so that a tubule and the cells herniating into it were similar in size and shape to a glomerulus. That these were dilated tubules and not altered glomeruli was demonstrated by serial sections through many lesions, which showed that both their proximal and distal ends were continuous with tubules. (Sections were cut at six micra-intervals; every third section was stained and examined.) Serial sections also revealed compression of these and adjacent tubules by the same interstitial infiltrate which at other levels herniated into their lumina.
5. In some tubules invaginated by mononuclear cells, the remaining lumen contained degenerating inflammatory debris, which, in contrast to the interstitial infiltrate, included many polymorphonuclear leukocytes. Occasional tubules without spherical projections of mononuclear cells contained similar degenerating inflammatory debris.
6. Within this debris were many elongated clefts left by crystalline material which had dissolved during tissue processing.
7. In each kidney just beneath the epithelium of the renal pelvis was a widespread, dense, inflammatory infiltrate consisting predominantly of small lymphocytes, but also histiocytes, plasma cells, and polymorphonuclear leukocytes (Figure 3). Within this infiltrate were small nodules composed primarily of histocytes.

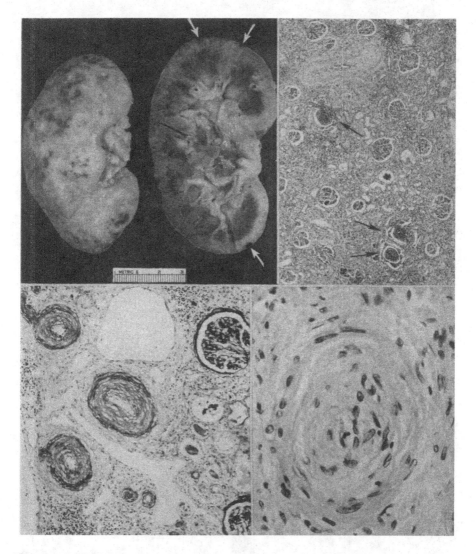

Figure 1 **Top left**, Punctate renal cortical hemorrhages (**arrows**). **Top right**, Dilated renal tubules (**arrows**) invaginated by mononuclear cells (hematoxylin and eosin, × 39). **Bottom left**, Renal arterioles and small arteries (PAS, × 99). **Bottom right**, A small renal artery (hematoxylin and eosin, × 400).

8. The renal medullae contained increased interstitial fibrous tissue, but no cellular infiltrates. Stains of the kidneys for spirochetes (Warthin-Starry), bacteria (Brown and Brenn), fungi (methenamine silver), and acid-fast bacteria (Ziehl-Neelsen) disclosed no organisms.

There were no changes suggesting syphilis in any organ, and the intima, media, and adventitia of the ascending aorta were normal.

COMMENT

Except for the interstitial nephritis, the clinical course and autopsy findings in this patient are typical of those in malignant hypertension. Cardiac tamponade

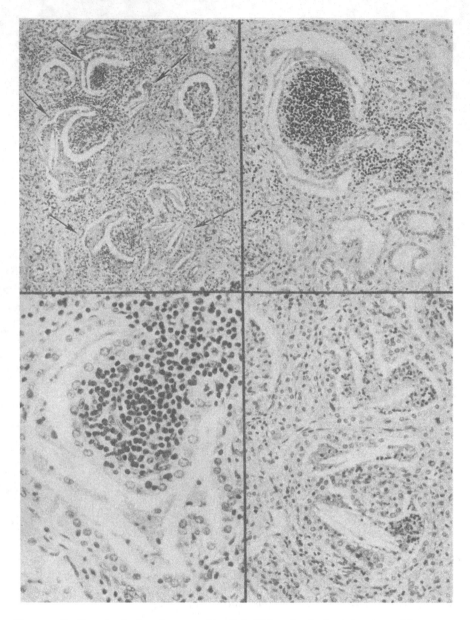

Figure 2 Renal tubular changes. **Top left,** Dilated tubules invaginated by mononuclear cells (**solid arrows**). The remainder of each tubular lumen and other tubular lumina (**dashed arrows**) contain degenerating cellular debris and crystal-clefts (hemertoxylin and eosin, × 99). **Top right,** (hematoxylin and eosin, × 160). **Bottom left,** (hematoxylin and eosin, × 400). **Bottom right,** (hematoxylin and eosin, × 230).

is an uncommon occurrence in uremia from any cause, but we have observed it in another patient with malignant hypertension in whom hemorrhage into the pericardial cavity complicated existing fibrinous pericarditis, as happened in the present patient.

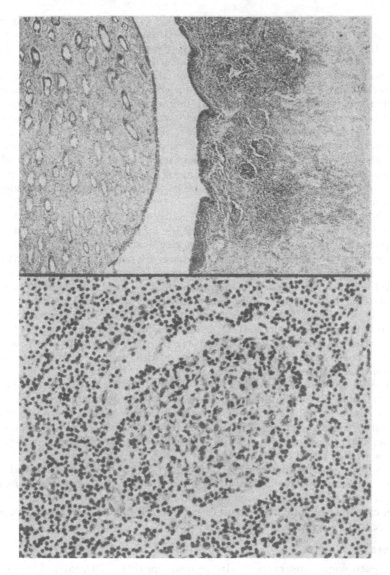

Figure 3 Renal pelvis. **Top,** Dense pleomorphic infiltrate, predominantly small lymphocytes, beneath the renal pelvic epithelium. Within this infiltrate are spherical nodules (hematoxylin and eosin, × 25). **Bottom,** An enlargement of one of the nodules, which is composed predominantly of histiocytes (hematoxylin and eosin, × 251).

The morphologically unique interstitial nephritis observed in the present patient is identical to that described by Rich, and the renal cortical lesions in Figure 1 and 2 are indistinguishable from those illustrated in his report,[1] He, however, did not mention inflammation beneath the renal pelvic epithelium. Rich postulated that the interstitial inflammation obstructed tubules by compression, thus enabling the herniating masses of cells in more proximal, dilated portions of the tubules to become quite large. Stasis, caused by obstruction, allowed the accumulation of inflammatory debris in which crystals formed. The histologic findings in the present patient support these postulates. Rich found that crystals were still present in the elongated clefts in frozen sections of kidney, and their shape, melting point, and staining characteristics suggested that they were composed of cholesterol. The nephritis was always focal, but its extent varied considerably in different patients. All 19 of Rich's patients had some abnormality on urinalysis. Ten of 14 had azotemia, and in seven of the 19 the interstitial nephritis was associated with some other renal disease. Because of frequently co-existing renal disease, or cardiac failure, Rich could not draw any definite conclusions about the functional significance of the lesions but commented that "renal insufficiency can be expected to result from this type of lesion only when it is very widespread, for it is primarily an interstitial nephritis . . . . " In the present patient, renal insufficiency can readily be explained on the basis of malignant nephrosclerosis alone.

Although the relation between the two is unknown, it is possible that the renal disease in the patient presented was responsible for the systemic hypertension. The changes in the systemic arteries, however, were typical of those seen in the malignant phase of essential hypertension and, like the parenchymal changes, appeared to be of similar severity in each kidney. The juxtaglomerular complexes appeared normal in both kidneys. Conversely, there is no evidence that the interstitial nephritis resulted from systemic hypertension, and to our knowledge, similar lesions have not been described in studies of hypertensive subjects. Nine of Rich's 15 patients (excluding the four with aortic regurgitation), however, had diastolic blood pressures of 95 mm Hg or greater; five of them were 120 mm Hg or more.[1] Bauer's patient had severe diastolic hypertension (130 to 160 mm Hg) and died with uremia after a clinical course similar to that of the present patient.[2]

Since all their patients had tertiary syphilis, Rich[1] and Bauer[2] ascribed the interstitial nephritis to syphilis, but spirochetes were never demonstrated in the kidneys. The present patient had neither clinical, serologic, nor necropsy evidence of syphilis. Allen[3] and Heptinstall[4] described similar renal lesions in patients with pyelonephritis. There were no clinical features suggesting chronic urinary tract infection in the present patient.

Although the interstitial nephritis first described by Rich and observed in the present patient is morphologically unique and easily distinguished from other forms of renal disease, its etiology may well be different in different patients, or it may be caused by a common but as yet unknown factor. The present patient provides evidence that the lesion is not specific for syphilis.

SUMMARY

Clinicopathologic observations in a nonsyphilitic, 26-year-old man who died of malignant hypertension are described. At autopsy, in addition to the usual changes of malignant nephrosclerosis, there was an unusual and morphologically unique interstitial nephritis which in the past has been attributed to syphilis.

GENERIC AND TRADE NAMES OF DRUGS

Methyldopa—*Aldomet.*
Ampicillin—*Penbritin, Polycillin.*
Cephalothin sodium—*Keflin.*
Furosemide—*Lasix.*

REFERENCES

1. Rich, A.R.: The Pathology of Nineteen Cases of a Peculiar and Specific Form of Nephritis Associated With Acquired Syphilis, *Bull Hopkins Hosp* 50:357–382 (June) 1932.
2. Bauer, J.T.: A Case of Peculiar Nephritis Associated With Acquired Syphilis, *Bull Ayer Clin Lab Penn Hosp* 3:1–6 (May) 1934.
3. Allen, A.C.: *The Kidney: Medical and Surgical Diseases*, ed 2, New York: Grune & Stratton, 1962, pp. 456–460.
4. Heptinstall, R.H.: *Pathology of the Kidney*, Boston: Little, Brown & Co., 1966, pp. 434–435.

Case 283 Medial Calcinosis of Mönckeberg

A Review of the Problem and a Description of a Patient with Involvement of Peripheral, Visceral and Coronary Arteries

Anthony S. Lachman, M.D. and Thomas L. Spray, M.D.
Bethesda, Maryland
Donald M. Kerwin, M.D. and Gerald I. Shugoll, M.D.*
Washington, D.C.
William C. Roberts, M.D.
Bethesda, Maryland

Massive medial calcific deposits (Mönckeberg's calcinosis) are described in the peripheral and visceral arteries, and similar but small-sized deposits in the coronary arteries of a 41 year old woman with diabetes mellitus. Although observed by roentgenogram fairly commonly during life in the muscular arteries of the legs in middle-aged men, medial calcinosis infrequently involves the visceral arteries and has never, to our knowledge, been documented in the coronary arteries. Although it may be associated with intimal atherosclerosis, medial calcinosis, per se, does not obstruct the lumens of the arteries and, therefore, does not lead to symptoms or signs of limb or organ ischemia. The cause of medial calcinosis remains a mystery, but it appears to affect people with diabetes more frequently than those without.

Although described in 1903,[1] calcification of the medial smooth muscle layer of arteries of the extremities (Mönckeberg's calcinosis) has received relatively little attention, particularly in recent years. The condition does not involve the intimal layer of the artery and, therefore, luminal narrowing is not a consequence.[1-5] Indeed, the lumen is held open by the rigid media. Therefore, organ or limb ischemia is not a consequence of this condition.[1-5] Because medial calcinosis may be a striking roentgenographic finding and because medial calcific deposits in sites other than the lower limbs are usually not recognized, the finding of severe medial calcinosis in the abdominal arteries and, to a lesser extent, in the coronary arteries in addition to those in the extremities prompted a description of our patient and a reexamination of this entity.

CASE REPORT

A 41 year old black woman, a habitual alcoholic, was asymptomatic until age 36 when exertional dyspnea developed. Examination disclosed systemic hypertension (blood pressure 180/100 mm Hg), azotemia (blood urea nitrogen 108 mg/100 ml) and anemia (hematocrit value 25 per cent). Although there was no evidence of carbohydrate intolerance (fasting blood glucose 107 mg/100 ml), a renal biopsy specimen disclosed a Kimmelstiel-Wilson type of glomerular lesion. Other members of her family had diabetes mellitus and systemic hypertension.

From the Pathology Branch, National Heart, Lung and Blood Institute, National Institutes of Health, Bethesda, Maryland; and the Departments of Pathology and Medicine, Georgetown University, Washington, D.C. Request for reprints should be addressed to Dr. William C. Roberts, Building 10A, Room 3E-30, National Institutes of Health, Bethesda, Maryland 20014. Manuscript accepted March 22, 1977.
* Present address: 5530 Wisconsin Avenue, Chevy Chase, Maryland 20015.

DOI: 10.1201/9781003408321-5

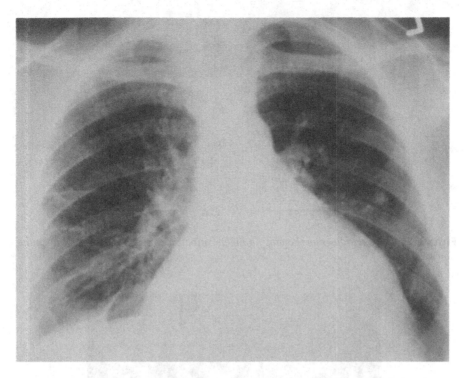

Figure 1 *Chest roentgenogram showing cardiomegaly, atelectasis and pleural effusion, and focal parenchymal pulmonary lesions in the patient described.*

By the age of 40 (four years later), congestive cardiac and renal failure (creatinine 7.0 mg/100 ml) had developed, and on three occasions she had required hospitalization for treatment of fluid retention. Mild carbohydrate intolerance was documented during these episodes but was controlled with diet alone. She remained in borderline compensated cardiac and renal failure but was readmitted to the hospital three months before death with a cold, dark and tender right lower leg. Examination revealed absence of pulses below the femoral artery on the right but good (1+ to 2+) pulsations in the femoral arteries and in the dorsalis pedis artery on the left. Chest roentgenograms showed cardiomegaly and a rightsided pleural effusion plus evidence for old calcified granulomatous disease (Figure 1). The electrocardiogram showed an indeterminate axis and interventricular conduction delay, and no evidence of myocardial damage (Figure 2). Roentgenograms of the abdomen, forearms and legs (Figure 3) showed diffuse multiple ring-type arterial calcific deposits which distinctly outlined the medium to small muscular arteries but did not involve the aorta. The serum calcium was 6.9 mg/100 ml, the serum phosphorus 6.3 mg/100 ml, and the total serum proteins were 6.8 g/100 ml. The patient's right leg remained cold and painful despite heparin therapy, the skin excoriated over the heel and great toe, and the leg was amputated above the knee. Examination of the excised leg showed marked narrowing of the lumen of the popliteal artery by atherosclerotic plaques. Peritoneal dialysis initially produced improvement in her renal and cardiac status, but generalized Staphylococcus aureus septicemia developed and she died despite antibiotic therapy.

At necropsy (75A1), the heart weighed 550 g. A diffuse fibrinous pericardial exudate was present. Both ventricular cavities were dilated, and the left ventricular

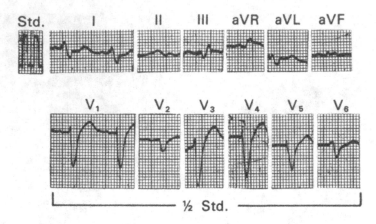

Figure 2 *Electrocardiogram showing an indeterminate axis and interventricular conduction delay.*

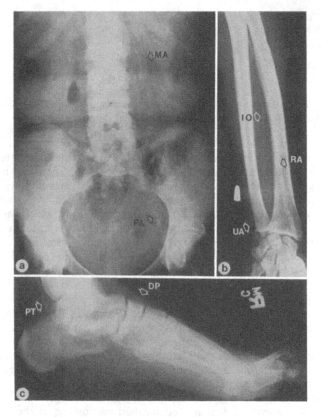

Figure 3 *Roentgenograms of the abdomen (**a**), forearm (**b**) and right foot (**c**) showing calcific deposits in the muscular arteries. **a**, abdominal film shows ring-like calcific deposits in the mesenteric (MA) and pelvic (PA) arteries. **b**, calcific deposits in the radial (RA), ulnar (UA) and interosseus (IO) arteries of the forearm. **c**, roentgenogram of the right foot showing ring-like calcific deposits in the dorsalis pedis (DP) and posterior tibial (PT) arteries.*

wall was thick (up to 2.0 cm). A transmural myocardial scar, extending almost from the base to the apex of the heart, involved the posterior wall of the left ventricle (Figure 4). No areas of myocardial necrosis were noted.

The coronary arteries contained heavy calcific deposits (Figure 5). Histologic examination of subserial sections of the major extramural coronary arteries showed marked atherosclerosis with luminal narrowing of more than 75 per cent in cross-sectional area of segments of the right and left circumflex branches by intimal plaques. The left anterior descending artery and its diagonal branches also contained calcified atherosclerotic plaques, but the lumens of these vessels were less than 50 per cent narrowed in cross-sectional area. In addition, calcific deposits were present in the media in the left anterior descending artery and its diagonal branches (Figure 5); portions of the media in these arteries were atrophied, and nuclei in residual smooth muscle cells stained poorly or not at all.

Postmortem roentgenograms of the mesenteric and renal (Figure 6), celiac, splenic (Figure 7) and iliac (Figure 8) arteries showed diffuse calcific deposits arranged in multiple rings. Unlike the coronary arteries, histologic examination showed that the calcific deposits in these arteries involved only the media; the internal elastic membrane remained intact, and the calcific deposits of the media often extended outward from the internal elastic membrane to involve only a portion of the media. The smooth muscle cells were indistinct, nuclear detail was absent in the areas of medial calcinosis, and the cytoplasm of the smooth muscle cells contained finely granular basophilic calcific deposits in the medial layer, but no intimal calcific deposits were present. Calcific deposits were also present in the aorta, but these were restricted to the intimal layer (Figure 8). No inflammatory cells were present in the media of any vessel examined, and frozen sections of the abdominal and iliac arteries stained for neutral lipids showed deposits of lipid material in the intima but none in the media.

Sections of the kidneys showed intercapillary glomerulosclerosis (Kimmelstiel-Wilson disease) (Figure 9), and the liver showed mild periportal fibrous and fatty

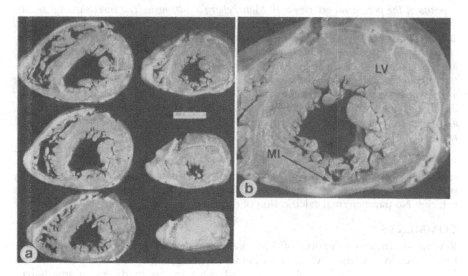

Figure 4 *Transverse slices of the cardiac ventricles (**a**) showing mild left ventricular hypertrophy and a transmural myocardial scar in the posterior left ventricular wall extending almost from the base to the apex. A close-up of one slice (**b**) showing left ventricular hypertrophy (LV) and the transmural scar (MI).*

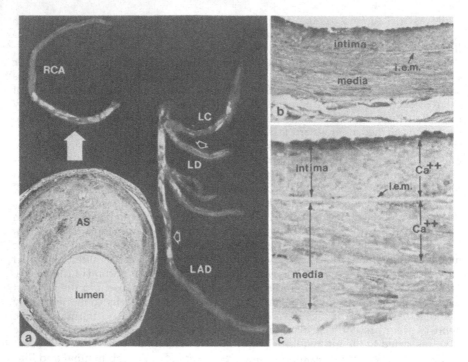

Figure 5 *Coronary arteries.* **a**, *postmortem roentgenogram showing intimal and medial calcific deposits in the coronary arteries. Typical atherosclerotic intimal calcific deposits are seen in the right (RCA), left anterior descending (LAD) and left circumflex (LC) coronary arteries. The first left diagonal coronary artery (LD) and portions of the LAD coronary artery, however, show calcific deposits (open arrows) which are similar to the ring-like calcific deposits of the peripheral arteries with Mönckeberg's calcinosis. The inset shows a section of proximal right coronary artery from the area shown by the large arrow. Typical intimal atherosclerosis (AS) with significant narrowing of the lumen of the vessel is present. Movat stain; original magnification × 20, reduced by 41 per cent.* **b**, *section of the LAD coronary artery from the area shown by the open arrow in a showing medial calcinosis in addition to the intimal atherosclerosis. i.e.m. = internal elastic membrane.* **c**, *high-power view of same area as in* **b** *showing medial calcinosis (Ca++) and loss of medial smooth muscle cellular detail in the inner one half of the media. Intimal atherosclerosis with calcific deposits (Ca++) also are seen. Hematoxylin and eosin stains; original magnification × 330 (b), × 860 (c), reduced by 41 per cent.*

infiltrates. The pancreas was grossly normal and histologic sections showed only mild hyaline changes of the islets of Langerhans and medial calcinosis of the arteries. No parenchymal calcification of the solid organs was noted.

COMMENTS

Review of previous reports of Mönckeberg's medial calcinosis discloses that this condition is usually an incidental roentgenologic or histologic finding. Roentgenographically, it is observed most often in the medium- to small-sized muscular arteries of the extremities of young to middle-aged (20 to 50 years) men. Its cause is unknown and its course is benign.[4-7] Circulatory impairment in association with the medial calcinosis is unusual[4,5]; when present, it is the result of an associated intimal process and not the medial disease. Medial calcinosis is

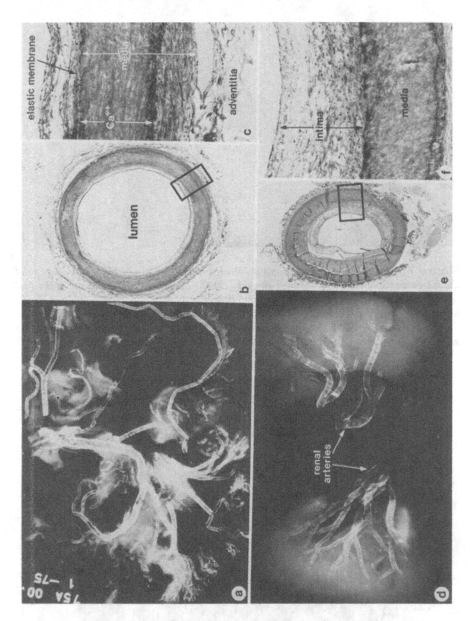

Figure 6 *Medial calcinosis of the abdominal arteries.* **a,** *postmortem roentgenogram of the superior mesenteric artery and its branches showing heavy ring-like calcific deposits.* **b,** *section of the superior mesenteric artery showing circumferential calcific deposits in the media but little intimal thickening and a widely patent lumen.* **c,** *higher-power view of area enclosed by box in b showing little intimal thickening, an intact internal elastic membrane and calcific deposits (Ca++) with loss of cellular detail of the smooth muscle of the inner two thirds of the media.* **d,** *postmortem roentgenogram of the renal arteries showing typical ring-like medial calcinosis.* **e,** *section of renal artery showing medial calcific deposits in addition to intimal fibrous thickening.* **f,** *higher-power view of area enclosed by box in e showing a thickened intima without calcific deposits and the granular, calcified media. Hematoxylin and eosin stains; original magnification × 20* **(b and e),** *× 140 (c and f). reduced by 35 per cent.*

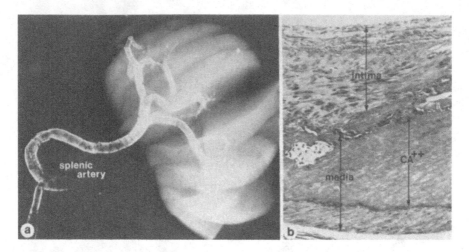

Figure 7 *Medial calcific deposits in the splenic artery. **a**, postmortem roentgenogram of the spleen and splenic artery showing ring-like calcific deposits along the length of the vessel. No parenchymal calcific deposits are seen. **b**, section of splenic artery showing moderate intimal thickening, and calcific deposits and loss of smooth muscle in the inner two thirds of the media. Despite moderate intimal thickening, the vessel was widely patent. Hematoxylin and eosin stain; original magnification × 140, reduced by 40 per cent.*

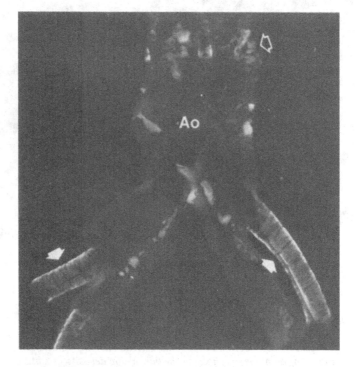

Figure 8 *Postmortem roentgenogram of the distal abdominal aorta (Ao) and iliac arteries. Intimal atherosclerotic calcific deposits are seen in the aorta (open arrow). In contrast, the iliac vessels show ring-like calcific deposits (closed arrows) and no intimal calcific deposits.*

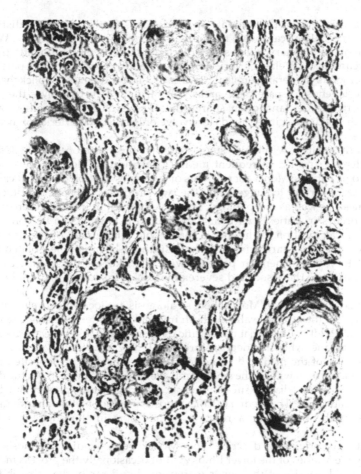

Figure 9 *Section of kidney showing eosinophilic nodular lesions of the glomerular lobules (arrow) typical of the Kimmelstiel-Wilson type of diabetic glomerulosclerosis. Hematoxylin and eosin stain; magnification × 130.*

diagnosed most commonly during roentgenologic examination of the extremities of patients with bone or joint disease or evidence of limb ischemia from atherosclerosis.[4,5] Although clinically medial calcinosis is observed (by roentgenogram) most commonly in men less than 50 years of age, necropsy studies of persons more than 50 years of age have shown an equal sex distribution of medial calcinosis in the peripheral arteries.[8]

The typical picture of Mönckeberg's calcinosis by roentgenogram is one of ring-like accumulations of calcium against a finely "granular" background.[4–6,9,10] The affected arteries thus resemble a chain of rings and have been compared to a "goose neck." When the medial calcific deposits are small in amount, the ring-like accumulations may not be apparent but the "granular" deposits may be visible and give a "pipe stem" roentgenographic appearance,[9] as seen in the left diagonal coronary artery of our patient (Figure 5). Atherosclerotic calcific deposits which are entirely in the intimal layer, in contrast, are irregular and patchy in distribution and do not have the ring-like or granular appearance as do medial calcific deposits.[9]

The distribution of the arterial calcific deposits further serves to distinguish Mönckeberg's medial calcinosis from atherosclerotic intimal calcinosis. With the exception of the coronary arteries, atherosclerosis affects predominantly the aorta and its arch arteries (all elastic arteries) and the arteries of the extremities, particularly those over joints (femoral, popliteal, brachial),[4,9] In contrast, the Mönckeberg type of calcinosis tends to spare these areas.[5,8] It virtually never involves the aorta or other elastic arteries and often spares the vessels of the extremities over the joints[9,11]; the medial calcinosis tends to involve only muscular arteries of medium to small size.

As early as 1856, Virchow[12] suggested that the common intimal lesions of atherosclerosis and the infrequent medial "petrification" lesions were separate morphologic entities; Mönckeberg, in his original description of medial calcinosis in 1903,[1] went further to suggest that the two processes differed in etiology and pathogenesis as well as morphology. The development of intimal atherosclerosis, when it occurs in patients with medial calcinosis, appears to be coincidental. In fact, the calcification of the media may "hold" the lumen of the artery open and prevent luminal narrowing and the resulting ischemia. The isolated reports of circulatory impairment in patients with Mönckeberg's sclerosis, as in our patient, are due to the associated severe atherosclerosis rather than to the medial calcification.[5]

The calcific deposits in Mönckeberg's calcinosis are located entirely within the medial layer of the arterial wall, and both internal and external elastic membranes are spared.[1,4,5,13] It is likely that the calcific deposits begin just beneath the internal elastic membrane; when the deposits are small, they are virtually always located in this portion of the media.[4,14] The calcium salts appear to be deposited initially between, rather than within, the smooth muscle cells of the media,[15] As the deposits increase in size, the adjacent smooth muscle cells degenerate, presumably because of pressure atrophy.[16] The medial calcific deposits produce neither an inflammatory response in the media nor a reaction of any sort in the adjacent intima or adventitia.

As it was originally described by Mönckeberg, medial calcinosis affects primarily the arteries of the lower limbs,[1,4–7] but occasionally the process may affect the peripheral arteries of the upper extremities,[4] and rarely the intra-abdominal arteries.[4,8,10,13,17–19] Of the latter, the renal and splenic arteries are the ones most often affected.[17–19] Medial calcinosis in the renal arteries appears to occur particularly in patients with diabetes mellitus.[17,18]

Diffuse, severe medial calcinosis involving the mesenteric arteries has not, to our knowledge, been reported previously. The extensive mesenteric arterial medial calcinosis without intimal calcinosis as occurred in our patient, therefore, is unique. Mesenteric arterial insufficiency is not a consequence of medial calcinosis of these arteries.

Although their involvement was suggested by Mönckeberg in his initial report,[1] coronary arterial medial calcinosis has not, to our knowledge, been documented previously. Although our patient did have medial calcific deposits in these arteries, the deposits were minimal and limited to only small portions of the left anterior descending coronary artery and its diagonal branch. The lumen of the coronary arteries involved by the medial calcific deposits were widely patent and, therefore, the medial deposits had no functional significance.

In contrast to the minimal extent of medial calcinosis in the extramural coronary arteries of our patient, extensive intimal calcific deposits of atherosclerotic origin were present. Indeed, the lumens of two of the three major epicardial coronary arteries in our patient were more than 75 per cent narrowed in cross-sectional area by old atherosclerotic plaques, and a transmural left ventricular scar was present.

During life, our patient never had clinical or electrocardiographic evidence of acute myocardial infarction. Interestingly, the lumens of the coronary branches (left anterior descending and left diagonal) containing the foci of medial calcinosis were less than 50 per cent narrowed in cross-sectional area, whereas the lumens in the two severely (more than 75 per cent) narrowed coronary arteries (right and left circumflex) contained no medial calcific deposits.

The cause of Mönckeberg's medial calcinosis remains unknown. Several reports have described medial calcification in experimental animals in association with certain agents, including vitamin D and adrenalin,[20-23] and it has been suggested that a prolonged vasotonic influence may produce the medial calcific deposits.[24] The medial calcific deposits in these studies, however, usually involve the aorta, an artery uninvolved by medial calcinosis in the human being. Furthermore, medial necrotic lesions often preceded the medial calcific deposits in these experiments, and foci of medial necrosis have not been observed as a precursor of medial calcinosis in man.

Although it is the most common type of medial calcinosis, Mönckeberg's calcinosis is not the only form of medial calcinosis. Calcific deposits occur frequently in the media of thyroidal or intrauterine arteries, but the internal elastic membrane is also the site of calcific deposition, an occurrence not observed in Mönckeberg's calcinosis.[24] Medial calcinosis in infancy is also quite different from Mönckeberg's calcinosis.[25]

The relationship between Mönckeberg's calcinosis and diabetes mellitus is not clear.[17,26] Medial calcinosis is well described in diabetic patients[6,10,17,18,26] and probably occurs as the earliest manifestation of diabetic microangiography.[26] The severity of the calcific deposits appears to be related to the duration of the metabolic disturbance and not to the severity of, or the control of, the diabetes.[6] The role played by the metabolic disturbances accompanying the renal failure in causing the medial calcinosis remains speculative. Calcium phosphorus imbalance with secondary hyperparathyroidism must be considered a possible factor. The absence of generalized soft tissue calcinosis in our patient, however, is against this as an important etiologic factor.

REFERENCES

1. Mönckeberg JG: Uber die Heine Mediaverkalkung der Extremitätenarterien und ihr Verhalten zur Arteriosklerose. *Virchows Arch [Pathol Anat]* 171: 141, 1903.
2. Mönckeberg JG: Mediaverkalkung und Arteriosklerose. *Virchows Arch [Pathol Anat]* 216: 408, 1914.
3. Moschocowitz E: *Vascular Sclerosis*, New York, Oxford University Press, 1942, p. 76.
4. Silbert S, Lippmann HI: Moenckeberg's sclerosis. A clinical entity. *J Mt Sinai Hosp NY* 12–13: 689, 1945.
5. Silbert S, Lippmann HI, Gordon E: Mönckeberg's arteriosclerosis. *JAMA* 151: 1176, 1953.
6. Ferrier TM: Radiologically demonstrable arterial calcification in diabetes mellitus. *Australas Ann Med* 13: 222, 1964.
7. Merlen JF: Les calcinoses des membres inférieurs. *Phlébologie* 28: 531, 1975.
8. Cavallero C, Martinazzi M, Turolla E, et al.: Etudes morphologiques de la maladie arteriélle de Mönckeberg (calcification de la média). *Revue de l'athérosclérose et des artériopathies périphériques. Arch Mal Coeur* 10 (suppl 1): 2, 1968.
9. Lindbom A: Arteriosclerosis and arterial thrombosis in the lower limb; roentgenological study. *Acta Radiol Suppl* 80, 1950.
10. Donner MW, McAfee JG: Roentgenographic manifestations of diabetes mellitus. *Am J Med Sci* 239: 622, 1960.

11. Mönckeberg JG: *Arterienverkalkung: Therapie d, Herzinsuffizienz*, Georg Thieme Verlag, 1924, p. 63.
12. Virchow R, cit Mönckeberg JG: Mediaverkalkung und Arteriosklerose. *Virchows Arch [Pathol Anat]* 216: 408, 1914. Verlag von Georg Reimer, Berlin.
13. Klotz O: Fracture of arteries. *J Med Res* 34: 495, 1916.
14. Jores L: Arterien. Handbuch der Pathologischen. *Anatomie* 2: 632, 1924.
15. Hueck W: Anatomisches zur Frage nach Wesen und Ursache der Arteriosklerose. *Munch Med Wochenschr* 67: 535, 1920.
16. Faber A: *Die Arteriosklerose*, Verlag von Gustav Fischer Jena, 1912, p. 81.
17. Reinhardt K: Nierenarterienverkalkung bei einer Diabetikerin mit Mönckeberg-Sklerose. *Fortschr Geb Roentgenstr Nuklearmed* 119: 363, 1973.
18. Seshanarayana KN, Keats TE: Intrarenal arterial calcification: roentgen appearance and significance. *Radiology* 95: 145, 1970.
19. Moritz AR: Arteriosclerosis of the abdominal vessels, chap 16. *Cowdry's Arteriosclerosis* (Blumenthal HT, ed), Springfield, IL, Charles C. Thomas, 1967.
20. Duguid JB: Vitamin D sclerosis in the rat's aorta. *J Pathol Bacteriol* 33: 697, 1930.
21. Friedman WF, Roberts WC: Vitamin D and the supravalvar aortic stenosis syndrome. The transplacental effects of vitamin D on the aorta of the rabbit. *Circulation* 34: 77, 1966.
22. Erb W: Experimentelle und Histologische studien über Arterienerkrankungen nach Adrenalininjektionen. *Arch Exp Pathol Pharmakol* 53: 173, 1905.
23. Cavallero C, Spagnoli LG, DiTondo U: Early mitochondrial calcifications in the rabbit aorta after adrenalin. *Virchows Arch [Pathol Anat Histol]* 362: 23, 1974.
24. Bhagwat RR, Mittal S, Monga JN: Medial calcification of intra-uterine arteries. *J Indian Med Assoc* 63: 77, 1974.
25. Moran JJ, Becker SM: Idiopathic arterial calcification of infancy. *Am J Clin Pathol* 31: 517, 1959.
26. Christensen NJ: Diabetic macroangiopathy: blood flow and radiological studies. *Adv Metab Disord Suppl* 2: 129, 1972.

Case 342 Sucking Action of the Left Ventricle

Demonstration of a Physiologic Principle by a Gunshot Wound Penetrating Only the Right Side of the Heart

William C. Roberts, MD, FACC, William J. Brownlee, MD,
Ancil A. Jones, MD and James L. Luke, MD
Bethesda, Maryland

This report describes a man who died after a gunshot wound that entered the right atrium and exited from the right ventricle without entering the cardiac septa or the left side of the heart. At necropsy, the left atrial appendage was found to be inverted and invaginated into the mitral orifice. The invagination of the left atrial appendage is viewed as anatomic evidence that a negative left ventricular pressure was created as the left ventricular volume rapidly decreased as a result of right-sided cardiac exsanguination. Previously reported experiments in animals demonstrating the sucking (negative pressure) action of the left ventricle during ventricular diastole are summarized. The prerequisite for creation of a negative pressure in the ventricles during diastole is an extreme diminution in left ventricular volume, in this case as a result of right-sided cardiac bleeding. Only a vacuum effect of the left ventricle during diastole can explain the inversion and invagination of the left atrial appendage in this patient.

Whether the human cardiac ventricles can create a negative pressure or have a suction-like action has been debated for years. This report is the first to present evidence that the human left ventricle does have the capacity under certain circumstances to create a negative pressure and to suck blood into it from the left atrium.

CASE REPORT

The bullet from a 0.38 caliber handgun penetrated the right side of the chest of a 27 year old man sitting in a car, killing him within minutes. At necropsy (Case 78–301), the right side of the chest contained large quantities of blood, and about 300 ml of blood was present in the pericardial sac which had been severed by the bullet at two sites (Figure 1). The projectile had entered the heart through the right atrial appendage and exited through the right ventricular outflow tract. The bullet did not enter the left side of the heart, and both atrial and ventricular septa were intact. The left side of the heart was completely devoid of blood, and the left atrial appendage was inverted and invaginated into the mitral orifice (Figure 1 and 2).

COMMENTS

Spontaneous invagination of the left atrial appendage into the mitral orifice has not been described previously to our knowledge, and its explanation provides new

From the Pathology Branch, National Heart, Lung, and Blood Institute, National Institutes of Health, Bethesda, Maryland, and The Office of the Chief Medical Examiner, Washington, D.C. Manuscript received December 5, 1978; revised manuscript received and accepted January 10, 1979.

Address for reprints: William C. Roberts, MD, Building 10A, Room 3E-30, National Institutes of Health, Bethesda, Maryland 20014.

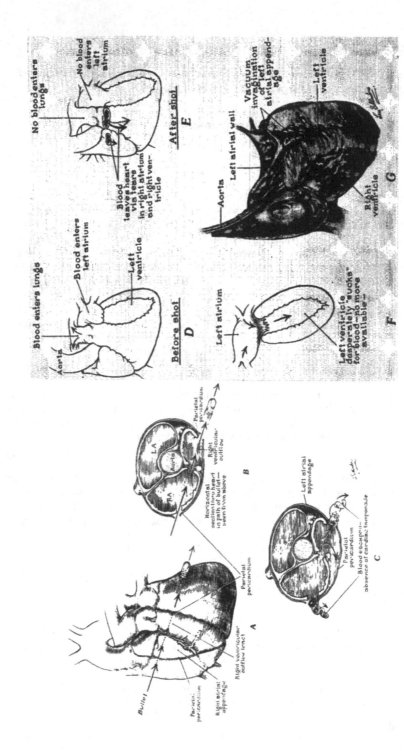

Figure 1 Diagrams illustrating the path of the bullet in the heart of the patient (A to E) and the resulting effects on the left atrium and left ventricle (F and G).

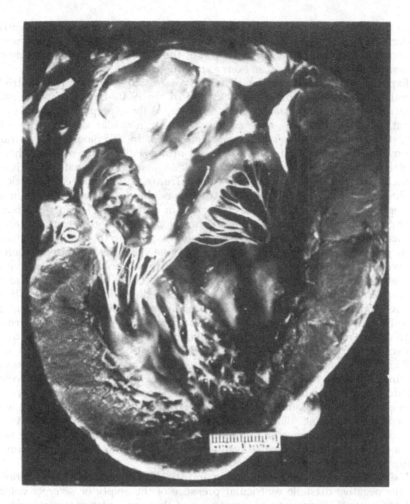

Figure 2 Opened left atrium, mitral valve and left ventricle showing the inverted left atrial appendage protruding into the mitral valve orifice.

insight into the physiologic dynamics of the human left ventricle. When the bullet perforations were made in the walls of the right atrium and ventricle, no blood thereafter entered the lungs. Tamponade was prevented because the perforations in the parietal pericardium provided egress for blood entering the pericardial sac from the right atrium and ventricle. After the cardiac wound, the only blood available to the left ventricle was that already present in the left-sided chambers and in the lungs. After emptying its chambers and the blood in the lungs, the left ventricle created a sucking action—actually a vacuum effect—that caused the left atrial appendage to invaginate and to be "pulled" through the mitral orifice toward the left ventricle.

For years, indeed centuries, it has been debated whether the cardiac ventricles filled entirely passively or filled to some extent by an active sucking action. In 1628, William Harvey[1] stated ". . . it is not true, as commonly believed, that the heart by its own action or distention draws blood into the ventricles . . . blood enters the ventricles, not by the suction or dilatation of the ventricles, but by the beat of the auricles." In 1922, Wiggers and Katz[2] demonstrated that it was not atrial contraction

39

which filled the ventricles, and in 1930 Katz,[3] utilizing the isolated turtle ventricle connected to a reservoir, demonstrated during relaxation that the pressure within the ventricle dropped below the zero level of the system, thus demonstrating that the mammalian ventricle ". . . can exert a sucking action . . ."

Experimental demonstration of negative pressures within the ventricles: Several experimental preparations described in the 1950's demonstrated negative pressures within the cardiac ventricles.[4-10] In all of these preparations and in our patient, negative pressures were created in the ventricular cavities only when the *ventricular end-systolic volumes were extremely small*. In 1955 Bloom[4] demonstrated, with motion pictures of the excised rat heart immersed in saline solution, that the left atrial walls descended into the mitral orifice (just as in our patient) with each ventricular diastole and that fluid was ejected from the aorta with each ventricular systole. Bloom concluded that the ventricle was able to fill only because it had developed a negative pressure. In 1956, Bloom and Ferris,[5,6] using the excised beating rat heart suspended in saline solution, found that with the atria intact the ventricular pressures were continuously negative (causing the atria to collapse, as in our patient, and thus preventing inflow into the ventricles). However, when the atria were excised, the ventricular diastolic pressure was only slightly negative and the systolic pressure in the ventricles was positive. These authors also found that in the open chest intact dog the right ventricular diastolic pressure was slightly negative and became progressively more negative as the inflow (from the superior and inferior vena cava and coronary sinus) was occluded. As the venous return was progressively more occluded, the ventricular pressure tracing approached that of the excised heart with intact atria. In 1956 Brecher[7] also recorded negative (−1.3 to −10.8 cm H_2O) ventricular diastolic pressures in the intact dog heart (submerged by filling the chest with saline solution) when the mitral orifice was temporarily occluded. Ventricular diastolic pressures in some animals became more negative when epinephrine was administered. Although the mitral orifice was occluded in his experiments, saline solution or blood flowed into the ventricle through a left ventricular cannula connected to a reservoir situated below the level of the heart. He concluded that the mammalian ventricle was capable of sucking blood from the atrium into its cavity.

Using the same experimental design and the dog, Brecher and Kissen[8] showed that the negative diastolic ventricular pressure of the empty or severely volume-depleted ventricle (from manual expression of the ventricular contents) gradually rose to 0 and finally became positive as fluid was progressively added to the ventricles. An average of 5 and 8 ml of fluid had to be added to the right and left ventricles, respectively, to raise the negative ventricular pressures to 0.

Fowler and associates[9] confirmed the observation of Brecher that obstruction to left ventricular inflow (produced by inflation of the bag of a Foley catheter inserted through the left atrial appendage) did indeed result in negative (−2.5 to −18 mm Hg) left ventricular diastolic pressures; obstruction to right ventricular inflow (produced by occluding the superior and inferior vena cava and coronary sinus) caused negative (−1 to −3 mm Hg) right ventricular diastolic pressures. As Brecher[10,11] observed, negative ventricular diastolic pressure did not develop immediately upon obstruction to filling, but rather after several heart beats. This observation indicates that the negative pressure occurs only after the heart has been reduced to a critical volume by expulsion of its contents in systole.

Role of hemorrhage from right ventricle: Fowler et al.[9] produced experimentally the identical situation that occurred spontaneously in our patient, namely, the effect of rapid bleeding from the right ventricle on left ventricular diastolic pressure. Rapid exsanguination was produced by inserting a rubber tube into the right ventricular cavity, the same site of bleeding as in our patient. During removal of 360 to 700 ml of blood in 89 to 236 seconds, the left ventricular diastolic pressures fell from control levels of 0 to +5 mm Hg to –2.5 to –6.5 mm Hg.

REFERENCES

1. Harvey W: *Exercitatio Anatomica De Motu Cordis et Sanguinis In Animalibus, 1628*. (English translation by Leake CD). Springfield, IL, Charles C Thomas, 1928, p. 33, 41.
2. Wiggers CJ, Katz LN: The contour of the ventricular volume curves under different conditions. *Am J Physiol* 58:439–475, 1922.
3. Katz LN: The role played by the ventricular relaxation process in filling the ventricle. *Am J Physiol* 95:542–553, 1930.
4. Bloom WL: Demonstration of diastolic filling of the beating excised heart (abstr). *Am J Physiol* 183:597, 1955.
5. Bloom WL, Ferris EB: Elastic recoil of the heart as a factor in diastolic filling. *Trans Assoc. Am Physicians* 69:200–206, 1956.
6. Bloom WL, Ferris EB: Negative ventricular diastolic pressure in beating heart studied *in vitro* and *in vivo*. *Proc Soc Exp Biol Med* 93:451–454, 1956.
7. Brecher G: Experimental evidence of ventricular diastolic suction. *Circ Res* 4:513–518, 1956.
8. Brecher GA, Kissen AT: Relation of negative intraventricular pressure to ventricular volume. *Circ Res* 5:157–162, 1957.
9. Fowler NO, Couves C, Bewick J: Effect of inflow obstruction and rapid bleeding on the ventricular diastolic pressure. *J Thorac Surg* 35:532–537, 1958.
10. Brecher GA: Critical review of recent work on ventricular diastolic suction. *Circ Res* 6:554–566, 1958.
11. Brecher GA, Kolder H, Horres AD: Ventricular volume of nonbeating excised dog hearts in the state of elastic equilibrium. *Circ Res* 19:1080–1085, 1966.

Case 384 Self-Induced Pulmonary Granulomatosis*

A Consequence of Intravenous Injection of Drugs Intended for Oral Use

Bruce F. Waller, M.D.; William J. Brownlee, M.D.; and William C. Roberts, M.D., F.C.C.P.

Dr. William C. Roberts: Herein we will discuss pulmonary and cardiac findings in a girl who injected into her systemic veins dissolved drugs originally intended for oral use. Dr. Brownlee will describe the patient.

Dr. William J. Brownlee: An 18-year-old white woman began injecting heroin intravenously at the age of 15 years, about 30 months before her death. About six months later, she began injecting regularly into her systemic veins various other drugs, including methylphenidate (Ritalin), after dissolving them in liquids. She noted periodic wheezing and exertional dyspnea about 12 months before death, and these symptoms gradually progressed thereafter. The patient died suddenly at home after an episode of severe dyspnea. She had never sought medical care.

At necropsy, the surfaces of both lungs appeared normal; but on sectioning, multiple small (about 1 to 2 mm) relatively firm lesions were present throughout all lobes. Histologically, these little nodules were granulomas containing refractile material typical of talc (Figure 1 and 2). The alveolar septa contained similar refractile material and also numerous inflammatory cells (Figure 3). In addition, the media and intima of many pulmonary arteries were thickened, and many small pulmonary arteries were totally obstructed by talc-containing granulomas (Figure 2). The heart, which weighed 440 gm, was typical of that observed in cor pulmonale; both the right atrial and right ventricular cavities were dilated, and their walls were quite thickened; the tricuspid valvular anulus was dilated.

Dr. Roberts: This girl obviously died from self-induced pulmonary granulomatosis, causing morphologic evidence of severe pulmonary hypertension. Because it holds the components of the pill together, talc is present in virtually all tablets; and, consequently, if tablets of nearly any variety are dissolved in a fluid and injected into systemic veins, rather than swallowed, pulmonary talc granulomas are the expected consequence. If few talc granulomas form, no functional consequence ensues. If numerous talc granulomas develop, the consequence is either obstruction of the lumina of many pulmonary arteries, producing pulmonary hypertension and cor pulmonale or interstitial pulmonary fibrosis or both. Although nearly all contain talc, the tablets most commonly used for intravenous injection after crushing and dissolving are methylphenidate (Ritalin) (as in our patient), methadone, tripalennamine (Pyribenzamine), propoxyphene hydrochloride (Darvon), phenmetrazine (Preludin), and amphetamines.

Dr. Waller, would you summarize the findings in previously reported necropsies of patients with pulmonary talc granulomatosis?

Dr. Bruce F. Waller: From 1950 to June 1979, at least 16 necropsies of patients with pulmonary talc granulomas from intravenous injection of dissolved tablets were reported (Table 1).[1-12] All patients were known to have repeatedly injected

* From the Pathology Branch, National Heart Lung, and Blood Institute, National Institutes of Health, Bethesda, Md, and the District of Columbia Medical Examiner's Office, Washington, DC.
Reprint requests: Dr. Roberts, National Institutes of Health, Bldg 10A, Room 3E30, Bethesda 20205

DOI: 10.1201/9781003408321-7

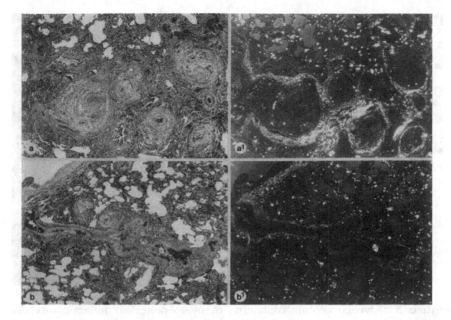

Figure 1 Multiple talc granulomas in pulmonary interstitium (*a* and *a*[1]) and within lumen of pulmonary artery (*b* and *b*[1]). Polarized sections (*a*[1] and *b*[1]) are from the same areas shown in *a* and *b*, respectively. Refractile material, for most part, represents talc (hematoxylin-eosin, original magnifications × 60 [*a* and *a*[1]] and × 22 [*b* and *b*[1]]).

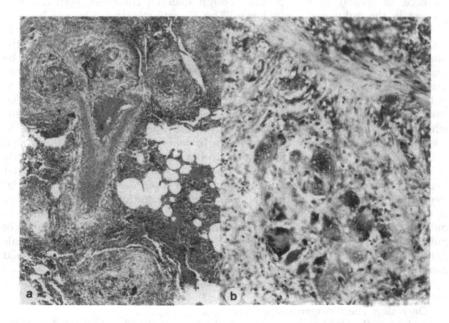

Figure 2 Talc granulomas located within pulmonary artery (*a*) and close-up of large granuloma adjacent to pulmonary artery (*b*) (hematoxylin-eosin, original magnifications × 100 [*a*] and × 220 [*b*]).

43

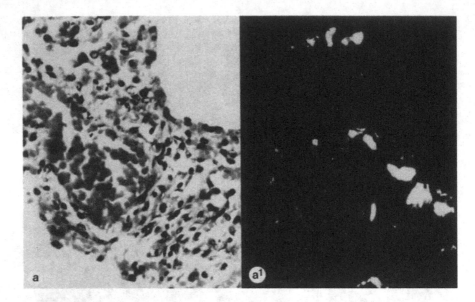

Figure 3 Alveolar septum containing many mononuclear inflammatory cells producing "active-appearing" alveolitis (*a*). Same section polarized is shown (*b*). Lumina of septal capillaries contain birefringent particles typical of talc (*b*) (hematoxylin-eosin, original magnification × 500).

intravenously drugs intended for oral use for periods ranging from 2 to 20 years (average, ten years). In each patient, foreign material consistent with talc was present in the pulmonary granulomas. The 16 patients ranged in age from 22 to 52 years (average, 31 years); 13 were men, and three were women. In all 16 patients the granulomas were present in both pulmonary interstitium and in the lumina of the pulmonary arteries. In 11 patients the interstitium appeared to be the predominant location; in four, the pulmonary arteries were the predominant location; and in one patient, it was not mentioned. The interstitial location led to pulmonary interstitial fibrosis, and the arterial location led to pulmonary arterial narrowing with changes consistent with pulmonary hypertension. The patients who had been taking dissolved tablets intravenously the longest tended to have the talc granulomas located primarily in the pulmonary interstitium, and those with the shortest duration of addiction tended to have the granulomas predominantly in the lumina of the pulmonary arteries. Morphologic evidence (right ventricular hypertrophy or pulmonary arterial changes or both) of pulmonary arterial hypertension was present in 13 of the 16 patients. In addition to the 16 necropsies, at least 13 living patients[1,5,11,13,14] have been reported to have talc granulomas in pulmonary biopsies. Of them, seven had pulmonary arterial changes indicative of pulmonary hypertension. Thus, of 29 previous reports of cases of pulmonary talc granulomas, 20 had morphologic evidence of pulmonary hypertension, and six had plexiform lesions indicating that the pulmonary hypertension was severe.[15]

Dr. Roberts: Dr. Waller, what does the roentgenogram of the chest disclose in patients with pulmonary talc granulomatosis?

Dr. Waller: The roentgenographic changes appear, to some extent at least to be dependent on the stage of the process at which the patient is examined. When the pulmonary granulomas are few in number, the pulmonary parenchyma is normal by radiographic examination. When the pulmonary granulomas are widespread

Table 1: Data from 16 necropsies of patients with pulmonary talc granulomas from intravenous injection of dissolved tablets

Reference	Patient's Sex and Age (yr)	Duration of Addiction, yr*			Pulmonary Granuloma**		Alveolitis†				Pulmonary Arteries‡			Weight of Heart, gm	RV Wall >5 mm§
		IV	Oral	Total	PA	I	Leu	PC	Lym	AH	MT	IT	PL		
Spain[1]	M, ...	...	...	...	+	++	+	-	-	-	0	0	0	...	+
Wendt et al[2]	F, 32	←2→	...	2	++	+	+	-	+	+	+	+	+	720	+
Burton et al[3]	M,25	...	...	...	+	++	-	-	-	+	0	0	0	400	+
Butz[4]	M, 29	...	...	...	++	+	+	-	+	+	+	+	0	375	+
Hahn et al[5]	M, 30	...	...	...	+	++	-	-	-	-	0	0	0	...	-
Hahn et al[5]	F, 28	...	...	...	+	++	-	-	-	-	0	0	+	...	+
Bainborough and Jerico[6]	M, 35	...	...	...	+	++	-	-	-	-	0	0	0	...	+
Douglas et al[7]	M, 52	←30→		30	+	++	-	-	-	-	0	0	0	...	-
	F, 28	←10→		10	+	++	-	-	-	-	0	0	0	...	+
	M, 42	←5→		5	+	+	-	-	-	-	+	+	+	...	+
Lewman[8]	M, 30	←7→		7	++	+	+	-	+	-	+	+	+	400	+
Groth et al[9]	M, 40	5	?	5	+	++	-	-	-	-	0	-	-	...	0
Genereux and Emson[10]	M, 52	←25→		25	+	++	-	-	+	-	0	0	0	...	+
	M, 32	←"Many"→		...	++	+	-	-	-	-	+	+	+	...	+
Arnett et al[11]	M, 22	←7→		7	++	+	-	-	+	-	+	+	+	550	+
Paré et al[12]	M, 25	5	1.5	6.5	+	++	-	-	-	-	-	-	-	...	-

* IV, intravenous.
** PA, pulmonary arteries; and I, interstitium.
† Leu, leukocytes; PC, plasma cells; Lym, lymphocytes; and AH, alveolar hemorrhage.
‡ MT, medial thickening; IT, intimal thickening; and PL, plexiform lesion.
§ RV, right ventricular.

and fatal, the pulmonary parenchyma by roentgenographic examination may still be normal.[4,12,16] Thus, a normal roentgenogram of the chest does not rule out the presence of extensive pulmonary talc granulomatosis. In a study of 17 living patients who administered intravenously at least 2,500 to 50,000 dissolved tablets of methadone during periods ranging from one to nine years, ten patients had normal and seven had abnormal chest roentgenograms.[12] The abnormalities consisted of widespread nodules measuring 1 mm or less in diameter (seven patients) and diminished pulmonary volumes (two patients). Surprisingly, pulmonary infarcts appear to be infrequent, despite the frequent total obliteration of the lumina of many pulmonary arteries. Of course, the patients with pulmonary hypertension may have dilated pulmonary trunks and right ventricular and right atrial cavities. The electrocardiogram in the latter patients also may provide evidence of right ventricular hypertrophy and right atrial abnormality.

Dr. Roberts: Dr. Waller, what alterations in pulmonary function occur in patients with pulmonary talc granulomatosis?

Dr. Waller: Relatively few reported necropsies of cases of fatal pulmonary granulomatosis were from patients who had pulmonary function tests during life, and most patients with pulmonary function tests have not had the pulmonary granulomatosis confirmed anatomically (biopsy or necropsy). Nevertheless, several patients who took dissolved tablets intravenously for long periods have undergone tests of pulmonary function.[12,14] The major functional abnormality is a slowed diffusion of air from the alveolar spaces to the alveolar capillaries (decreased diffusing capacity). A second abnormality described is an increased period of time to expel a certain amount of pulmonary air (diminished forced expiratory volume in one second and diminished midexpiratory flow rate). These latter disturbances may result in an increased pulmonary volume (*ie,* hyperinflation). Whether or not this diminished expiratory flow rate and increased residual pulmonary volume are the result of the pulmonary granulomatosis or whether they are the result of associated cigarette smoking, which is extremely common in the drug addicts, is unclear. Surprisingly, despite the extensive distribution of the pulmonary talc granulomas, systemic arterial hypoxia is usually absent; or at least, cyanosis, except terminally, is uncommon. *Dyspnea* is the usual symptom resulting from the pulmonary talc granulomatosis. Again, clinical evidences of pulmonary infarcts are not reported.

Dr. Roberts: I have a few comments regarding pulmonary morphologic findings in patients with talc granulomatosis. As shown in Figure 1, numerous birefringent particles may be present throughout the pulmonary parenchyma. These birefringent particles are more numerous in alveolar septa not containing granulomas than in the granulomas *per se.* The alveolar septa usually contain many mononuclear inflammatory cells, producing a very "active"-appearing diffuse *alveolitis* as a consequence of the talc granulomatosis (Figure 3). The inflammatory cells generally consist of lymphocytes, plasma cells, and eosinophils; or at least, this was the finding in our patient. In our patient, large numbers of plasma cells and eosinophils were present in many alveolar septa. The alveolitis is consistent with the pulmonary functional abnormality of slowed perfusion of air from alveolar space to alveolar capillary. There has been very little comment regarding alveolitis in previous reports on pulmonary talc granulomatosis. Another infrequently mentioned abnormality in the lungs of these patients is the presence of hemosiderin-laden macrophages within the alveolar spaces. We interpret this abnormality, which was quite extensive in our patient, as resulting from a rupture of the membranes of alveolar capillaries, allowing extravasation of erythrocytes and other blood products into the alveolar spaces (Figure 4). Thus, it might be possible to find hemosiderin or iron deposits in

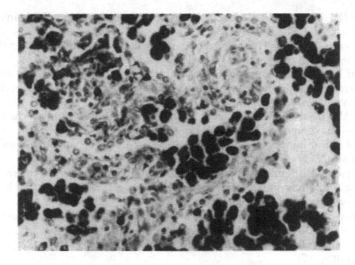

Figure 4 Hemosiderin-laden macrophages located within alveolar spaces (Mallory's stain for iron, original magnification × 400).

the pulmonary expectorates; however, talc spicules or granulomas are infrequent in the alveolar spaces.

I have one final comment regarding diagnosis. Some patients with pulmonary talc granulomatosis initially have evidence of severe pulmonary hypertension. A male patient with pulmonary talcosis, who was previously studied by us,[11] was initially diagnosed as having primary or idiopathic pulmonary hypertension. The finding of evidence of severe pulmonary hypertension in a man should arouse suspicion of the possibility of pulmonary talc granulomatosis as the cause of the pulmonary hypertension, because most patients with primary pulmonary hypertension are women, and most patients with pulmonary talc granulomatosis are men.

REFERENCES

1. Spain DM: Patterns of pulmonary fibrosis as related to pulmonary function. *Ann Intern Med* 33:1150–1163, 1950.
2. Wendt VE, Puro HE, Shapiro J, et al: Angiothrombotic pulmonary hypertension in addicts: "Blue velvet" addiction. *JAMA* 188:755–757, 1964.
3. Burton JF, Zawadzki ES, Wetherell HR, et al: Mainliners and blue velvet. *J Forensic Sci* 10:466–472, 1965.
4. Butz WC: Pulmonary arteriole foreign body granulomata associated with angiomatoids resulting from the intravenous injection of oral medications, e.g., propxyphene hydrochloride (Darvon®). *J Forensic Sci* 14:317–325, 1969.
5. Hahn HH, Schweid AL, Beaty HN: Complications of injecting dissolved methylphenidate tablets. *Arch Intern Med* 123:656–659, 1969.
6. Bainborough AR, Jerico KWF: Cor pulmonale secondary to talc granulomata in the lungs of a drug addict. *Can Med Assoc J* 103:1297–1298, 1970.
7. Douglas FG, Kafilmont KJ, Patt NL: Foreign particle embolism in drug addicts. *Ann Intern Med* 75:865–872, 1971.
8. Lewman LV: Fatal pulmonary hypertension from intravenous injection of methylphenidate (Ritalin) tablets. *Hum Pathol* 3:67–70, 1972.

9. Groth DH, Mackay GR, Crable JV, et al: Intravenous injection of talc in a narcotics addict. *Arch Pathol* 94:171178, 1972.
10. Genereux GP, Emson HE: Talc granulomatosis and angiothrombotic pulmonary hypertension in drug addicts. *J Can Assoc Radiol* 25:87–93, 1974.
11. Arnett EN, Battle WE, Russe JV, et al: Intravenous infection of talc-containing drugs intended for oral use: A cause of pulmonary granulomatosis and pulmonary hypertension. *Am J Med* 60:711–717, 1976.
12. Paré JAP, Fraser RG, Hogg JC, et al: Pulmonary "mainline" granulomatosis; talcosis of intravenous methadone abuse. *Medicine* 58:229–239, 1979.
13. Szwed JJ: Pulmonary angiothrombosis caused by "blue velvet" addiction. *Ann Intern Med* 73:771–774, 1970.
14. Robertson CH, Reynolds J, Wilson JE III: Pulmonary hypertension and foreign body granulomatosis, in intravenous drug abusers: Documentation by cardiac catheterization and lung biopsy. *Ann J Med* 61:657–663, 1976.
15. Virmani R, Roberts WC: Pulmonary arteries in congenital heart disease: A structure-function analysis. *Cardiovasc Clin* 10:455–499, 1979.
16. Hopkins GB, Taylor DG: Pulmonary talc granulomatosis. *Ann Rev Respir Dis* 101:101–108, 1970.

Case 412 Right Ventricular Outflow Obstruction from Thrombus with Small Peripheral Pulmonary Emboli*

Bruce F. Waller, M.D.; Patrick J. Dean, M.D.; Oscar Mann, M.D.; Jeffrey H. Rosen, M.D.; and William C. Roberts, M.D., F.C.C.P.

A patient is described with clinical features of massive pulmonary embolism and a normal pulmonary angiogram. At necropsy, a large thrombus obstructed right ventricular outflow. A right atrial or right ventricular angiogram is suggested in patients suspected of having pulmonary embolism when a pulmonary angiogram shows the pulmonary trunk and main right and left pulmonary arteries to be normal.

This report calls attention to the necessity of performing right sided cardiac angiographic studies when pulmonary angiograms are normal in patients suspected of having pulmonary embolism.

CASE REPORT

A 40-year-old white woman who died in August 1979, had granulomatous ileitis (Crohn's disease) diagnosed in October 1966 (13 years before death). An ileocolostomy was carried out in 1973 because of ileal obstruction; she continued, however, to have episodic abdominal pain, diarrhea, and arthritis. Prednisone (12.5 to 20 mg daily) was begun in 1974 and continued until death. She also took estrogen orally and intramuscularly (after oophorectomy) during her last five years, during which time the white blood cell count was usually about 19,000 mm^3 and the platelet count, about 600,000 cu mm.

In August 1979 (three days before death), abdominal pain was severe and an abdominal radiograph showed subdiaphragmatic "air." Laparotomy disclosed an ileal perforation and it was closed. Postoperatively, she was hypovolemic, dyspneic and hypoxemic. A few hours after operation, while on the respirator, she became cyanotic and her heart stopped ("straight-line" on the electrocardiogram). She was resuscitated and a pulmonary angiogram was performed (14 hours before death); it was normal. Thereafter, cyanosis, hypotension, and atrial and ventricular arrhythmias occurred. A few minutes before death, the neck and face swelled, the skin became cyanotic, and the pulmonary arterial systolic pressure fell precipitously (Swan-Ganz catheter). She could not be resuscitated.

At necropsy, the heart weighed 220 grams and both right and left ventricular cavities were of normal size. In the right ventricular outflow tract attached primarily to chordae tendineae was a thrombus, measuring about 5 × 1 × 1 cm and it extended into the pulmonary trunk (Figure 1 and 2). Small thrombi also were attached to each tricuspid valve leaflet (Figure 2) and to each pulmonic valve cusp (Figure 1 and 2). Histologically, the large thrombus consisted nearly entirely of fibrin. The pulmonary trunk and main right and left pulmonary arteries were free of thrombus.

* From the Pathology Branch, National Heart, Lung, and Blood Institute, National Institutes of Health, Bethesda, Md; The Cardiology Division, Department of Medicine, and the Pathology Department, Georgetown University Medical Center, Washington, D.C.
Reprint requests: Dr. Roberts, Building 10A, Room 3E30, NIH, Bethesda 20205

DOI: 10.1201/9781003408321-8

49

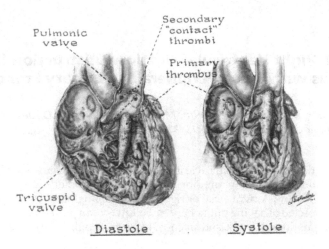

Figure 1 Drawing of opened right atrial and ventricular cavities in ventricular diastole (*left*) and systole (*right*) showing a large thrombus in the right ventricular outflow tract. Small thrombi also are present on the tricuspid valve leaflets and the pulmonic cusps.

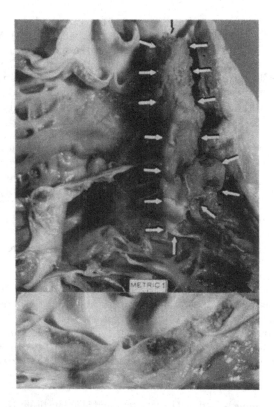

Figure 2 Photograph of the thrombus (*arrows*) in the right ventricular outflow tract (*upper*) and of the pulmonic valve cusps (*lower*) after removal of the thrombus. (Photographs by Margaret M. M. Moore).

Small thrombi were present in the peripheral intrapulmonary pulmonary arteries but no pulmonary infarcts were present. Many alveoli were filled with serous fluid.

COMMENTS

The above-described patient had right ventricular outflow obstruction from thrombus, the cause of which is unclear but probably the result of longterm use of prednisone and estrogen and the presence of thrombocytosis. The sudden respiratory arrest suggested "massive" pulmonary embolism clinically, but when the pulmonary arterial angiogram was normal this diagnosis was dismissed. A right atrial or right ventricular angiogram, however, almost certainly would have demonstrated the mass in the right ventricular outflow tract. Right atrial or right ventricular angiography is suggested in patients clinically suspected of having pulmonary embolism when injection of contrast material into the pulmonary trunk or main right or left pulmonary arteries discloses no filling defects in these vessels.

Case 431 Prolonged QT Interval-Ventricular Tachycardia Syndrome from Massive Rapid Weight Loss Utilizing the Liquid-Protein-Modified-Fast Diet

Sudden Death with Sinus Node Ganglionitis and Neuritis

Robert J. Siegel, M.D., William R. Cabeen, Jr., M.D., and William C. Roberts, M.D. Bethesda, Md., and Santa Monica, Calif.

Prolongation of the QT interval, ventricular tachycardia (VT), and sudden death are now well-recognized consequences of rapid massive weight loss utilizing the liquid-protein-modified-fast (LPMF) diet.[1,2] The mechanism of the conduction disturbances in these patients has not been determined and, to our knowledge, study of the sinus and atrioventricular (AV) nodes at necropsy has not been carried out. Histologic studies in several patients with prolongation of the QT interval and VT unassociated with dieting, however, have disclosed inflammatory cells in and around ganglia and nerves adjacent to the sinus node.[3-5]

To determine if ganglionitis and neuritis in the sinus node area were associated with sudden death from ventricular arhythmias caused by LPMF dieting, we examined serial sections of the sinus and AV nodes and AV bundle in a 33-year-old white woman who, during her last 6 months of life, lost 45 kg (from 109 to 64 kg) while utilizing the LPMF diet. During this long period of dieting she felt well until about 7 days before death when she became "weak," dizzy, and noted "skipped heart beats." These symptoms worsened and on the day of death she had transient substernal chest pain associated with sweating and dizziness. Shortly thereafter she was hospitalized. Her systemic blood pressure was 110/80 mm Hg. Precordial examination disclosed no abnormalities. The neck veins were flat and there was no subcutaneous edema. ECGs recorded during the final 10 hours showed widespread ST-T wave changes, prolonged QT interval, frequent ventricular premature complexes with bigeminy, and finally VT (Figure 1).

At necropsy, the heart weighed 250 gm and it appeared normal grossly. Histologic sections of the right and left ventricular free walls and ventricular septum disclosed polymorphonuclear and mononuclear interstitial myocarditis (Figure 2). Sections of the sinus node disclosed it to be normal, but a number of adjacent ganglions and nerves were surrounded by mononuclear inflammatory cells (Figure 3). Additionally, some of the ganglion cells were degenerated (Figure 3). No abnormalities were found in the AV node or bundle or in the proximal right and left bundle branches.

Thus the finding of ganglionitis and neuritis in the sinus node area of our patient demonstrates that LPMF dieting-induced prolongation of the QT interval and ventricular arrhythmias also is associated with a cardiac conduction tissue abnormality similar to that observed in nondieting induced prolonged QT

From the Pathology Branch, National Heart, Lung, and Blood Institute, National Institutes of Health; and the Department of Medicine, Saint John's Hospital and Health Center.

Received for publication March 13,1981; accepted March 18, 1981.

Reprint requests: William C. Roberts, M.D., Chief, Pathology Branch, NHLBI-NIH, Bldg. 10A, Room 3E-30, Bethesda, MD 20205.

DOI: 10.1201/9781003408321-9

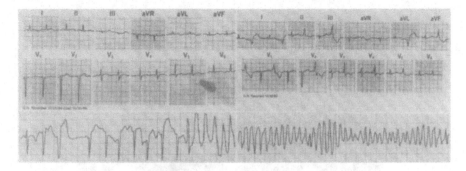

Figure 1 *Top left*, ECG recorded 10 hours before death showing sinus rhythm, low voltage, a prolonged $QT_C{}^1$ (0.485 second) and widespread ST-T wave changes. *Top right*, ECG recorded 6 hours before death showing ventricular bigeminy. *Bottom left*, Rhythm strip demonstrating ventricular tachycardia initiated by a ventricular premature complex occurring at the end of a T wave. *Bottom right*, Atypical ventricular tachycardia or "torsades de pointes" which was recurrent and refractory to therapy.[6]

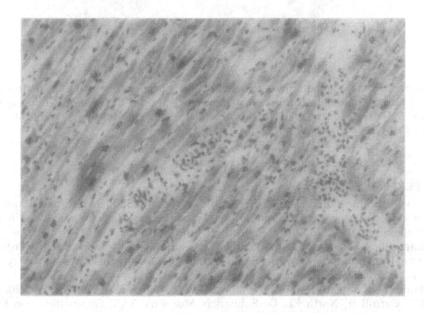

Figure 2 Photomicrograph of portion of left ventricular myocardium showing polymorphonuclear and mononuclear interstitial infiltrates (myocarditis). (Hematoxylin and eosin stain; original magnification × 170.)

interval-VT syndromes. The cause of the inflammation around the ganglions and nerves adjacent to the sinus node and in the ventricular wall interstitium (myocarditis) remains undetermined, but the later finding has been observed in other LPMF dieters.[1]

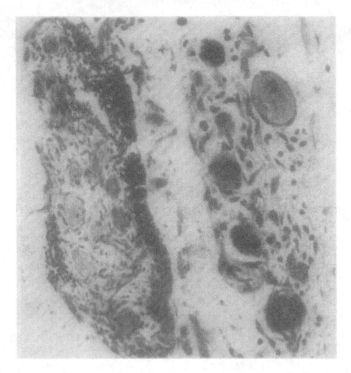

Figure 3 Photomicrographs of two cardiac ganglia adjacent to the sinus node. *Left panel*, Cardiac ganglion surrounded by mononuclear cells. *Right panel*, Multiple ganglion cells are degenerated. (Hematoxylin and eosin stains; original magnifications ×272 (*left*), and ×430 (*right*).

REFERENCES

1. Isner JM, Sours HE, Paris AL, Ferrans VJ, Roberts WC: Sudden, unexpected death in avid dieters using the liquid-protein-modified-fast diet. Observations in 17 patients and the role of the prolonged QT interval. *Circulation* **60**:1401, 1979.
2. Lantigua RA, Amatruda JM, Biddle TL, Forbes GB, Lockwood DH: Cardiac arrhythmias associated with a liquid protein diet for the treatment of obesity. *N Engl J Med* **303**:735,1980.
3. James TN, Froggatt P, Atkinson WJ, Lurie PR, McNamara DG, Miller WW, Schloss GT, Carroll JF, North RL: De Subitancis Mortibus. XXX. Observations on the pathophysiology of the long QT syndromes with special reference to the neuropathology of the heart. *Circulation* **57**:1221, 1978.
4. James TN, Zipes DP, Finegan RE, Eisele JW, Carter JE: Cardiac ganglionitis associated with sudden unexpected death. *Ann Intern Med* **91**:727, 1979.
5. James TV, MacLean WA: Paroxysmal ventricular arrhythmias and familial sudden death associated with neural lesions in the heart. *Chest* **78**:24,1980.
6. Singh BN, Gaarder TD, Kanegae T, Goldstein M, Montgomerie JZ, Mills H: Liquid protein diets and torsade de pointes. *JAMA* **240**:115, 1978.

Case 438 Systolic Clicks Caused by Rocks in the Right Heart Chambers

Bruce F. Waller, M.D., and William C. Roberts, M.D.
Bethesda, Md.

Precordial systolic clicks usually result from prolapse of the mitral and/or tricuspid valve leaflets.[1] Clicks have been produced, however, by catheters inserted into the right side of the heart.[2,3] Another hitherto unreported cause of systolic clicks are calcified masses in the right side of the heart. Such was the case in an 8-year-old boy who died of acute myelogenous leukemia after a 17-month course. About 10 months before death, multiple precordial systolic clicks were heard and recorded (Figure 1), loudest along the right sternal border, and several calcified masses were visible on a chest radiograph (Figure 2). The systolic clicks and calcified masses on chest radiograph remained unchanged thereafter until death. At necropsy, several large calcified masses were present in both the right atrial and right ventricular cavities and the tricuspid and mitral valves were anatomically normal (Figure 3). The clicks appear to have resulted from contact of one calcified mass with another in a manner similar to that shown in Figure 4. The cause of the calcified masses is undetermined.

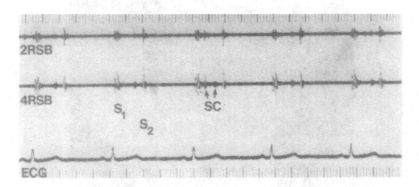

Figure 1 Phonocardiogram obtained 10 months before death showing multiple systolic clicks *(SC)*. ECG = electrocardiogram; *RSB* = right sternal border; S_1 = first heart sound; S_2 = second heart sound.

From the Pathology Branch, National Heart, Lung and Blood Institute, National Institutes of Health.

Received for publication Apr. 9, 1981; accepted Apr. 14, 1981.

Reprint requests: William C. Roberts, M.D., Pathology Branch, Bldg. 10-A, Room 3E-30, National Heart, Lung and Blood Institute, NIH, Bethesda, MD 20205.

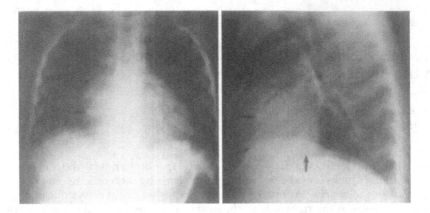

Figure 2 Posteroanterior (*left*) and lateral (*right*) chest radiographs obtained 10 months before death showing multiple calcific deposits (*arrows*).

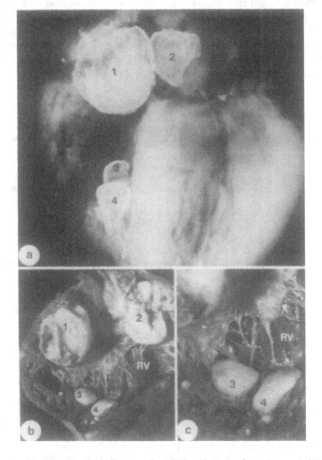

Figure 3 *a*, Postmortem radiograph of the heart showing multiple calcified masses. *b*, Opened right atrial (*RA*) and right ventricular (*RV*) cavities. *c*, Close-up of two calcified masses. The *numbers* label the same calcified masses in each photograph.

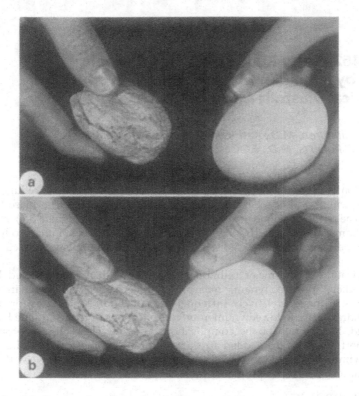

Figure 4   Mechanism by which "rocks" cause clicks.

REFERENCES

1. Jeresaty RM: Mitral valve prolapse-click syndrome. *Progr Cardiovasc Dis* **15**:623, 1973.
2. Murdock MP, Meyers BA, Bacos JM: Auscultatory clicks produced by pacemaker catheters. *Ann Intern Med* **68**:1320, 1968.
3. Isner JM, Horton J, Ronan JA: Systolic click from a Swan-Ganz catheter: Phonoechocardiographic depiction of the underlying mechanism. *Am J Cardiol* **43**:1046, 1979.

Case 462 Acute Rupture of the Pulmonic Valve by a Balloon-tipped Catheter Producing a Musical Diastolic Murmur*

Keith M. Lindgren, M.D.; Kathleen McShane, M.D.; and
William C. Roberts, M.D., F.C.C.P.

Attention is called to the development of severe pulmonic-valve regurgitation during withdrawal of a balloon-tipped catheter that had been in place for six days. The resulting pulmonic regurgitation produced a loud (grade 5/6), musical diastolic murmur recorded by phonocardiogram at the time of its initial production. Autopsy disclosed a noninfected tear in one of the three pulmonic valve cusps.

Catheterization of the major pulmonary arteries with a flow-directed balloon-tipped catheter for hemodynamic measurement has gained wide usage in critically ill patients. Although relatively infrequent when certain guidelines for insertion and withdrawal are followed,[1] numerous complications of the technique have been described. Recognition of the complications requires close clinical observation. This report describes the sudden appearance of a loud musical diastolic murmur during withdrawal of a Swan-Ganz catheter across the pulmonic valve with autopsy confirmation of a tear in a pulmonic valve cusp.

CASE REPORT

A 59-year-old man was admitted to Washington Adventist Hospital with recurrent acute myocardial infarction complicated by severe congestive heart failure. Physical examination and phonocardiogram documented a late systolic crescendo murmur and prominent third and fourth heart sounds. No diastolic murmur was heard or recorded. On the fourth hospital day, a No. 6 double lumen, balloon-tipped catheter (Edwards, Swan-Ganz) was inserted and advanced to the pulmonary wedge position under pressure monitoring. No difficulty was encountered. With the balloon deflated, sampling was done on pullback from pulmonary trunk, to right ventricle, right atrium and superior vena cava to exclude a ventricular septal defect. The catheter was again advanced with the balloon inflated and with pressures monitored to wedge position. Chest roentgenogram confirmed the location of the catheter in the pulmonary artery to the right lower lobe. The right-sided pressures (in mm Hg) were: right atrial mean, 18; right ventricular, 60/22; pulmonary arterial 60/30; and pulmonary arterial wedge mean, 30, with V waves of 40. Auscultatory findings were unchanged.

After nitroprusside infusion, the pulmonary arterial wedge mean pressure fell to 22 mm Hg and the pulmonary arterial pressure to 45/20 mm Hg. Six days after the balloon-tipped catheter had been inserted, an early diastolic crescendo-decrescendo grade 2/6 murmur was heard along the left sternal border. On the assumption that the catheter induced pulmonic regurgitation, the catheter was

* From the Department of Cardiology, Washington Adventist Hospital, Takoma Park, Md, and the Pathology Branch, National Heart, Lung, and Blood Institute, National Institutes of Health, Bethesda.

Reprint requests: Dr. Lindgren, 7600 Carroll Avenue, Takoma Park, Maryland 20012

DOI: 10.1201/9781003408321-11

removed with the balloon deflated while recording a phonocardiogram from the third left intercostal space. As the catheter was withdrawn, the diastolic murmur became consistently grade 4 to 5/6 in intensity with pure frequency (100 cycles/sec) and a honking musical character (Figure 1 and 2). The patient experienced no immediate untoward effects. Six days after the balloon-tipped catheter had been removed, he developed *Escherichia coli* septicemia. The congestive heart failure worsened, and four days later he died.

At autopsy, a tear was present in one of the three pulmonic valve cusps (Figure 3). No inflammatory cells or microorganisms were observed in the pulmonic valve cusps. The other three cardiac valves were normal. The heart weighed 420 g, and both acute and healed left ventricular myocardial infarcts were present. The posteromedial papillary muscle was severely scarred. The kidneys contained many abscesses with gram-negative organisms.

COMMENTS

The patient described is unique for two major reasons: (1) pulmonic valve regurgitation was documented to have been produced by a catheter, and such occurrence has been published, to our knowledge, in only one previous report, and (2) the resulting pulmonic valve regurgitation produced a precordial murmur of unusual character and intensity, both of which were documented by phonocardiogram. Before removal of the catheter, a murmur was heard and recorded which corresponded to the typical murmur of pulmonic regurgitation without pulmonary hypertension; *ie*, a crescendo-decrescendo murmur of low-to-moderate frequency and intensity beginning shortly

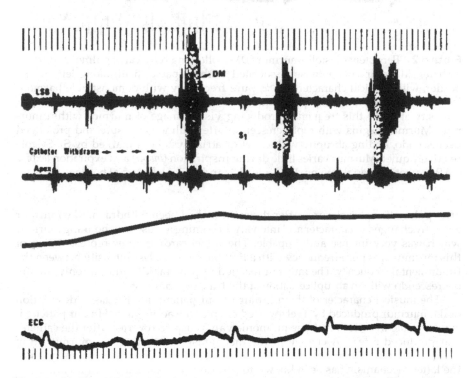

Figure 1 On withdrawal of catheter from pulmonary trunk into right ventricle, diamond-shaped diastolic murmur (DM) is abruptly transformed into very intense musical murmur, generally decrescendo. LSB = left sternal border.

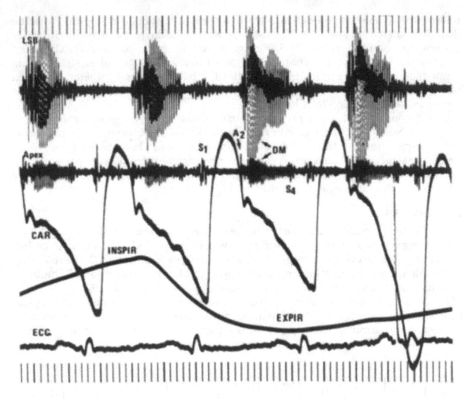

Figure 2 Persistent diastolic murmur (DM) following removal of pulmonary artery catheter. Murmur very intense (associated with palpable thrill) along left sternal border, with musical characteristic: *ie,* pure frequency with demonstrable harmonics. Most intense vibrations approximately 100 cycles/psec, with harmonic of lesser intensity at twice this frequency producing visual image of murmur within murmur. Murmur begins with rapid crescendo after pulmonic closure and prolonged decrescendo, ending abruptly with onset of atrial systole as marked by S_4. Systole relatively quiet. Murmur varies little during inspiration (*inspir*) and expiration (*expir*). CAR = carotid arterial tracing; ECG = lead 2, and LSB = left sternal border.

after pulmonic valve closure. After the catheter had been withdrawn, the murmur abruptly changed in character and intensity, becoming a musical or honking murmur which was very intense and palpable. The phonocardiographic representation of this murmur was pure frequency with a first harmonic of less intensity between the fundamental frequency. The murmur reached its peak rapidly and was only slightly decrescendo with an abrupt cessation at the time of atrial systole.

The musical character of the murmur in our patient fits the classic description of the murmur produced by a retroverted cusp of the aortic valve.[2] In our patient, it is reasonable to believe that one pulmonic valve cusp retroverted after the catheter had produced a tear. A change in the mechanism generating the murmur from a regurgitant jet to a retroverted cusp accounts for the change in intensity, since the latter mechanism has been known to produce "the loudest murmurs known to medicine."[2] The abrupt termination of the murmur at atrial systole can be explained by the rise in right ventricular pressure which occurs at this point, often reversing the gradient from pulmonary artery to right ventricle.

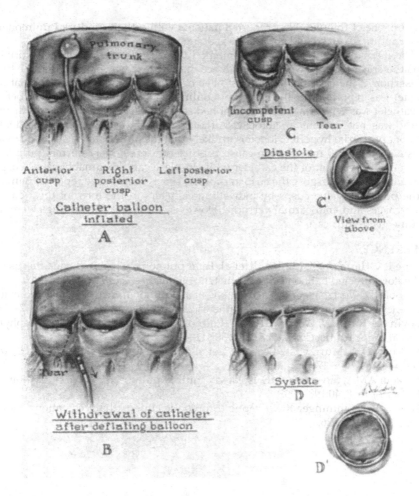

Figure 3 Pulmonic valve at autopsy with probable catheter location and resulting cuspal tear.

Musical diastolic murmurs have usually been associated with aortic regurgitation and the high pressure in the left side of the heart. Thus, documentation of a loud, palpable, musical murmur from pulmonic valve regurgitation with only mild elevation of pulmonary pressure supports the fact that the acoustic mechanism of the murmur is more important than the pressure gradient associated with it. In our patient, assuming that the gradient did not change with removal of the catheter, the retroversion of the cusp apparently resulted in increase in intensity of the murmur and its unique characteristics. That the intensity of the musical murmur does not directly parallel the gradient across the valve during the cardiac cycle also can be explained by a valve flap which varies its location in the regurgitant stream throughout diastole, sometimes actually increasing the diastolic murmur in later diastole.

Despite the intensity of the murmur of catheter-induced pulmonic valve rupture in our patient, he appeared to suffer no immediate untoward effects. Similar benign consequences of pulmonic valve regurgitation have been reported by others.[3] In addition, one of the two other reported patients with catheter-induced pulmonary valve rupture survived and apparently is doing well.[4]

The mechanism by which the pulmonic valve cusp in our patient was torn by the catheter is unclear. There is no evidence that the tear was produced at the time of insertion of the catheter, but it must have occurred during the six days that the catheter was in place, since the murmur of pulmonic regurgitation was heard before the catheter was withdrawn. The patient had septicemia, but infective endocarditis clearly was not present at autopsy. Although our patient did have moderate pulmonary arterial hypertension, it is unlikely that the pulmonary arterial diastolic pressure of 30 to 40 mm Hg can cause rupture of a previously normal pulmonic valve cusp. Movement of the catheter while in place can presumably cause cuspal weakening and predispose the cusp to rupture, since others[5] have reported damage to the pulmonic valve cusps by indwelling catheters in the form of focal cuspal hemorrhages and endocardial verrucae. However, these specific findings were not documented in this case.

REFERENCES

1. Pape LA, Haffajee CI, Markis JE, et al. Fatal pulmonary hemorrhage after use of the flow-directed balloon-tipped catheter. *Ann Intern Med* 1979; 90:344–347.
2. O'Toole JD, Wortzbacher JJ, Wearner NE, et al. Pulmonary valve injury and insufficiency during pulmonary artery catheterization. *N Engl J Med* 1979; 30:1167–1168.
3. Levin HS, Runco V, Wooley CF, et al. Pulmonic regurgitation following staphylococcal endocarditis. *Circulation* 1964; 30:411–416.
4. McKusick VA, Murray GE, Peeler RG, et al. Musical murmurs. *Bull Johns Hopkins Hosp* 1955; 97:136–176.
5. Faruqui AMA, Silverman ME. Isolated acquired pulmonary valve regurgitation. *Br Heart J* 1978; 40:198–200.
6. Greene JF, Comminger KC. Aseptic thrombotic endocardial vegetations. *JAMA* 1973; 225:1525–1526.

Case 653 *Aspergillus Fumigatus* Thrombi Causing Total Occlusion of Both Coronary Arterial Ostia, All Four Major Epicardial Coronary Arteries and Coronary Sinus and Associated with Purulent Pericarditis

*Elizabeth M. Ross, MD, Abe M. Macher, MD
and William C. Roberts, MD*

Cardiac aspergillosis, rarely diagnosed premortem, occurs in immunosuppressed patients, particularly in those with hematologic and lymphoreticular malignancies or in those having had an organ transplant.[1-3] Endocarditis, myocarditis and thrombi of coronary vessels have been described. We report a patient with fungal occlusion of both coronary arterial ostia, the lumens of all 4 major epicardial coronary arteries and the coronary sinus with associated diffuse fungal pericarditis.

A 31-year-old man, who had lymphoblastic lymphoma during his last 33 months of life, was treated with chemotherapy and cranial irradiation. He had 3 bone marrow relapses between initial chemotherapy and his final relapse 27 months later (6 months before death). He was hospitalized 2 months before death because of granulocytopenia, fever and pulmonary infiltrates. He received broad-spectrum antibiotic therapy, amphotericin and rifampin without response. Clinical evidence of cardiac dysfunction never developed. Results of the electrocardiogram and M-mode and cross-sectional echocardiograms were normal. Results of all fungal culture tests were negative.

Necropsy showed disseminated aspergillosis with multiple fungal pulmonary infarcts. Aspergillus fumigatus was cultured from lung tissue at necropsy. The heart weighed 490 g. Both coronary ostia were occluded by fungal thrombi (Figure 1 and 2). The thrombus in the left coronary ostium extended into the lumens of the left anterior descending and left circumflex coronary arteries. The lumen of coronary sinus was filled with fungal thrombus. There were no myocardial or endocardial lesions. Histologic sections, stained by Gomori-methanamine-silver method, showed numerous dichotomously branching fungi consistent with aspergillus species within the thrombi (Figure 2). The epicardium of the heart was covered with fibrin containing hyphal organisms.

To our knowledge, neither occlusion of both coronary ostia nor occlusion of a coronary sinus by thrombi—either infected or noninfected—have been described previously.

From the Pathology Branch, National Heart, Lung, and Blood Institute, and the Laboratory of Pathology, National Cancer Institute, National Institutes of Health, Bethesda, Maryland 20205. Manuscript received and accepted April 8, 1985.

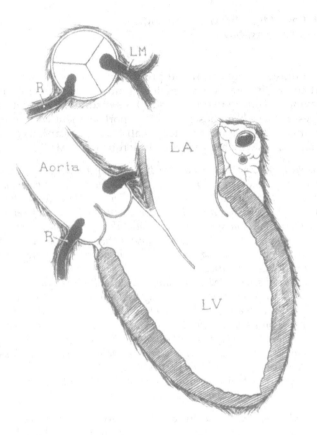

Figure 1 Drawing of the heart in the patient described showing fungal thrombi occluding both coronary ostia and the lumen of the coronary sinus. Fibrin and hyphal organisms cover the pericardial surfaces. LA = left atrium; LM = left main artery; LV = left ventricle; R = right coronary artery.

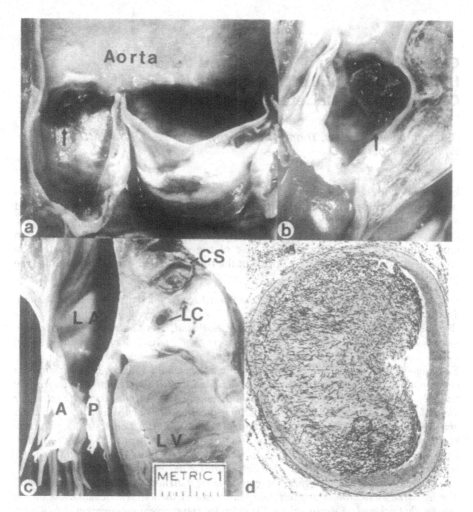

Figure 2 The heart of the patient described. **a**, fungal thrombus (**arrow**) occluding the ostium of the right coronary artery. **b**, fungal thrombus (**arrow**) occluding the ostium of the left main coronary artery. **c**, longitudinal section showing occlusion by fungal thrombus of both the left circumflex (LC) coronary artery and the coronary sinus (CS). **d**, photomicrograph of cross section of left anterior descending coronary artery just after its origin from the left main artery. The dark-staining structures are fungal hyphae consistent with aspergillus species. A = anterior mitral leaflet; LA = left atrial cavity; LV = left ventricular wall; P = posterior mitral leaflet. Gomori-silver stain ×27, reduced 30%.

REFERENCES

1. Young RC, Bennett JE, Vogel CL, Carbone PP, DeVita VT. Aspergillosis: the spectrum of the disease in 98 patients. *Medicine* 1970;49:147–173.
2. Rubinstein E, Noriego ER, Simberkoff MS, Holzman R, Rahal JJ. Fungal endocarditis: analysis of 24 cases and review of the literature. *Medicine* 1975;54:331–344.
3. Walsh TJ, Hutchins GM, Bulkley BH, Mendelsohn G. Fungal infections of the heart: analysis of 51 autopsy cases. *Am J Cardiol* 1980;45:357–366.

Case 703 Pulmonary Arterial and Venous Hypertension and Left Ventricular Calcification of Undetermined Etiology

Deborah J. Barbour, MD, Thomas V. Inglesby, MD, Joel A. Roth, MD and William C. Roberts, MD

In patients with severe pulmonary hypertension, the cause can nearly always be determined clinically or, if not, by necropsy examination. We recently studied a young woman with severe pulmonary hypertension and, despite cardiac catheterization, echocardiography, radionuclide angiography, pulmonary function studies, and, finally, necropsy, the cause of the severe pulmonary hypertension could not be determined. A description of the findings in this unusual patient is the purpose of this report.

M.B., a 20-year-old white woman, was well until age 14 years, when exertional dyspnea developed and gradually worsened. At age 18, she had several respiratory infections (Figure 1). *She was evaluated 2 months before death and severe pulmonary hypertension was found. Cyanosis was absent and her lungs were clear. Precordial murmurs were absent; S_2 was loud, the interval between A_2 and P_2 did not vary with respiration, and both S_3 and S_4 gallops were present. The electrocardiogram is shown in* Figure 2. *A radionuclide angiogram revealed right ventricular enlargement and the left ventricular ejection fraction was 52%. On echocardiogram, the left atrial dimension was 42 mm, the left ventricular dimensions were 45 mm in diastole and 22 mm in systole; left ventricular wall thickness and motion and the cardiac valves were normal. Pulmonary function tests showed severe impairment of diffusion capacity, mild obstruction and a vital capacity 58% of predicted. Data obtained at cardiac catheterization are summarized in* Table 1. *Plans were made for combined heart and lung transplantation but she died of pneumonia while waiting.*

At necropsy, the heart weighed 360 g and the right atrium and ventricle were dilated. The left atrial endocardium was diffusely thickened and the left ventricular endocardium was focally thickened. A dense, calcific bar extended transversely for approximately 4.5 cm in the ventricular septum and protruded approximately 1 cm into the left ventricular cavity (Figure 3). *Several left ventricular trabeculae also were calcified. The valves and coronary arteries were normal. Histologic sections of myocardium disclosed only myocyte hypertrophy.*

Atherosclerotic plaques were present in the intima of the pulmonary trunk and in the extraparenchymal pulmonary arteries (Figure 4). *Histologic examination of both ascending aorta and pulmonary trunk (stained for elastic tissue) showed normal configuration of the elastic fibers in the pulmonary trunk (adult pattern).[1] Plexiform lesions were absent in all 16 sections of lung examined. The pulmonary veins were thickened and dilated, the alveolar septae were focally fibrotic and many but not all of the muscular pulmonary arteries had thickened media and in a few the intima was thickened by fibrous tissue. Many hemosiderin laden macrophages were present in alveolar spaces and the alveolar lining cells were cuboidal in shape and increased in number. The interlobular septa were thickened by fluid, fibrous tissue and dilated lymphatic channels.*

From the Pathology Branch, National Heart, Lung, and Blood Institute, National Institutes of Health, Bethesda, Maryland, and the Departments of Medicine (Cardiology) and Pathology, Overlook Hospital, Summit, New Jersey. Manuscript received and accepted March 6, 1986.

DOI: 10.1201/9781003408321-13

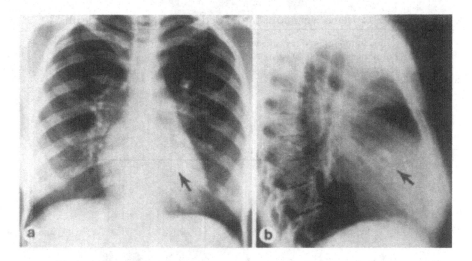

Figure 1 Posteroanterior and lateral chest radiographs taken 19 months before the patient's death showing mild cardiomegaly and an intracardiac calcific density (*arrows*) variously interpreted at the time as involving the aortic or mitral valve but which, at necropsy, was present in the ventricular septum.

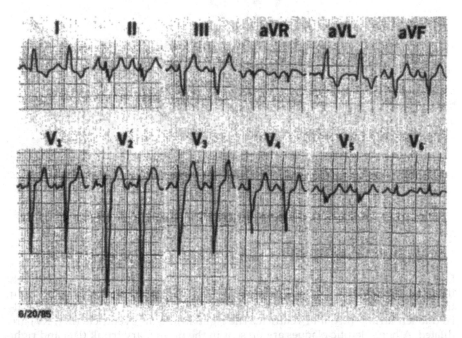

Figure 2 Twelve-lead electrocardiogram taken 3 months before death. The QRS axis is leftward (–40°), there is an intraventricular conduction delay and right atrial abnormality.

Table 1: Hemodynamic data recorded two months before death

Pressures (mm Hg) (s/d = peak systole/end diastole)	
Pulmonary artery (PA) (s/d)	145/62
Right ventricle (s/d)	130/16
Right atrium (mean)	9
PA wedge (mean)	22
Left ventricle (s/d)	100/20
Systemic artery (s/d)	100/68
Cardiac index (liters/min/m^2)	1.9
Pulmonary vascular resistance (dynes s cm^{-5})	200

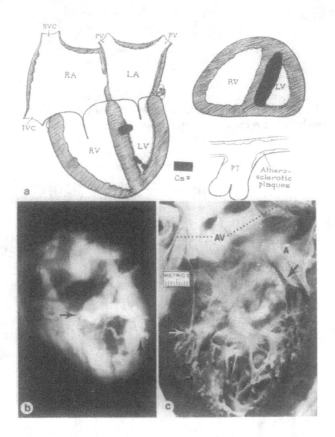

Figure 3 Heart. *a* (*left*), schematic representation of longitudinal section through the heart showing calcific bar on ventricular septum and calcified trabeculae within the left ventricular (LV) cavity. *Stippling* indicates thickened endocardium localized to left atrium (LA) and ventricle. The right atrium and ventricle (RA, RV) are dilated. Atherosclerotic plaques are present in the pulmonary trunk (PT) and right and left main pulmonary arteries. *b*, radiograph of the heart at necropsy showing a dense calcific bar (*between arrows*) extending across the ventricular septum and several calcified left ventricular trabeculae, *c*, a long axial cut showing the left ventricular aspect of the ventricular septum, opened aortic valve (AV) and anterior (A) mitral leaflet. The calcific bar (*between arrows*) extends across the ventricular septum. IVC = inferior vena cava; PV = pulmonary valve; SVC = superior vena cava.

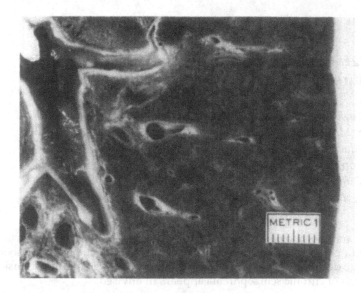

Figure 4 Close-up view of a longitudinal section of the lung showing a thickened large pulmonary artery. The aorta was free of atherosclerosis.

During life this patient was believed to have primary pulmonary hypertension, but at necropsy no plexiform lesions were present in the lungs, a finding essential for this diagnosis.[2] The medial thickening of the pulmonary arteries is simply an anatomic manifestation of severe pulmonary hypertension and not an indication of its cause. Study at necropsy of histologic sections of the wall of the pulmonary trunk indicated an adult configuration of the medial elastic fibers, a finding that indicates that the pulmonary hypertension was acquired rather than having persisted from birth.[1] The calcific bar in the ventricular septum and left ventricular free wall, of course, is not observed in patients with primary pulmonary hypertension, but again, its cause was not revealed by anatomic study. Thus, both the cause of the severe pulmonary arterial and venous hypertension and of the cardiac ventricular calcific deposit remain unexplained.

REFERENCES

1. Heath D, Wood EH, DuShane JW, Edwards JE. The structure of the pulmonary trunk at different ages and in cases of pulmonary hypetension and pulmonary stenosis. *J Path Bact* 1959;77:443–456.
2. Wagenvoort CA, Wagenvoort N. Primary pulmonary hypertension: a pathologic study of the lung vessels in 156 clinically diagnosed cases. *Circulation* 1970:42:1183–1184.

Case 728 Fatal Water Intoxication, Schizophrenia, and Diuretic Therapy for Systemic Hypertension

Stewart Levine, M.D.* and Bruce M. McManus, M.D., Ph.D.
Bethesda, Maryland
Brian D. Blackbourne, M.D.
Washington, D.C.
William C. Roberts, M.D.
Bethesda, Maryland

Clinical and morphologic findings are described in a 37-year-old hypertensive man with chronic schizophrenia who had two well-documented episodes of water intoxication. The use of diuretics for control of systemic hypertension in the setting of chronic schizophrenia appears ill-advised.

Water intoxication occurs when body fluids become dilute and body tissues edematous, and results from either excessive hypotonic fluid intake or excessive hypertonic fluid loss. The resulting symptoms include headache, anorexia, blurred vision, confusion, aphasia, delirium, seizure, and muscle weakness.[1] At least six patients with fatal acute water intoxication have been described,[2-6] and death was usually attributed to cerebral edema. This report describes clinical and morphologic observations in another patient who had two episodes of acute water intoxication, the last one fatal, and it emphasizes consequences of inappropriate therapy.

CASE REPORT

A 37-year-old man with chronic undifferentiated schizophrenia who died on October 24, 1980, had two episodes of severe acute water intoxication, one 28 months before death and the second one fatal (**Table 1**). The quantity of water drunk during the first episode of water intoxication is unclear, but the resulting serum electrolyte values and urine specific gravity were similar to those found during his second and fatal episode (**Table 1**). He consumed about 96 glasses of water daily (equivalent to 17 ml/minute) for several days before death. During each episode of acute water intoxication, he was unsteady in gait, lethargic, and had a seizure shortly after hospitalization on each occasion. Because of these findings, he had sought hospitalization at his psychiatric hospital. During his final acute episode, he was transferred to the intensive care unit of a neighboring hospital several hours before death. On admission, it was learned that he had taken

From the Pathology Branch, National Heart, Lung, and Blood Institute, National Institutes of Health, Bethesda, Maryland, and the Medical Examiner's Office, District of Columbia, Washington, D.C. Requests for reprints should be addressed to either Dr. Stewart Levine or Dr. William C. Roberts, Building 10A, Room 3E30, National Institutes of Health, Bethesda, Maryland 20205. Manuscript submitted July 23, 1985, and accepted August 30, 1985.
* Current address: 935 Intercostal Drive, Fort Lauderdale, Florida 33304.

DOI: 10.1201/9781003408321-14

Table 1: Various laboratory values at four different times in the patient described

	August 1971 (age 29)	June 1978 (age 35)	February 1979 (age 36)	October 1980 (age 37)
Sodium (meq/liter)	138	110	138	108
Potassium (meq/liter)	3.7	2.6	4.1	2.3
Chloride (meq/liter)	105	71	105	69
Bicarbonate (meq/liter)	25	15	28	27
Blood urea nitrogen (mg/dl)	14	8	16	3
Serum osmolarity (mOsm/kg)		267		
Urine osmolarity (mOsm/kg)		92		
Urine specific gravity	1.013	1.006	1.010	1.006
Water intake (liters/day)	4	—	4	24
Urine output (ml)		3,900 in 8 hours		5,300 in 2 hours
Blood pressure (mm Hg)	120/80	180/100		160/90
Total cholesterol (mg/dl)	225			
Triglycerides (mg/dl)	48			

Table 2: Amount of cross-sectional area narrowing in each 5 mm segment of the four major epicardlal coronary arteries in the patient described

Coronary Artery	Number of 5 mm Segments	Percent of Cross-Sectional Area Narrowing by Atherosclerotic Plaque				
		0–25	26–50	51–75	76–95	>95
Left main	1	1	—	—	—	—
Left anterior descending	23	7	1	7	8	0
Left circumflex	12	4	2	5	1	0
Right	28	0	7	16	5	0
Total (percent)	64	12(19)	10(16)	28 (43)	14(22)	0(0)

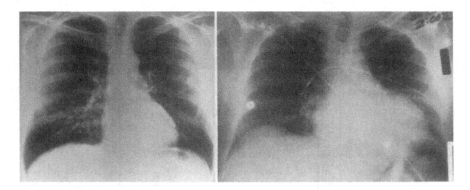

Figure 1 *Anteroposterior chest radiographs.* **Left,** *taken several months before death.* **Right,** *taken five hours before death.*

hydrochlorothiazide for systemic hypertension for the last 30 months and had been taking phenothiazine drugs (fluphenazine or thioridazine) for his psychotic condition for several years. Chest radiography (Figure 1) showed an enlarged cardiac silhouette and pulmonary venous congestion. Electrocardiography (Figure 2) disclosed Q waves in leads III and aVF, prominent U waves, a prolonged Q-T interval, and an intraventricular conduction delay. Despite administration of saline and potassium in solution, the patient had an epileptic seizure followed by refractory ventricular fibrillation.

At necropsy, the epicardium was smooth and glistening. The heart weighed 510 g. The right, left main, left anterior descending, and left circumflex coronary arteries were divided into 5 mm segments, and a histologic section was prepared from each segment. Of the 62 sections of coronary artery, 14 (23 percent) were narrowed more than 75 percent in cross-sectional area by atherosclerotic plaque (**Table 2**). The right ventricular cavity was markedly dilated and the left ventricular cavity was moderately dilated. The four valves were normal. The ventricular walls were free of foci of fibrosis and necrosis.

COMMENTS

The most common causes of water intoxication include[7]: (1) improper fluid and electrolyte administration; (2) medication affecting release of antidiuretic hormone; (3) diuretic agents, which reduce the kidney's ability to conserve sodium or excrete free water; (4) the syndrome of inappropriate antidiuretic hormone

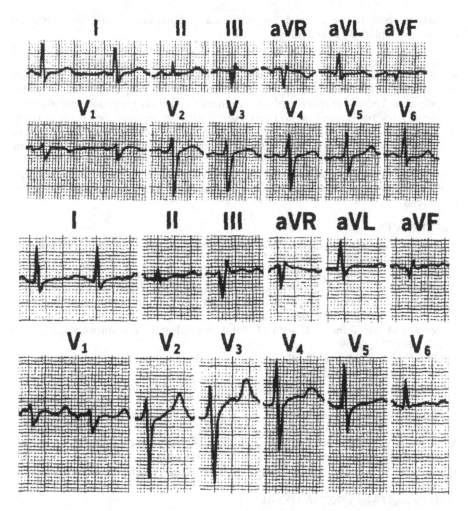

Figure 2 *Electrocardiograms. The **top** one was recorded on April 30, 1980, and the **bottom** one on October 24, 1980, five hours before death.*

release associated with a variety of diseases; and (5) excessive water intake alone (psychogenic polydipsia). Excessive beer intake also may cause "water" intoxication.[8] The diagnosis is confirmed by lowered urine and serum osmolarities along with hyponatremia. A fall in the blood urea nitrogen level also may be indicative of acute water intoxication. Most patients become symptomatic when the serum sodium level falls below 120 meq/liter. Hypokalemia occurs frequently in association with water intoxication and may give rise to electrocardiographic abnormalities, including prominent U waves, a prolonged Q-T interval, and nonspecific S-T segment and T wave changes.

In mild cases of water intoxication, treatment consists of fluid restriction. In more severe cases, hypertonic saline may be administered to correct the serum osmolality, promote a water diuresis, and lessen cellular edema. Treatment with isotonic saline should be avoided as such therapy will further increase the already expanded extracellular fluid volume and will not significantly increase the serum sodium concentration.[1] Electrolytes, particularly potassium, must be monitored closely and replaced as needed.

Most reported cases of water intoxication resulting from excessive water intake have occurred in patients with psychiatric disorders. Many patients were taking phenothiazine drugs, which may promote excessive thirst through parasympathetic mechanisms, thereby further increasing their risk of water intoxication. The use of thiazide diuretics in these patients may cause more severe hyponatremia by increasing sodium excretion with relative decrease in urine volume.[9] Indeed, diuretic therapy may have played a role in the development of water intoxication in the patient presented herein. Therefore, psychiatric patients being treated for systemic hypertension with diuretic agents must be followed closely for signs of water intoxication. If such signs develop, diuretic therapy may be contraindicated and alternative methods of blood pressure control employed.

REFERENCES

1. Wynn V, Rob CG: Water intoxication. Differential diagnosis of the hypotonic syndromes. *Lancet* 1954; I: 587–594.
2. Helwig FC, Schultz CB, Curry DE: Water intoxication: report of a fatal human case with clinical, pathological, and experimental studies. *JAMA* 1935; 104; 1569–1575.
3. Raskind M: Psychosis, polydipsia, and water intoxication. Report of a fatal case. *Arch Gen Psychiatry* 1974; 30; 112–114.
4. Rendall M, McGrane D, Cuesta M: Fatal compulsive water intoxication. *JAMA* 1978; 240: 2557–2559.
5. DiMaio VJM, DiMaio SJ: Fatal water intoxication in a case of psychogenic polydipsia. *Forensic Sci* 1980; 25: 332–335.
6. Blotcky MJ, Grossman I, Looney JG: Psychogenic water intoxication: a fatality. *Tex Med* 1980; 76: 58–59.
7. Crumpacker RW, Kriel RL: Voluntary water intoxication in normal infants. *Neurology* 1973; 23: 1251–1255.
8. Demanet JC, Bonnyns M, Bleiberg H, Stevens-Rocmans C: Coma due to water intoxication in beer drinkers. *Lancet* 1971; II: 1115–1117.
9. Kennedy RM, Earley LE: Profound hyponatremia resulting from a thiazide-induced decrease in urinary diluting capacity in a patient with primary polydipsia. *N Engl J Med* 1970; 282: 1185–1186.

Case 834 Cardiac Consequences of Massive Acetaminophen Overdose

Jessica M. Mann, MD, Marie Pierre-Louis, MD, Peter J. Kragel, MD, Amy H. Kragel, MD, and William C. Roberts, MD

Ingestion of >10 g of acetaminophen is a well-known cause of hepatic necrosis, but cardiac toxicity with this drug is uncommon.[1-3] Herein we describe cardiac findings in a patient who took 35 g of acetaminophen and died 8 days later.

WS, a 31-year-old white man with a previous suicide attempt (radial artery incision) at age 30, had a history of alcohol abuse but no other drug abuse. On March 30, 1988, he ingested 35 g of acetaminophen (70 Extra-Strength 500 mg Tylenol caplets). On April 2, 1988, he was hospitalized because of vomiting. The blood pressure was 95/40 mm Hg. No precordial murmurs or rubs were heard, and he had no bowel sounds. On electrocardiogram, the heart rate was 125 beats/min and nonspecific ST-T changes were present (Figure 1). A chest x-ray was normal. Laboratory values are listed in Table 1. He was lethargic, went into hepatorenal failure on his second hospital day and died 8 days after the acetaminophen ingestion.

At necropsy, the heart weighed 415 g. Both ventricular cavities were mildly dilated. Portions of the left and right ventricular free walls and ventricular septum were yellow (Figure 2). On hematoxylin-eosin-stained sections, the myocardial fibers in these yellow areas contained numerous small vesicles of fat confirmed by the Sudan black stain (Figure 3). Electron microscopy showed myocytes containing numerous lipid vacuoles (Figure 4). The coronary arteries and cardiac valves were normal. Sections of liver showed massive necrosis and collapsed architecture. The few remaining viable hepatocytes as well as ghosts of necrotic hepatocytes showed microvesicular fatty change.

In 1968, Pimstone et al[1] described a 26-year-old woman who took 60 to 80 tablets of paracetamol and died 8 days after ingestion. At necropsy, subendocardial hemorrhage was present in the left ventricular wall. Histologic sections of the myocardium showed interstitial edema, foci of necrosis and a significant amount of polymorphonuclear leukocytes. In 1971, Sanerkin[2] reported a 15-year-old girl who died 40 hours after ingestion of 16.2 g of paracetamol. At necropsy, the wall of the left ventricle was focally purple, and sections of the discolored areas showed focal necrosis and intramyocardial fat. Sanerkin[2] also described similar changes. In 1987, Wakeel et al[3] described a 15-year-old girl who died 80 hours after ingestion of an unspecified quantity of paracetamol. At necropsy, the left ventricular cavity was dilated and its myocardium was pale and soft. Histologic sections showed myocardial necrosis and focal infiltrates of polymorphonuclear leukocytes with some mast cells.

Our patient appears to be the first reported with extensive intramyocardial fat after ingestion of massive doses of acetaminophen. The mechanism of the fatty degeneration of the myocytes cells is unclear.

From the Pathology Branch, National Heart, Lung, and Blood Institute, National Institutes of Health, Bethesda, Maryland 20892, the Pathology Department, District of Columbia Medical Examiner's Office, Washington, DC, and the Uniformed Services University of the Health Sciences, Pathology Department, Bethesda. Manuscript received November 18, 1988; revised manuscript received and accepted January 26, 1989.

DOI: 10.1201/9781003408321-15

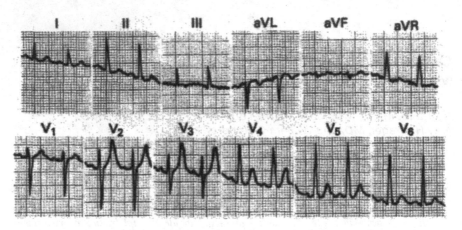

Figure 1 Electrocardiogram taken 4 days after acetaminophen ingestion. Heart rate is 125 beats/min; tall T waves are present in leads V_2 and V_3. The serum potassium was 3.7 mmol/liter. The PR interval measures 120 ms and the total QRS amplitude in the 12 leads is 155 mm (10 mm = 1 mv).

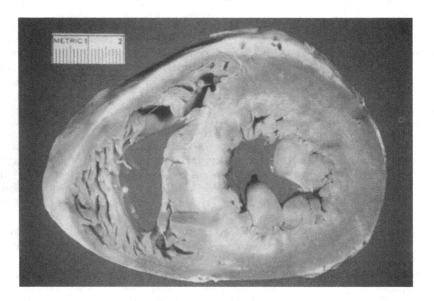

Figure 2 Transverse section of the cardiac ventricles showing the areas of extensive fatty change. The ventricular septum is more severely involved than the left ventricular free wall. The *photograph on facing page* also shows extensive fatty change of the moderator band and some involvement of the anterior wall of the right ventricle.

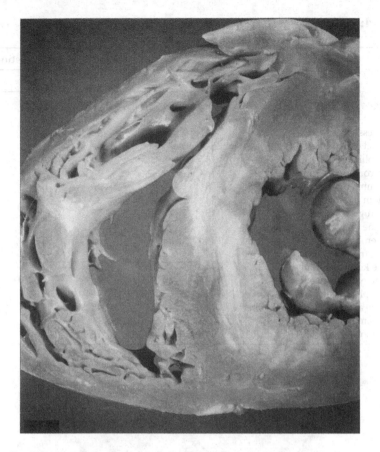

Figure 2 Continued. Scale same as in Figure 2 on facing page.

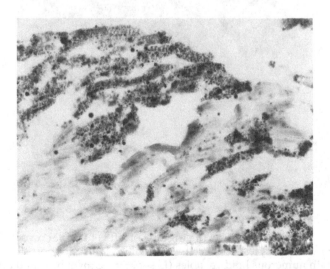

Figure 3 Histologic section stained for fat by the Sudan black method showing vesicles of fat in many myocardial fibers. Original magnification × 260 (no reduction).

77

Table 1: Laboratory results four to eight days after ingestion of 35 g of acetaminophen

	Days after Acetaminophen Ingestion				
	4	5	6	7	8
pH	7.0	7.5	7.5	7.3	7.3
pO$_2$	65	143	95	67	60
Base excess	–21	–5	4.5	–8	–7
Red blood cell count (×10^6/mm^3)	5.35	3.65	3.4 '	2.4	3.4
Hemoglobin (g/dl)	16.5	11.3	10.5	7.4	10.7
Platelet count (×10^3/mm^3)	167	—	47	52	23
Prothrombin time (seconds)	78	35	46	30	31
Potassium (mmol/liter)	3.7	3.4	3.5	3.1	5.0
Urea nitrogen (mg/dl)	13	17	35	30	8
Creatinine (mg/dl)	3.6	5.1	7.3	—	12.3
Cholesterol (mg/dl)	68	73	69	—	65
Bilirubin (mg/dl)	5.3	6.7	7.1	—	13.9
Creatine kinase (U/liter)	1410	3191	3234	8371	—
Lactic dehydrogenase (U/liter)	69793	37571	19759	15710	12080
Alkaline phosphatase (U/liter)	255	179	—	161	120
Aspartate aminotransferase (U/liter)	18726	7659	4529	2394	375
Alanine aminotransferase (U/liter)	9394	7910	—	2435	1444
Acetaminophen (μg/ml)	68	48	26	—	—

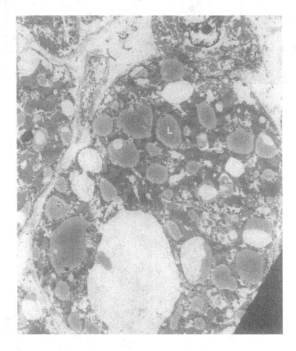

Figure 4 Transmission electron micrograph of left ventricular myocardium showing portions of 5 myocytes. The 2 cells in which a significant portion of cytoplasm is seen contain numerous lipid vacuoles (L) separating myofibrils and other cellular organelles. (Uranyl acetate and lead citrate, original magnification X 2800, reduced by 58%).

REFERENCES

1. Pimstone BL, Uys CJ. Liver necrosis and myocardiopathy following paracetamol overdosage. *S Afr Med J* 1968;42:259–262.
2. Sanerkin NG. Acute myocardial necrosis in paracetamol poisoning. *Br Med J* 1971;3:478.
3. Wakeel RA, Davies HT, Williams JD. Toxic myocarditis in paracetamol poisoning. *Br Med J* 1987;295:1097.

Case 867 Cholesterol Pericarditis and Cardiac Tamponade with Congenital Hypothyroidism in Adulthood

Peter C. Van Buren, MD,* and William C. Roberts, MD. Bethesda, Md.

Although initially considered rare at necropsy,[1] pericardial effusions are found by echocardiogram in about 30% of adults with hypothyroidism.[2,3] The effusions are usually small, measuring <5 mm in thickness or <200 ml in volume. In contrast to the frequency of small pericardial effusions in adults with hypothyroidism, large pericardial effusions are rare and associated tamponade is extremely rare.[4-14] Such was the case, however, in the patient to be described herein.

G.L., a 34-year-old black woman, was found to have diabetes mellitus and systemic hypertension at age 30. She had reached only the eighth grade in school. She had never menstruated. She was in her usual state of health until about 4 months before death, when she noted weakness, lethargy, pedal edema, exertional and nocturnal dyspnea. When hospitalized 3.5 weeks before death, she was stocky, had a round face, enlarged ear lobes, and short arms and legs. She was lethargic and mentally slow. The blood pressure was 150/100 mm Hg, and the pulse was 88 beats/min. Her hairline had receded and her hair was brittle. The eye lids were puffy. The thyroid gland was not palpable. The heart sounds were distant and no precordial murmurs were heard. The external genitalia and breasts were juvenile in size. The legs were edematous (3+/4+). The deep tendon reflexes were diminished. The skin was coarse and dry. The blood hematocrit was 32% (erythrocytes were normochromic and normocytic); prothrombin time was 17 seconds; serum creatinine was 1.4 mmol/L; blood urea nitrogen was 44 mg/dl; uric acid was 11 mg/dl; fasting glucose was 140 mg/dl; serum total cholesterol was 355 mg/dl; resin T_3 uptake was 17%; protein iodine was 1.4 µg/dl; and T_4 was 1.2 µg/dl. The thyroid function tests were consistent with hypothyroidism. The tuberculin skin test was negative. Chest radiograph revealed a globular-shaped cardiac silhouette and clear lung fields. The electrocardiogram showed low voltage. A carbon dioxide angiogram was consistent with an 18 mm thick pericardial effusion.

The patient was started on L-triiodothyronine, incrementally increased to 25 mg/day. Urinary output decreased despite diuretic use. On hospital day 8, she developed pleuritic chest pain, increased dyspnea, pulsus paradoxus of 10 mm Hg, and the blood pressure fell to 130/80 mm Hg. A third heart sound now was audible. Electrocardiogram showed ST segment elevation in leads V_1 to V_5. On hospital day 10 she developed a pulsus paradoxus of 15 mm Hg with associated marked orthopnea. Pericardiocentesis yielded 500 ml of golden cloudy fluid containing 6300/

From the Pathology Branch, National Heart, Lung, and Blood Institute, National Institutes of Health.

Reprint requests: William C. Roberts, MD, Pathology Branch, NHLBI-NIH, Bldg. 10, Room 2N258, Bethesda, MD 20892.

* Resident, Department of Medicine, Georgetown University Medical Center, Washington, DC.

4/4/18131

DOI: 10.1201/9781003408321-16

mm³ leukocytes with 96% granulocytes; cholesterol was 162 mg/dl; total protein was 6.1 gm/dl; and lactate dehydrogenase was 1780 units/ml. A pericardiocentesis catheter was placed and 2 L of fluid were drained during the next 5 days. The patient underwent renal angiography to evaluate her worsening renal function. She subsequently became anuric, and died 16 days later.

At necropsy, the heart weighed 400 gm. After incising the thickened parietal pericardium, focal yellow deposits were seen over the epicardium (Figure 1). Histologically, these yellow deposits were collections of foam cells that stained positively for lipid (oil-red O) and within some collections were many cholesterol clefts (Figure 2). The four valves were normal except for foam cells on the anterior mitral leaflet. The right, left anterior descending, and left circumflex coronary arteries were narrowed at some point >75% in cross-sectional area by atherosclerotic plaque. These four major (also includes left main) coronary arteries were divided into 5 mm long segments and a histologic section was prepared from each 5 mm segment and stained by the Movat method. Of the 35 segments, one (3%) was narrowed 0% to 25% in cross-sectional area; eight (24%) were narrowed 26% to 50%; 16 (46%) were narrowed 51% to 75%, and 10 (27%) were narrowed 76 % to 95 % in cross-sectional area by atherosclerotic plaque. Many atherosclerotic plaques contained foam cells with cholesterol clefts (Figure 3). Every 5 mm segment contained atherosclerotic plaque. Both ventricular cavities were of normal size, and the ventricular walls were free of lesions. The thyroid gland weighed <10 gm, few follicles were present, and the fibrous tissue in it was extensive. The left kidney weighed only 8 gm, consisted mainly of fibrous tissue, and the left main renal artery was totally occluded; the right kidney weighed 260 gm, about 25% of it was grossly infarcted, and many glomeruli and tubules were necrotic (Figure 4).

Several features (round facies, short extremities, and juvenile external genitalia) strongly suggest that the aforementioned patient had hypothyroidism from birth. The pericardial changes in congenital hypothyroidism (cretinism) have not been

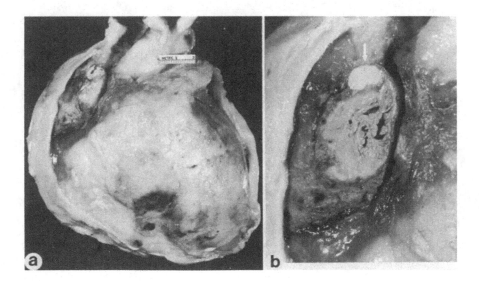

Figure 1 Exterior of heart after excision of the parietal pericardium anteriorly in the patient described, a, Many yellow lipid deposits are present over the epicardium. b, Close-up view of the right atrial appendage after excision of its tip showing a lipid deposit (*arrow*) over the epicardium.

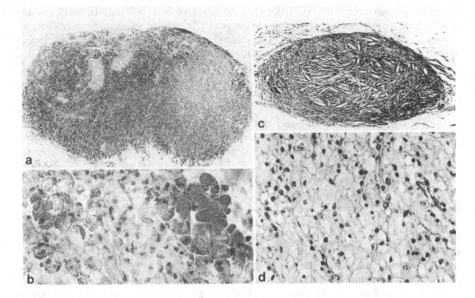

Figure 2 Photomicrographs of lipid deposits over the epicardium. **a**, Oil-red O stain of the lipid deposit just cephalad to the right atrial appendage and shown in Figure la (original magnification ×16). **b**, Close-up of oil-red O stain showing lipid within the cells of the deposit shown in **a** (original magnification ×400). **c**, Another epicardial lipid deposit, but this one is loaded with cholesterol clefts (hematoxylin and eosin stain; original magnification ×50). **d**, Close-up view of the foam cells from the lipid deposit shown in **c** (hematoxylin and eosin stain; original magnification ×400).

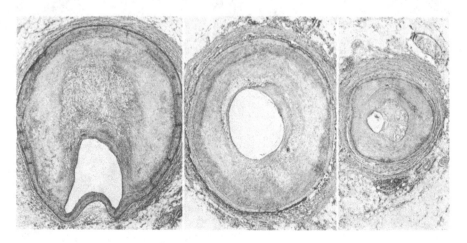

Figure 3 Photomicrographs of sections of the right coronary artery (*left* and *middle*) and a posterior descending branch (*right*) showing collections of foam cells (*left* and *middle*) and mainly fibrous tissue (posterior descending) in the atherosclerotic plaque. (Movat stains; each original magnification ×31.)

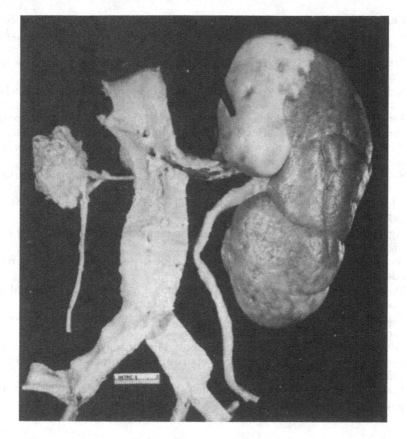

Figure 4   Photograph of opened abdominal aorta and proximal common iliac arteries, minute left kidney, and large but infarcted right kidney that also had a thrombus in the right main renal artery.

described previously. Similar pathologic findings, however, were described in a 54-year-old woman with untreated hypothyroidism.[5] Most pericardial effusions resolve after the initiation of thyroid hormone supplementation.[2,3] At least two reported patients had persistent effusion with tamponade despite thyroid replacement hormone.[7,14] The lipid deposits on the epicardium in our patient were similar to portions of the coronary atherosclerotic plaques and appear to be the consequence of the severe hypercholesterolemia. The pericardial lipid deposits, such as present in our patient and as reported by others[12] in hypothyroidism, have not been observed to our knowledge in patients with hypercholesterolemia not associated with hypothyroidism, such as homozygous or heterozygous familial hypercholesterolemia.

REFERENCES

1 Watanakunakom C, Hodges RE, Evans TC. Myxedema, a study of 400 cases. *Arch Intern Med* 1965;116:183–190.
2. Hardisty CA, Naik DR, Munro DS. Pericardial effusion in hypothyroidism. *Clin Endocrinol* 1980;13:349–354.

3. Kerber RE, Sherman B. Echocardiographic evaluation of pericardial effusion in myxedema, incidence and biochemical and clinical correlation. *Circulation* 1975;52:823–827.

4. Manolis AS, Varriale P, Ostrowski RM. Hypothyroid cardiac tamponade. *Arch Intern Med* 1987;147:1167–1169.

5. Kelly JK, Butt JC. Fatal myxedema pericarditis in a Christian Scientist. *Am J Clin Pathol* 1986;86:113–116.

6. King BF, Kreipke DL, Holden RW, Jackson VP, Tarver RD. Cardiac tamponade from chronic pericardial effusion in hypothyroidism. *Indiana Med* 1989;79:32–34.

7. Arvan S. Pericardial tamponade in a patient with treated myxedema. *Arch Intern Med* 1983;143:1983–1984.

8. Smolar EN, Rubin JE, Avramides A, Carter AC. Cardiac tamponade in primary myxedema and review of the literature. *Am J Med Sci* 1976;272:345–352.

9. Alsever RN, Stjernholm MR. Cardiac tamponade in myxedema. *Am J Med Sci* 1976;269:117–121.

10. Agarwal BL, Mital VN, Misra DN. Cardiac tamponade in myxoedema. *J Indian Med* 1974;63:25–28.

11. Sharma SK, Bordia A. Cardiac tamponade due to pericardial effusion in myxoedema. *Indian Heart J* 1969;10:210–216.

12. Davis PJ, Sheldon J. Myxedema with cardiac tamponade and pericardial effusion of "gold paint" appearance. *Arch Intern Med* 1967;120:615–619.

13. Martin L, Spathis GS. Case of myxoedema with a huge pericardial effusion and cardiac tamponade. *Br Med J* 1965;2:83–85.

14. Silverstone FA. Recurrent heart failure with tamponade due to pericardial effusion; improvement following pleural-pericardial fenestration. *Ann Intern Med* 1955;42:937–941.

15. Brawley RK, Vasko JS, Morrow AG. Cholesterol pericarditis; considerations of its pathogenesis and treatment. *Am J Med* 1966;41:235–248.

Case 1021 Radiation-Induced Cardiovascular Disease Including Stenosis of Coronary Ostium, Coronary and Carotid Arteries, and Aortic Valve

Leigh Anne C. Harvey, MD, Pathology Resident; Samuel J. DeMaio, MD, Cardiology Division; and William C. Roberts, MD, Baylor Cardiovascular Institute

Clinical and necropsy findings are described in a 42-year-old man who received mediastinal irradiation (about 40 Gy) for Hodgkin's disease when he was 24 years old. He subsequently developed virtually every cardiovascular manifestation of radiation heart disease, including constrictive pericardial disease, complete occlusion of the ostium of a coronary artery, severe narrowing of the right coronary artery and of both carotid arteries, complete heart block (infranodal), hemodynamically confirmed aortic valve stenosis, and transmural right ventricular infarction.

Before the 1940s, the heart was considered a "radioresistant" organ. With the introduction of megavoltage radiotherapy for treatment of neoplasms, it became apparent that the heart could indeed be damaged by high-dose radiation, and numerous reports have documented such damage. The portion of the heart most frequently affected is the pericardium, the visceral and parietal aspects of which may eventually become thickened and adherent and cause myocardial constriction.[1-4] The coronary arteries reside in the subepicardial adipose tissue; their lumens may be narrowed by atherosclerotic plaques, the development of which is greatly accelerated by irradiation. The myocardial wall frequently contains an increased amount of fibrous tissue, but usually no grossly visible myocardial lesions are seen in patients with radiation heart disease. Mural and valvular endocardium typically is focally thickened by fibrous tissue.[4] Because the thickening is focal, the valvular involvement generally does not cause valvular dysfunction; if dysfunction does occur, it usually is pure regurgitation. Recently, we studied a man at necropsy who had received large-dose mediastinal irradiation 18 years earlier and 17 years later had hemodynamically demonstrated aortic valve stenosis, complete occlusion of a coronary ostium, coronary and carotid arterial stenosis, and other evidences of radiation-induced damage to vascular structures. A description of the extensive damage in this patient is the purpose of this report.

CASE DESCRIPTION

W.P., a 42-year-old white man who died on May 17, 1993, was well until age 24 years (1975) when he was found to have Hodgkin's disease, stage IA, with large supraclavicular and mediastinal lymph nodes. Following splenectomy he received approximately 40 Gy of irradiation to the upper mediastinum, lower neck, and axillary areas ("upper mantle"). At age 29 (1980), he developed clinical evidence of constrictive pericardial disease and underwent "total" pericardiectomy. The symptoms of cardiac dysfunction were relieved by this procedure.

He was then well until age 40 (April 1991, 25 months before death) when he developed respiratory symptoms, and pulmonary function tests disclosed evidence of both restrictive and obstructive pulmonary disease. During the next 2 years, he also had recurring acute pulmonary infections (cytomegalovirus, *Pseudomonas*) and pleural effusions. In April 1992, he had the

DOI: 10.1201/9781003408321- 17

first of several episodes of syncope. Examination in August 1992 disclosed a grade 3/6 harsh systolic murmur and a grade 2/6 blowing diastolic murmur over the precordium, loudest in the basal area. Echocardiogram disclosed thickening of the cusps of both mitral and aortic valves with poor mobility of the aortic valve cusps. Electrocardiogram showed sinus rhythm and complete right bundle branch block and later, complete heart block.

Cardiac catheterization on September 30, 1992, disclosed the following pressures in mm Hg: pulmonary artery, 19/10; right ventricle, 23/3; right atrium, mean 9; pulmonary arterial wedge, mean 6; left ventricle, 124/13; and aorta, 87/52, yielding on pullback of the catheter a peak systolic pressure gradient of 37 mm Hg between the left ventricle and aorta. The calculated aortic valve area was 1.2 cm^2 and the valve index, 0.59 cm^2/m^2. By left ventriculogram, the ejection fraction was 64%. Injection of contrast material into the left main coronary artery disclosed no narrowing of this artery or of the left anterior descending or left circumflex arteries The ostium of the right coronary artery could not be cannulated.

On October 1, 1992, an electrophysiologic study disclosed atrioventricular nodal block distal to the atrioventricular bundle. Wenckebach block occurred at atrial pacing with a cycle length of 490 milliseconds, and 2:1 block occurred at a cycle length of 470 milliseconds. Extra stimuli in the right ventricular outflow tract readily induced sustained monomorphic ventricular tachycardia that was easily terminated by burst pacing. An automatic pacer cardioverter-defibrillator was implanted.

The patient returned home and was treated daily with furosemide and enalapril. He remained in satisfactory condition until early May 1993, when a pacemaker lead was noted to have fractured. Following insertion of a new lead 7 days before death, he developed recurrent and progressive pulmonary insufficiency, his heart rate slowed, and he was found unresponsive in electromechanical dissociation.

Between September 28 and November 3, 1992, the serum total cholesterol was measured on at least 6 different occasions and ranged from 66 to 164 mg/dL (mean 121, median 129).

MORPHOLOGIC FINDINGS

At necropsy, the pleural spaces contained large, loculated effusions; the lungs were focally but extensively fibrotic; and histologic sections were compatible with chronic radiation pneumonitis. The epicardium was adherent by fibrous tissue to the surrounding structures. The heart weighed 420 g. Both atria were moderately dilated, and both ventricles were mildly dilated. The leaflets of all 4 cardiac valves were thickened by fibrous tissue, the mitral and aortic valves far more than the right-sided valves, and both left-sided valves also contained calcific deposits. The aortic valve cusps contained heavy calcific deposits on their aortic aspects; 1 cusp was made totally immobile by the deposits and was fixed in a ventricular diastolic position, and the mobility of the other 2 cusps also was limited (Figure 1). The adventitia of the sinus and proximal tubular portions of ascending aorta was severely thickened by dense, fibrous tissue, as was the adventitia about the arteries arising from the aortic arch (Figure 2). The ostium of the right coronary artery was totally occluded by plaque. Small calcific deposits were present locally in all major epicardial coronary arteries. The lumen of the right coronary artery proximally was virtually totally occluded by plaque, and the left anterior descending coronary artery was narrowed up to 75% in cross-sectional area by plaque. Histologically, the adventitia of the major epicardial coronary arteries was thickened severely by dense fibrous tissue. No grossly visible foci of fibrosis or necrosis were noted in the left ventricular free wall or ventricular septum; in contrast, portions of the right ventricular wall, in its outflow tract, were completely replaced by fibrous tissue (Figure 1).

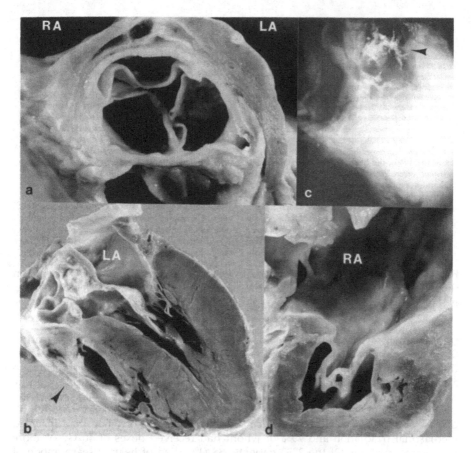

Figure 1 Photographs of the heart in the patient described. (a) Aortic valve from above. The cusps are thickened by fibrous tissue, and calcific deposits are present on the aortic aspects. LA = left atrial cavity, RA = right atrial cavity. (b) Long axis view showing the calcific deposits in the aortic valve. The arrow points to the right ventricular wall in the outflow tract, which is essentially replaced by fibrous tissue. (c) Radiograph of the heart showing heavy calcific deposits in the aortic valve cusps and also calcium at the posteromedial commissure area of the mitral valve. (d) Thickened tricuspid valve cusps and thickened mural endocardium of both right ventricle and right atrium.

DISCUSSION

The heretofore described patient had evidence of radiation-induced heart disease. He had Hodgkin's disease at age 24 and received high doses of radiation to the mediastinum, including the heart. Five years later, he developed constrictive pericardial disease, and 17 years later, he developed a severe degree of heart block and hemodynamically confirmed aortic valve stenosis. At necropsy, he had typical morphologic features of radiation heart disease, including obliterative fibrous pericardial disease; fibrous replacement of the right ventricular wall (in its outflow tract) without grossly visible fibrosis of the left ventricular wall; obliteration of the aortic ostium of the right coronary artery; severe narrowing by plaque of the

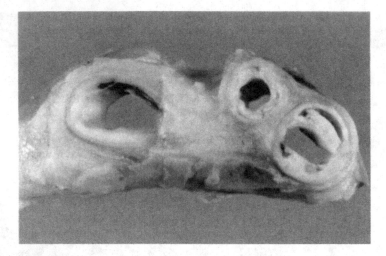

Figure 2 Great arteries arising from the aortic arch. The innominate artery is on the left and the left subclavian is on the right. All 3 contain atherosclerotic plaque. Doppler echocardiogram had shown considerable narrowing of both carotid arteries.

right coronary artery, with severe and extensive adventitial fibrosis (not a feature of atherosclerotic coronary artery disease) of all epicardial coronary arteries and thoracic aorta; focal fibrous thickening of the mural endocardium of the right atrium and right ventricle; and thickening of the valve cusps, particularly those of the aortic and mitral valves.

Hancock and associates[5] recently analyzed 2232 patients treated for Hodgkin's disease at Stanford University Medical Center, 2001 (90%) of whom had received mediastinal irradiation and 79% of whom had received doses of 40 Gy or more to the mediastinum. Of the 2232 patients, 88 (4%) died of heart disease: mode of death was acute myocardial infarction in 42 (48%), sudden coronary death (outside the hospital) in 13 (15%), ischemic cardiomyopathy in 11 (12%), radiation-induced pericardial disease in 14 (16%), valvular heart disease in 7 (8%), and doxorubicin-induced cardiomyopathy in 1 patient (1%). Of the 7 patients with valvular heart disease, 2 had infective endocarditis, 1 had a congenital valve abnormality, and 3 had aortic valve replacement. None of the 7 patients with valvular heart disease had a necropsy; or if so, the findings were not described, and therefore it is unclear if the valvular involvement was related to irradiation. The average interval between treatment for Hodgkin's disease and death from acute myocardial infarction or sudden unexpected cardiac arrest was 10.3 years (at an average age of 49 years), and from other types of cardiac disease, 11.3 years (at an average age of 51 years). The younger the patient at the time of radiation treatment, the greater was the risk of developing cardiac disease.

A number of case reports have described valvular abnormalities detected clinically many years after mediastinal irradiation, usually for Hodgkin's disease. In the 1991 publication by Carlson and associates,[6] 35 previously reported cases (7–19) with valvular abnormalities were tabulated, and 3 additional patients were described.[6] Subsequently, Suzuki and colleagues[20] reported an additional case. Of the total of 39 patients, 11 patients had echocardiographic evidence of thickening of the mitral (7 patients) or aortic valve (3 patients), or both (1 patient), without apparent valvular dysfunction; 6 patients had evidence of mitral regurgitation, 4 of aortic regurgitation, and 4 of both; 11 patients had evidence of aortic valve stenosis, including 5 with associated mitral regurgitation; 2 patients had pulmonic valve stenosis; and 1 had subpulmonic stenosis. None of the 39 patients had clinical evidence of mitral stenosis, and only 1 was reported to have associated tricuspid regurgitation. Seven of the 39 patients had attempted or actual replacement of the mitral (1 patient) or aortic (5 patients) valves, or both (1 patient), and 6 of these 7 patients had some degree of aortic valve stenosis.[6,11,15,17,18]

Although narrowing of the major epicardial coronary arteries is a well-recognized complication of mediastinal irradiation, severe stenosis or total occlusion of a coronary ostium by this process, as occurred in our patient, is less recognized. Pilliere and colleagues[21] tabulated 11 reported patients with single coronary ostial stenosis following mediastinal radiotherapy, and at least 2 such patients with bilateral coronary ostial stenosis have been reported.[22,23] Orzan and associates[24] performed coronary angiography late after mediastinal irradiation in 15 patients, and 10 had evidence of coronary ostial stenosis, 9 of whom also had extensive involvement of other cardiac structures. Only 8 of the 15 patients had clinical evidence of myocardial ischemia.

Although myocardial lesions, usually interstitial myocardial fibrosis, are a recognized consequence of high-dose mediastinal irradiation, transmural right ventricular replacement fibrosis (right ventricular infarction), as occurred in our patient, has not been described previously as a consequence of this process.

High degrees of atrioventricular block, as occurred in our patient, are uncommon consequences of mediastinal irradiation. Orzan and associates[25] described 4 patients aged 31 to 46 years who developed complete heart block 13 to 20 years after therapeutic mediastinal irradiation for Hodgkin's disease. They also tabulated 18 previously reported patients with complete heart block from the same mechanism. Of these 18 patients, 11 were under 50 years of age when the complete heart block appeared, as occurred in our patient. The level of the atrioventricular block was infranodal in all but 2 patients with complete heart block. All patients with atrioventricular block of a high degree had other recognized consequences of radiation heart disease.

REFERENCES

1. Cohn KE, Stewart JR, Fajardo LF, Hancock EW: Heart disease following radiation. *Medicine* 1967;46:281–298.
2. Fajardo LF, Stewart JR, Cohn KE: Morphology of radiation-induced heart disease. *Arch Pathol* 1968;86:512–519.
3. Ruckdeschel JC, Chang P, Martin RG, Byhardt RW, O'Connell MJ, Sutherland JC, Wiernik PH: Radiation-related pericardial effusions in patients with Hodgkin's disease. *Medicine* 1975;54:245–259.
4. Brosius FC III, Waller BF, Roberts WC: Radiation heart disease: analysis of 16 young (aged 15 to 33 years) necropsy patients who received over 3500 rads to the heart. *Am J Med* 1981;70:519–530.
5. Hancock SL, Tucker MA, Hoppe RT: Factors affecting late mortality from heart disease after treatment of Hodgkin's disease. *JAMA* 1993;270:1949–1955.
6. Carlson RG, Mayfield WR, Normann S, Alexander JA. Radiation-associated valvular disease. *Chest* 1991;99:538–545.
7. Stewart JR, Cohn KE, Fajardo LF, Hancock EW, Kaplan HS: Radiation-induced heart disease: a study of 25 patients. *Radiology* 1967;89:302–310.
8. Steinberg I: Effusive-constrictive radiation pericarditis: two cases illustrating value of angiocardiography in diagnosis. *Am J Cardiol* 1967;19:434–439.
9. Morton DL, Glancy DL, Joseph WL, Adkins PC: Management of patients with radiation-induced pericarditis with effusion: a note on the development of aortic regurgitation in two of them. *Chest* 1973;64:291–297.

10. Fouchard J, Joly J, Rousseau J, Herreman F: Pericardite constrictive et myocardite post-radiotherapique avec: insuffisance mitrale. *Semaine des Hopitaux* 1978;54:1283–1287.

11. Warda M, Khan A, Massumi A, Mathur V, Klima T, Hall RJ: Radiation-induced valvular dysfunction. *J Am Coll Cardiol* 1983;2:180–185.

12. Detrano RC, Yiannikas J, Salcedo EE: Two-dimensional echocardiographic assessment of radiation-induced valvular heart disease. *Am Heart J* 1984;107:584–585.

13. Perrault DJ, Levy M, Herman JD, Burns BJ, Bar Schlomo BZ, Drunk MN, Wu WQ, McLaughlin PR, Gilbert BW: Echocardiographic abnormalities following cardiac radiation. *J Clin Oncol* 1985;3:546–551.

14. Pohjola-Sintonen S, Totterman KJ, Salmo M, Siltanen P: Late cardiac effects of mediastinal radiotherapy in patients with Hodgkin's disease. *Cancer* 1987;60:31–37.

15. Lederman GS, Sheldon TA, Chaffey JT, Herman TS, Gelman RS, Coleman CN: Cardiac disease after mediastinal irradiation for seminoma. *Cancer* 1987;60:772–776.

16. Moncure AC, Mark EJ: A 38-year-old woman with a history of radiation treatment for a malignant tumor in the right hemithorax and persistent chest pain and pleural abnormality. *N Engl J Med* 1987;316:1075–1083.

17. McEniery PT, Dorosti K, Schiavone WA, Pedrick TJ, Sheldon WC: Clinical and angiographic features of coronary artery disease after chest irradiation. *Am J Cardiol* 1987;60:1020–1024.

18. Hancock SL, Hoppe RT, Horning SJ, Rosenberg SA: Intercurrent death after Hodgkin disease therapy in radiotherapy and adjuvant MOPP trials. *Ann Intern Med* 1988;109:183–189.

19. Mauch P, Tarbell N, Weinstein H, Silver B, Goffman T, Osteen R, Zajac A, Coleman CN, Canellos G, Rosenthal D: Stage IA and IIA supradiaphragmatic Hodgkin's disease: prognostic factors in surgically staged patients treated with mantle and paraaortic irradiation. *J Clin Oncol* 1988;6:1576–1583.

20. Suzuki M, Hamada M, Matsumoto Y, Hiwada K, Osuka Y. Aortic valvular disease and right coronary artery stenosis induced by mediastinal irradiation: report of a case. *Japanese Circ J* 1993;57:467–471.

21. Pilliére R, Luquel L, Brun D, Jault F, Gandjbakhch I, Bourdarias JP: Ostial stenosis of the left main coronary artery after mediastinal radiotherapy: a case report. *Arch Mal Coeur Vaiss* 1991;84:869–872.

22. Deloche A, Bellin J, Hennetier J, Carpentier A: Post-irradiation coronary ostial stenosis treated by bilateral ostial endarterectomy. *Presse Med* 1987;16:780–781.

23. Stegaru-Hellring B, Keller H, Bode G, Usadel KM, Wallwork J: Ostium stenosis of both coronary arteries and latent hypothyroidism as sequelae of radiotherapy in Hodgkin disease. *Z Kardiol* 1985;74:458–488.

24. Orzan F, Brusca A, Conte MR, Presbitero P, Figliomeni MC: Severe coronary artery disease after radiation therapy of the chest and mediastinum: clinical presentation and treatment. *Br Heart J* 1993;69:496–500.

25. Orzan F, Brusca A, Gaita F, Giustetto C, Figliomeni MC, Libero L: Associated cardiac lesions in patients with radiation-induced complete heart block. *Int J Cardiol* 1993;39:151–156.

Case 1030 Long Asymptomatic Survival with A Bullet Adjacent to the Left Main Coronary Artery, the Only Site of Atherosclerotic Plaque in the Coronary Tree

Jamshid Shirani, MD, Abarmard M. Zafari, MD, Vincent E. Hill, MD, and William C. Roberts, MD Bethesda, Md.

Most people with a bullet penetrating the parietal pericardium die immediately. We describe a man who had a bullet lodged next to his left main coronary artery (LMCA) for 24 years and died of an unrelated cause. The bullet also stimulated atherosclerotic plaque formation in the LMCA.

A 55-year-old man died suddenly at home of heroin overdose. He had had systemic hypertension for many years. At age 31 years he was shot in the chest with a handgun. He had no immediate or late sequelae, and the bullet (0.22-inch caliber) was left in place. At necropsy (19–12–1285), the heart weighed 570 gm. A 1 × 0.6 × 0.6 cm bullet was lodged in the epicardium immediately anterior to the LMCA. It was partially covered by fibrous and adipose tissues (Figure 1). The ventricular walls were free of foci of fibrosis or necrosis. The major epicardial coronary arteries were free of atherosclerosis except for a portion of the LMCA immediately adjacent to the bullet, and it contained atherosclerotic plaque (Figure 1). The epicardium was normal and without adhesions.

Bullets and penetrating metallic fragments lodged within or in the vicinity of the heart can be tolerated if signs of cardiac dysfunction are absent immediately after the injury.[1-3] In our patient no symptoms of cardiac dysfunction or myocardial ischemia were present in the 24 years after the gunshot; no pericardial adhesions were present, although the bullet had entered the pericardial space. An atherosclerotic plaque was present in the wall of the LMCA immediately adjacent to the bullet. No other area of the major epicardial coronary arteries was so involved. Thus external trauma to the major epicardial coronary arteries may initiate atherosclerosis, which can be exclusively limited to the area of injury.

REFERENCES

1. Bland EF, Beebe GW. Missiles in the heart: a 20-year follow up report of World War II cases. N Engl J Med 1966;274:1039–1046.
2. Symbas PN, Vlasis-Hale SE, Picone AL, Hatcher CR. Missiles in the heart. Ann Thorac Surg 1989;48:192–194.
3. Decker HR. Foreign bodies in the heart and pericardium—should they be removed? J Thoracic Surg 1939;9:62–79.

From the Pathology Branch, National Heart, Lung, and Blood Institute, National Institutes of Health.

Present address: William C. Roberts, MD, Baylor Cardiovascular Institute, Baylor University Medical Center, 3500 Gaston Avenue, Dallas, TX 75246.

AM HEART J 1994;128:1043–1044.

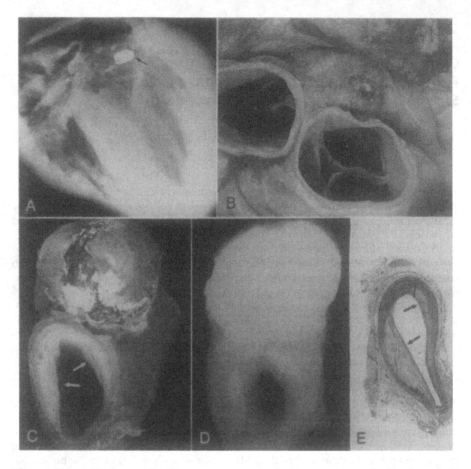

Figure 1 **A**, Radiograph of heart at necropsy shows radiopaque bullet (*arrow*). **B**, View of aorta (*mid left*) and pulmonary trunk (*mid lower*), with bullet adjacent to LMCA. **C**, Transverse cut of opened LMCA; *arrows* point to atherosclerotic plaques with bullet above. **D**, Radiograph of specimen at lower left. **E**, *Arrows* show atherosclerotic plaque in LMCA (Movat stain, original magnification × 50).

Case 1207 Cardiac Transplantation 40 Years After a Stab Wound to the Heart

William C. Roberts, MD, Sabrina D. Phillips, MD, Juan M. Escobar, MD, and John E. Capehart, MD

A 62-year-old man underwent cardiac transplantation in November 2000. In 1959, at the age of 22, he was stabbed in the chest with an 8" butcher knife that was "inserted to the handle." He survived the stabbing and went to the hospital but was discharged within an hour or so without any intervention. He functioned well the next 48 hours. Then, while changing a flat tire on his car, he suddenly began feeling very ill and was taken to a local hospital, where he was found to have a widened cardiac silhouette. He underwent a "7-hour cardiac operation" via a left lateral thoracotomy. His pericardial sac was filled with blood, and a perforating wound in the right ventricular wall was closed. No other details of the cardiac procedure are available. Following recovery from the operation, he felt well again until 1990, when he noted the onset of exertional dyspnea and decreased stamina.

During the next 6 years, the dyspnea slowly but progressively worsened and, in 1996 at age 59, he underwent evaluation by a cardiologist. Cardiac catheterization disclosed angiographically normal epicardial coronary arteries and a left ventricular ejection fraction of approximately 25%. Echocardiogram disclosed left ventricular dimensions of 6.3 cm in end diastole and 5.7 cm in peak systole. A diagnosis of idiopathic dilated cardiomyopathy was made, and appropriate therapy was instituted. A dual-chamber transvenous pacemaker was inserted because of complete heart block, which apparently had been present for decades.

In March 1999, the patient was reevaluated because of further worsening of symptoms of heart failure. At that time, his pulmonary arterial pressure was 55/22 mg Hg; mean pulmonary artery wedge pressure, 15 mm Hg; body mass index, 30 kg/m^2; and blood pressure, 135/90 mm Hg. On cardiopulmonary stress test, he was able to exercise for only 2 minutes and 14 seconds on a Naughton protocol, achieving a peak exercise oxygen consumption of 10 cc/kg/min. At baseline, his heart rate was 64, and at peak exercise, it was still only 64 beats a minute. The minute ventilation went from 15 to 46 L per minute (79% of predicted), despite the fact that the heart rate did not change. The room air blood gases disclosed a pH of 7.46; partial pressure of carbon dioxide, 39; partial pressure of oxygen, 58; forced expiratory volume in 1 second, 1.7; and forced vital capacity, 2.71. At this time, the patient was on enalapril, hydrochlorothiazide, allopurinol, spironolactone, digoxin, and aspirin. He had had systemic hypertension for many years before being on any hypertensive therapy. He smoked 20 cigarettes daily for about 40 years.

Because of progressive worsening of the heart failure, cardiac transplantation was performed. The procedure went smoothly. The excised heart weighed 707 g, and a number of adhesions were present on the epicardial surface. Both ventricular cavities were quite dilated (*Figure, next page*). A small scar was present in the anterior

From the Division of Cardiology, Department of Medicine (Roberts, Phillips, and Escobar), and the Department of Cardiothoracic Surgery (Capehart), Baylor University Medical Center, Dallas, Texas.

Corresponding author: William C. Roberts, MD, Baylor Cardiovascular Institute, Baylor University Medical Center, 3500 Gaston Avenue, Dallas, Texas 75246.

DOI: 10.1201/9781003408321-19

wall of the right ventricle, and a large transmural scar was present in the most basal portion of the ventricular septum in its central portion (*Figure*). There was no scarring in the left ventricular free wall. The 4 cardiac valves were normal. The epicardial coronary arteries were large and virtually devoid of atherosclerotic plaques.

• • •

The unusual finding in the heart was the large transmural scar in the ventricular septum and a smaller scar in the right ventricular free wall. The stab wound to the heart 40 years earlier led to a 2-day delay of hemopericardium and an emergency cardiac operation. The details of the operation 40 years ago are not available, but no sutures or prosthetic material was present in the ventricular septum, indicating that no procedure was done within the heart. It is likely, however, that the knife penetrated not only the right ventricular free wall but also the ventricular septum, producing a ventricular septal defect in the muscular portion of the ventricular septum. The ventricular septal defect later closed, because the ventricular septum was intact and no precordial murmur had ever been heard. The heart failure was probably a combination of 40 years of complete heart block, causing considerable

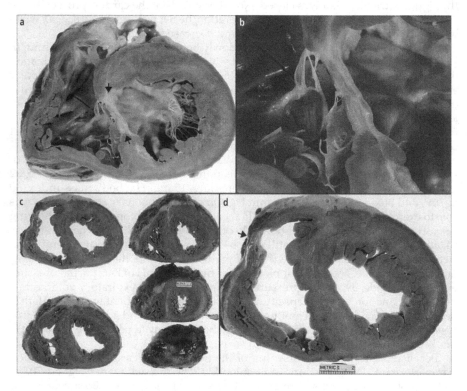

Figure 1 The heart removed for transplant. **(a)** The base of the heart, showing a large transmural scar in the mid portion of the ventricular septum (between the arrows) and dilated right and left ventricular cavities. **(b)** A close-up view of the large scar in the ventricular septum. **(c)** Transverse cuts of the more apical portions of the left ventricular cavity, showing the walls to be thickened and the cavities to be mildly to moderately dilated. **(d)** A magnification of a slice from (a); the arrow points to where the knife entered the anterior wall of the right ventricle.

dilatation of both ventricular cavities with superimposed systemic hypertension for many years. The area of the atrioventricular bundle was extensively scarred.

In summary, we describe a patient who underwent cardiac transplantation because of heart failure and was found to have a large scar in his ventricular septum and fibrosis of his atrioventricular nodal area, suggesting that he had complete heart block for 40 years. The ventricular dilatation likely was the result of both complete heart block and superimposed systemic hypertension.

Case 1222 Dyspnea with Hemoglobin SC Disease

Linda S. Bang, MD, Robert D. Black, MD, Shelley A. Hall, MD, and William C. Roberts, MD

CASE PRESENTATION

LINDA S. BANG, MD: A 41-year-old African American woman with sickle cell disease presented to the Baylor University Medical Center emergency department with dyspnea and dry cough for 3 weeks and back, leg, and chest pain for 2 to 3 days. The hemoglobin SC disease had been first diagnosed during pregnancy. Pleural tuberculosis with a left-sided effusion had been diagnosed 2 years earlier, and she had been treated with 4 antituberculosis medications. She also had had kidney stones and gallstones in the past. Her only operation was a hernia repair at age 38. Medications included rofecoxib, amitriptyline, and a recently completed 10-day course of trimethoprim and sulfamethoxazole for presumed tuberculous pleuritis. She worked for a laboratory, was separated, and had one daughter, who was well. She smoked about 10 cigarettes a day, drank alcohol occasionally, and denied intravenous drug use.

In the emergency department, her temperature was 97.4°F (36.4°C); heart rate, 121 beats per minute; respirations, 24 breaths per minute; and blood pressure, 110/80 mm Hg. Oxygen saturation was 87% on room air and 95% on oxygen via nasal canula. The pupils were equal and reactive to light. She had no precordial murmurs, rubs, or gallops. The lungs were clear to auscultation. No abdominal abnormalities were noted. The extremities showed no clubbing, cyanosis, or edema. The patient was alert and oriented with no focal deficits. Results of laboratory tests ordered in the emergency department are summarized in the *Table*.

After treatment with supplemental oxygen, intravenous fluids, and ketorolac tromethamine, the patient felt better and had decreased dyspnea and pain. When she walked, her oxygen saturation fell to 88%, and she became dyspneic, restless, and agitated and had a tonic-clonic seizure. She was given lorazepam and 100% oxygen via nonrebreathing mask; she soon became bradycardic, diaphoretic, apneic, and pulseless. Cardiopulmonary resuscitation was initiated and she was intubated. Approximately 10 minutes later, heartbeats returned, and she was transferred to the coronary care unit. Her blood pressure was 127/77 mm Hg, her heart rate was 112 beats per minute, and she was unresponsive and intubated. The pupils were reactive, the neck was supple, and she had jugular venous distention to the angle of the jaw. She had a right parasternal lift and bilateral pulmonary wheezes. The abdomen was soft and slightly distended. The bowel sounds were normal. The extremities were cool but pedal pulses were satisfactory.

An electrocardiogram showed sinus tachycardia with right bundle branch block, right atrial enlargement, and right ventricular hypertrophy with strain. A computed tomography (CT) scan of the head disclosed no abnormalities.

From the Department of Internal Medicine (Bang), Divisions of Pulmonary Medicine (Black) and Cardiology (Hall), and the Department of Pathology and the Baylor Heart and Vascular Center (Roberts), Baylor University Medical Center, Dallas, Texas.

Corresponding author: Robert D. Black, MD, 3600 Gaston Avenue, Suite 806, Dallas, Texas 75246.

DOI: 10.1201/9781003408321-20

Table 1: Summary of laboratory values

	Emergency department	Coronary care unit	
Test	10:00 PM	7:00 AM	1:00 PM
pH	7.45	6.96	7.16
PCO$_2$	28	30	26
PO$_2$	65	266	95
O$_2$ saturation (%)	94	98	95
Sodium (mEq/L)	136	143	141
Potassium (mEq/L)	5.1	7.2	3.9
Chloride (mEq/L)	106	110	109
Bicarbonate (mEq/L)	17	10	9
Blood urea nitrogen (mg/dL)	16	16	20
Creatinine (mg/dL)	1.0	1.0	1.7
Glucose (mg/dL)	121	280	383
Calcium (mg/dL)	9.0	8.5	9.4
White blood cells (×10^3/µL)	9.3	9.9	ND
Hematocrit (%)	28	20.7	29
Platelets (×10^3/µL)	116	68	ND
Reticulocyte count (%)	9.3	ND	ND
Total bilirubin (mg/dL)	1.6	0.9	ND
Alkaline phosphatase (U/L)	88	92	ND
Aspartate aminotransferase (U/L)	65	86	ND
Alanine aminotransferase (U/L)	31	48	ND
Troponin I (ng/mL)	<0.1	0.1	1.6
Creatine phosphokinase (U/L)	ND	53	706
Prothrombin time (sec)	ND	12.2	19.1
Partial thromboplastin time (sec)	ND	38.9	48.4

ND indicates not done.

Additional laboratory tests were done after the patient arrived in the coronary care unit (*Table*). The peripheral smear showed rare hemoglobin C crystals, rare sickle cells, occasional schistocytes, and target cells. The sickle cell preparation yielded a positive result, and hemoglobin electrophoresis disclosed 51% hemoglobin S and 49% hemoglobin C. Tests for rheumatoid factor, HIV, and pregnancy were negative. The fibrinogen level was 75 mg/dL, thrombin time was >120 seconds, D-dimers were elevated at 3.2 to 6.4 µg/mL, and fibrin split products were >20 µg/mL. Urinalysis results included positive tests for protein, glucose, blood, and leukocyte esterase. Microscopic examination revealed 3 to 5 white blood cells and 30 to 50 red blood cells per high-power field. Urine cultures grew *Escherichia coli* and *Citrobacter freundii*; 1 of 2 blood culture bottles grew *Corynebacterium* sp. Sputum culture grew coagulase-positive staphylococcus.

The patient was given a dopamine infusion, a bicarbonate infusion, 4 units of packed red blood cells, 2 units of fresh frozen plasma, and cefepime and clindamycin intravenously. A few hours later, her systolic blood pressure fell to 60 mm Hg. Norepinephrine was given, another pulseless electrical activity arrest occurred, and she died.

IMAGING STUDIES

LINDA S. BANG, MD: The chest radiograph taken in the emergency department showed that the pulmonary trunk, both right and left main pulmonary arteries, and heart were dilated. The lung fields were clear. A spiral CT scan showed no emboli, but an infiltrate was present in the right upper lobe. An abdominal and lower extremity sonogram showed gallstones, a thickened gallbladder wall, and dilated hepatic veins and inferior vena cava. The fluid-filled bowel loops were mildly dilated. The spleen was not visualized. There were no deep venous thrombi.

SHELLEY A. HALL, MD: The patient's 2-dimensional echocardiogram showed normal left ventricular function, a very dilated right side of the heart, an enlarged pulmonary trunk, and tricuspid regurgitation. The maximum pulmonary artery systolic pressure was estimated to be 120 mm Hg. The valves were all structurally normal.

DIFFERENTIAL DIAGNOSIS

ROBERT D. BLACK, MD: This 41-year-old African American woman with hemoglobin SC disease had recurrent cough; dyspnea; and chest, back, and leg pain consistent with a vaso-occlusive crisis involving the lungs, vertebral bodies, and long bones of the legs. She was wheezing and developed progressive hypoxemia. She was anemic. The peripheral blood smear demonstrated sickle cells, and hemoglobin electrophoresis confirmed the diagnosis of hemoglobin SC disease. A CT scan showed a right upper lobe segmental infiltrate and interstitial infiltrates. She had markedly enlarged pulmonary arteries, consistent with pulmonary hypertension, but no evidence of pulmonary emboli. The electrocardiogram showed findings of right ventricular hypertrophy and strain, and the CT and echocardiogram indicated that she had chronic pulmonary hypertension. The pulmonary trunk was 40 mm in greatest diameter, an indication of significant pulmonary hypertension. She developed respiratory failure requiring mechanical ventilation, refractory metabolic acidosis, and refractory hypotension. She died within 24 hours of admission.

Possibly relevant findings in this case include a urinary tract infection, which could be a source of sepsis. Sputum culture was positive for coagulase-positive staphylococcus, and the patient could have had staphylococcal pneumonia. She had a history of the tuberculous pleuritis, which should have been adequately treated. The positive blood culture probably represented a skin contaminant.

The most prominent feature of this case is that of severe pulmonary hypertension. The World Health Organization classification of pulmonary hypertension provides a framework for discussion of differential diagnoses. *Primary pulmonary hypertension* is an uncommon disease that occurs primarily in women in the third and fourth decades of life. Primary pulmonary hypertension, however, is a diagnosis of exclusion, and this patient had multiple potential secondary causes. Approximately 2% of cases of cirrhosis with portal hypertension are complicated by pulmonary hypertension. When the 2 coexist, the condition is known as *portopulmonary hypertension*. This patient had some mild elevation of liver function studies, but she had no evidence of cirrhosis.

The ingestion of any type of *anorexic agent* has been associated with a 6-fold increase in the risk of pulmonary hypertension. No information about this patient's body habitus or weight was given, but there was no history of ingestion of appetite suppressants. Pulmonary venous hypertension can be excluded since the echocardiogram showed no evidence of left ventricular dysfunction or left-sided valvular heart disease.

Pulmonary hypertension associated with *disorders of the respiratory system or hypoxemia* is a consideration, as the patient was a smoker and had evidence of interstitial lung disease. However, pulmonary pressures in the systemic range would be very uncommon, even in the most severe cases of obstructive lung disease and pulmonary fibrosis.

The most likely etiology of this patient's chronic pulmonary hypertension is *chronic thromboembolic disease*, related to either proximal pulmonary artery obstruction by recurrent pulmonary emboli or, more likely, obstruction of more distal vessels by in situ thrombosis and fat embolism associated with sickle cell disease.

An important question in this case is whether the CT scan was sufficient to exclude a clinically important pulmonary embolism. Until recently, there was some debate about the usefulness and accuracy of this technique. A review in the *Mayo Clinic Proceedings* reported that CT angiography using the pulmonary embolism protocol (also called helical or spiral CT) is an accurate, noninvasive method to diagnose pulmonary embolism at the main lobar and segmental pulmonary artery levels.[1] The main criticism of this technique is that it may miss pulmonary emboli in more distal vessels at the subsegmental level. Standard pulmonary angiograms also will miss some of these smaller emboli. CT angiography has a reported sensitivity and specificity of 90% in the diagnosis of clinically significant pulmonary emboli. Although 5% to 10% of the studies are nondiagnostic, the same problem exists with standard pulmonary angiography.

Ryu et al reported that the interobserver agreement between readers of CT angiography was significantly better than the agreement between readers of ventilation/perfusion (V/Q) scans.[1] A significant advantage of CT angiography is that it may provide an alternative diagnosis to pulmonary embolism, such as pneumonia, pleural effusion, adenopathy, or lung cancer.

Several outcome studies confirm the safety of withholding treatment in patients with negative CT scans.[2-4] In a retrospective review of 143 patients, 113 patients had a negative CT scan.[2] Of this group, 100 patients were followed up for 6 months, and investigators found no significant morbidity or mortality that could be attributed to pulmonary embolism.

A subsequent, somewhat larger retrospective review identified 126 patients who had a negative CT scan and compared their 6-month follow-up with that of >350 patients who had a V/Q scan.[3] Only 1 of 78 patients who had a negative CT scan was found to have a microscopic pulmonary embolism at autopsy. It is unclear whether embolism contributed to the patient's death. A significant number of patients who had very low or low probability V/Q scans were subsequently found to have pulmonary embolism and deep vein thrombi. Garg et al concluded that helical CT was effective in excluding clinically significant pulmonary emboli.

The largest and most recent study was a prospective comparison of patients who had negative CT scans with those who had normal or low probability V/Q scans.[4] Evidence for subsequent pulmonary emboli was found in only 1% of the patients who had a negative CT scan. This finding is comparable to that found in patients with a negative standard pulmonary angiogram. These studies show that helical CT is reliable for excluding clinically important pulmonary emboli.

This patient did not have CT scan evidence of acute or chronic pulmonary emboli. The etiology of her pulmonary hypertension relates primarily to her underlying disease process, sickle cell disease, which is caused by a group of hemoglobinopathies that are characterized by a single amino acid substitution in the beta globin chain. In hemoglobin S, the most common type of abnormality, valine is substituted for glutamic acid. In hemoglobin C, lysine is substituted at the same position. Patients who have hemoglobin S and hemoglobin A, typically in a 40%:60% ratio, have sickle cell trait. Although usually a benign condition, sickle cell trait has been associated with an increased risk of sudden death in military recruits undergoing vigorous training and in those who exercise vigorously at high altitudes. Patients with homozygous hemoglobin S disease, or sickle cell anemia, have the severest form of the disease. Compound heterozygosity for hemoglobin S and C is referred to as hemoglobin SC disease. The severity of hemoglobin SC disease is somewhere between the severity of sickle cell anemia and that of sickle cell trait.

The abnormal hemoglobin S tetramer is poorly soluble when it is deoxygenated. As a result, the deoxyhemoglobin S forms elongated, ropelike fibers that distort the red cell and cause sickling, which leads to decreased red cell deformability. While this polymerization is critical, an increased expression of adhesion molecules also contributes to the vaso-occlusive process. Several adhesion molecules have been identified; the most important one on the endothelium is named vascular cell adhesion molecule 1 (VCAM-1). The α_4/β_1 adhesion molecule is specific for the red cell membrane.[5]

Although hemoglobin C does not undergo polymerization, the presence of hemoglobin C results in increased potassium and chloride transport out of the cell. The loss of potassium chloride causes dehydration of the red cell and a relative increase in the concentration of hemoglobin S, which results in a greater propensity for polymerization and sickling.[6] Hypoxemia and acidosis also increase polymerization, and these factors may have relevance in this case.

This patient suffered from *pulmonary complications of sickle cell disease*, which ultimately caused her demise. One of the more commonly reported pulmonary complications is pneumonia. Patients with sickle cell disease have an increased risk of infection because of their functional asplenia. Although pneumonia is very common in children with sickle cell disease, especially those <5 years of age, it is an uncommon complicating or precipitating factor for vaso-occlusive crisis in adults. Adult patients more often have pulmonary infarction due to in situ thrombosis, and they may suffer from embolic phenomena due to fat emboli and bone marrow infarction. These 2 processes result in what has been termed the acute chest syndrome.

The *acute chest syndrome in sickle cell disease* is defined by the National Acute Chest Syndrome Study Group as the onset of a new pulmonary infiltrate associated with chest pain, fever, tachypnea, and wheezing or cough.[7] Among patients with sickle cell disease, acute chest syndrome is the most common form of acute pulmonary disease, occurring in 50% of all patients throughout their lifetime. It is the most common reported cause of death in patients hospitalized with vaso-occlusive crisis and is a significant risk factor for early mortality in these patients, accounting for 25% of premature deaths.

Microvascular infarction of the pulmonary parenchyma as a result of in situ sickling, occlusion, and thrombosis is the hallmark of the acute chest syndrome. The vaso-occlusive crisis begins with regional hypoxemia and the polymerization of hemoglobin S. Polymerization of hemoglobin S, red cell sickling, and increased expression of VCAM-1 lead to vaso-occlusive phenomena in various organs, particularly the bone marrow and lungs. Microvascular occlusion with bone marrow infarction can then lead to fat embolism. Concentrations of secretory phospholipase A_2 have been shown to be elevated in patients with vasoocclusive crises, resulting in the liberation of free fatty acids from the bone marrow fat, which in turn leads to additional lung injury. Pulmonary infection can be a contributing factor. The pain associated with vertebral body infarction or rib infarction can lead to hypoventilation and atelectasis, which contribute to the increase in shunt and worsening regional hypoxemia.[5,8]

Studies supporting this model of the acute chest syndrome report increased plasma concentrations of VCAM-1 in patients during a crisis.[5] Decreased concentrations of nitric oxide metabolites have been demonstrated as well, and nitric oxide has been shown in vitro to down-regulate the expression of VCAM-1. Patients with sickle cell disease who take hydroxyurea have a reduced expression of VCAM-1. Long-term hydroxyurea treatment has been shown to reduce the incidence of acute chest syndrome by 50%.

The National Acute Chest Syndrome Study Group analyzed 671 episodes of acute chest syndrome in 538 patients.[7] A specific cause of acute chest syndrome was extensively investigated with blood cultures, bronchoscopy, and serology. The most common causes were fat and bone marrow embolism and infection, although infection was more common in the younger age group. When an infection was identified, the most common causative organisms were *Chlamydia, Mycoplasma, Staphylococcus,* and *Streptococcus.* The study showed that 13% of patients required mechanical ventilation, and 22% of the adults had some type of neurological event, many of them being seizures. Among the adults in the study, there was a 9% mortality rate, which was attributed to fat embolism, cor pulmonale, or infection.

Repeated episodes of acute chest syndrome and repeated insults to the pulmonary circulation can lead to what has been termed *sickle cell chronic lung disease,* manifested by pulmonary hypertension and cor pulmonale in association with restrictive lung disease.[9] Autopsy studies show obliteration of the pulmonary vascular bed, smooth muscle hypertrophy, and parenchymal fibrosis. The risk factors identified for the development of this syndrome over time are recurrent episodes of acute chest syndrome and vaso-occlusive crises. There is also a strong correlation with aseptic bone necrosis.

In a longitudinal study of 128 patients with the diagnosis of sickle cell chronic lung disease, patients were observed to progress through 4 stages of disease.[9] These stages ranged from mild (mild chest pain and cough with mild pulmonary function study abnormalities but normal oxygenation and a mildly abnormal radiograph) to severe (prolonged, severe chest pain; dyspnea at rest; hypoxemia; severe pulmonary fibrosis; and severe pulmonary hypertension). In this study, the average survival after diagnosis was 5 years. Survival was reduced when compared with that of patients with hemoglobin SS disease who did not have the chronic lung disease. The investigators noted a high incidence of myocardial infarction without documented coronary artery disease; the etiology is unknown but may be related to right ventricular ischemia. The most significant risk factor for the development of sickle cell chronic lung disease was the total number of acute chest syndrome episodes that the patient had experienced.

To summarize, this patient had hemoglobin SC disease and evidence of recurrent chest syndrome. She probably had *sickle cell chronic lung disease,* as demonstrated by severe pulmonary hypertension and cor pulmonale and CT evidence of pulmonary fibrosis. Her acute illness was likely precipitated as an acute chest syndrome and vaso-occlusive crisis; she may have had staphylococcal pneumonia, although it is uncommon among adults. Urine culture results indicate possible urosepsis. The immediate cause of death was progressive right ventricular failure leading to refractory acidemia and pulseless electrical activity.

I predict that the autopsy findings will show chronic pulmonary hypertension with obliteration of the vascular bed, both the plexogenic and thrombotic pulmonary arteriopathy. Fat emboli may be present. I would expect evidence of pulmonary fibrosis, based on the CT findings. The right upper lobe infiltrate could represent pulmonary infarction or possibly staphylococcal pneumonia. Right ventricular hypertrophy and dilatation are likely, but I would not expect proximal thromboemboli. I will include the possibility of myocardial infarction simply because of the data from the previous study.

PATHOLOGY REPORT
WILLIAM C. ROBERTS, MD: The right pleural cavity contained 90 mL of straw-colored fluid, and the left had 20 mL of similar fluid. Numerous fibrous pleural adhesions were present bilaterally. No intrapulmonary masses, infarcts, or

infiltrates were present. The walls of the elastic and muscular pulmonary arteries were thickened, an indication of pulmonary hypertension.[10] Many muscular pulmonary arteries also had thickened intima, which led to narrowing of many lumens (Figure 1). No plexiform lesions were present. A few muscular pulmonary arteries contained multiluminal channels, an indication of previous organization of thrombus or embolus (Figure 2). A rare muscular pulmonary artery contained a fibrin thrombus (Figure 3). Many alveolar capillaries were packed with erythrocytes, but it was not possible to determine whether some were sickled. No bone marrow emboli were found.

The heart weighed 410 g. The right ventricular cavity was quite dilated (Figure 4) and its wall thick, typical findings of chronic cor pulmonale. The left ventricular wall and cavity were normal, as were the 4 cardiac valves and the epicardial coronary arteries. No myocardial lesions were present. No emboli were noted in the major pulmonary arteries, and no intracardiac thrombi were present.

In summary, the patient had morphologic evidence of chronic pulmonary hypertension that probably was reversible as evidenced by the absence of plexiform lesions. The presence of a rare thrombus (or embolus) in the small pulmonary arteries suggests that these thrombi were recurring and that many had organized into intimal fibrous lesions and some into multiluminal channels. No parenchymal lung disease was apparent. The heart was typical of chronic cor pulmonale.

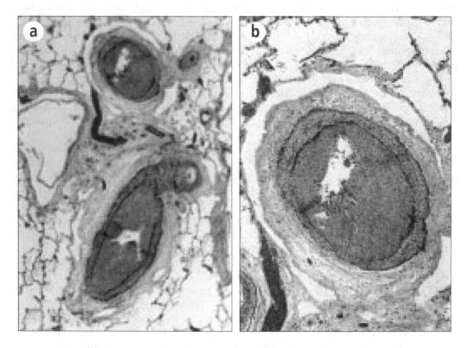

Figure 1 Photomicrographs of the lung in the patient described. (a) View of 2 muscular pulmonary arteries adjacent to a bronchus. The medial walls are thickened, and the intima contains fibrous tissue that has greatly narrowed the lumens. (b) A close-up view of one of the muscular pulmonary arteries shown in (a). Movat stains, ×40 (a); ×100 (b).

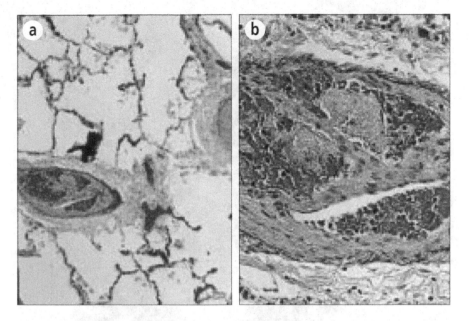

Figure 2 Photomicrograph of the lung showing a muscular pulmonary artery containing multiple luminal channels. **(a)** Low-power view. **(b)** Close-up view showing multiluminal channels containing red cells and a small fibrin clump in 2 of the channels. Movat stains, ×40 (a); ×100 (b).

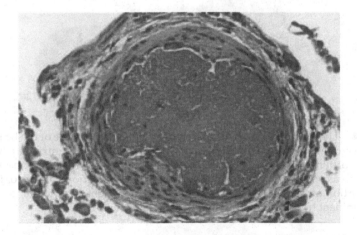

Figure 3 Photomicrograph of a small pulmonary arteriole containing a fibrin thrombus. Hematoxylin and eosin stain, ×400.

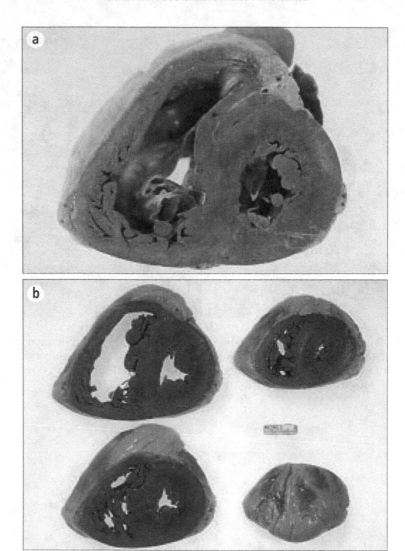

Figure 4 The heart in the patient described. **(a)** View of the base of the heart showing a very dilated right ventricular cavity and a thick right ventricular wall. The
anterior portion of the ventricular septum is thicker than the left ventricular free
wall, an occasional finding in cor pulmonale. **(b)** Cross-sectional views of the more
apical portion of the heart, again showing a dilated right ventricular cavity with
very prominent trabeculae in the right ventricular cavity.

REFERENCES

1. Ryu JH, Swensen SJ, Olson EJ, Pellikka PA. Diagnosis of pulmonary embolism
   with use of computed tomographic angiography. *Mayo Clin Proc* 2001;76:59–65.
2. Lomis NN, Yoon HC, Moran AG, Miller FJ. Clinical outcomes of patients after a
   negative spiral CT pulmonary arteriogram in the evaluation of acute pulmonary
   embolism. *J Vasc Interv Radiol* 1999;10:707–712.

3. Garg K, Sieler H, Welsh CH, Johnston RJ, Russ PD. Clinical validity of helical CT being interpreted as negative for pulmonary embolism: implications for patient treatment. *AJR Am J Roentgenol* 1999;172:1627–1631.
4. Goodman LR, Lipchik RJ, Kuzo RS, Liu Y, McAuliffe TL, O'Brien DJ. Subsequent pulmonary embolism: risk after a negative helical CT pulmonary angiogram— prospective comparison with scintigraphy. *Radiology* 2000;215:535–542.
5. Gladwin MT, Rodgers GP. Pathogenesis and treatment of acute chest syndrome of sickle-cell anaemia. *Lancet* 2000;355:1476–1478.
6. Bunn HF, Noguchi CT, Hofrichter J, Schechter GP, Schechter AN, Eaton WA. Molecular and cellular pathogenesis of hemoglobin SC disease. *Proc Natl Acad Sci U S A* 1982;79:7527–7531.
7. Vichinsky EP, Neumayr LD, Earles AN, Williams R, Lennette ET, Dean D, Nickerson B, Orringer E, McKie V, Bellevue R, Daeschner C, Manci EA. Causes and outcomes of the acute chest syndrome in sickle cell disease. National Acute Chest Syndrome Study Group. *N Engl J Med* 2000;342:1855–1865.
8. Maitre B, Habibi A, Roudot-Thoraval F, Bachir D, Belghiti DD, Galacteros F, Godeau B. Acute chest syndrome in adults with sickle cell disease. *Chest* 2000;117:1386–1392.
9. Powars D, Weidman JA, Odom-Maryon T, Niland JC, Johnson C. Sickle cell chronic lung disease: prior morbidity and the risk of pulmonary failure. *Medicine (Baltimore)* 1988;67:66–76.
10. Roberts WC. A simple histologic classification of pulmonary arterial hypertension. *Am J Cardiol* 1986;58:385–386.

Case 1251 Isolated Ventricular Septal Defect Caused by Nonpenetrating Trauma to the Chest

Dean T. Mason, MD, and William C. Roberts, MD

> *These ruptures happen oftenest from violent blows; then the individual who is attacked, passes from a state of perfect health to that of incurable disease, and in general soon mortal . . . .*
>
> —J. N. CORVISART, 1806[1]

Nonpenetrating trauma to the chest often results in injury to the heart, which may vary in severity from immediately fatal cardiac rupture to asymptomatic cardiac bruises. Contusion of the myocardium, as evidenced by electrocardiographic abnormalities, has been the most common lesion found clinically, and rupture of the myocardium has been the most common injury found at autopsy following nonpenetrating chest trauma. The rupture usually involves the free wall of either or both ventricles and rapidly leads to death. On occasion, the ventricular septum is ruptured without perforation of a ventricular free wall. This report describes a patient who survived isolated rupture of the ventricular septum following blunt trauma to the chest and summarizes pertinent features of some cases that have been reported.

• • •

A 24-year-old laborer was in excellent health until October 1960, when he was involved in an automobile accident. He struck his chest against the steering wheel after hitting the rear of a truck and was knocked unconscious. Upon awakening approximately 1 hour later, he heard and felt a "purring" sensation over his precordium and was hospitalized. The patient had had no previous history of cardiac disease, and no precordial murmur had ever been detected. His most recent physical examination had taken place in July 1959 upon discharge from the Armed Services.

On admission, several superficial cuts and bruises were present on his face, knees, and chest wall. His blood pressure was 110/75 mm Hg; heart rate, 80 beats per minute; and temperature, 38.4°C (101°F), which became normal after 3 days. Precordial examination disclosed a prominent systolic thrill and a grade 5/6 harsh holosystolic murmur, loudest along the left sternal border but audible over the entire anterior chest, back, and left axilla (Figure 1). A grade 1/6 presystolic rumble was heard along the lower left sternal border and at the apex. Admission chest radiograph (Figure 2) showed a normal-sized heart, an enlarged pulmonary arterial segment, increased pulmonary vascularity, and an incomplete fracture of the left fourth rib. Repeat chest radiograph 15 days later revealed an increase in the size of the cardiac silhouette. Serial electrocardiograms (Figure 3) showed

From the Department of Medicine, The Johns Hopkins Hospital, Baltimore, Maryland. Dr. Mason is now in El Macero, California. Dr. Roberts is now with the Baylor Heart and Vascular Institute, Baylor University Medical Center, Dallas, Texas.

Corresponding author: Dean T. Mason, MD, 44725 Country Club Drive, El Macero, California 95618.

DOI: 10.1201/9781003408321-21

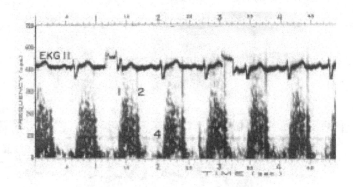

Figure 1 Spectral phonocardiogram recorded at the apex and lead II of the electrocardiogram taken at the first hospitalization in October 1960.

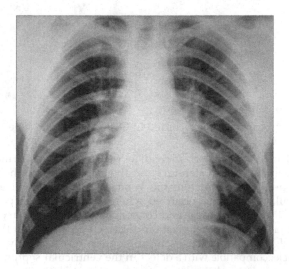

Figure 2 Chest radiograph at the first hospitalization in October 1960.

left axis deviation and changes compatible with anterior wall acute myocardial infarction. The hematocrit was 51%, and the white blood cell count, 13,500/mm³. Leukocytosis (13,500–19,000) remained throughout his 23 days in the hospital. The corrected erythrocyte sedimentation rate ranged from 28 to 34 mm in 1 hour. Over a 4-day period, aspartate aminotransferase levels changed from 58 to 70 and then to 17 units. Throughout the hospitalization, the patient continued to be aware of a noise in his anterior chest. At no time, however, did he have chest pain or signs or symptoms of congestive cardiac failure.

The patient was readmitted to the hospital in June 1961 for cardiac catheterization. During the 8-month interval he had worked as a hard laborer, lifting sheetrock on houses. At no time had he experienced dyspnea, chest pain, palpitations, or limitation of any sort. Physical examination was entirely unchanged. Chest radiograph revealed a slight decrease in cardiac size compared with the radiograph of November 1960. Repeat electrocardiogram continued to show left axis deviation and small R waves in the initial precordial leads, but the T waves in the precordial leads now had reverted to an upright position (Figure 3).

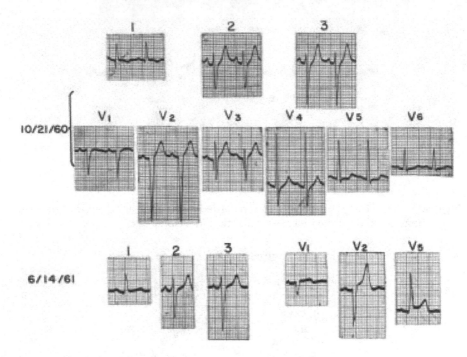

Figure 3   Electrocardiograms recorded in October 1960 and June 1961.

Right-sided cardiac catheterization disclosed a right ventricular pressure of 37/2 mm Hg, with an oxygen step-up from the right atrium to the right ventricle. No oxygen step-up was seen from the vena cavae to the right atrium. Several runs of ventricular tachycardia occurred when the catheter was positioned in the outflow tract of the right ventricle, and consequently the pulmonary trunk was not entered. Retrograde aortic catheterization disclosed a pressure in the left ventricle of 103/10 mm Hg. A left ventricular cineangiogram revealed early opacification of the right ventricle, compatible with a defect in the ventricular septum, and moderate regurgitation into a normal-sized left atrium, compatible with rupture of one or several mitral chordae tendineae. Because the left-to-right shunt was relatively small and the patient was asymptomatic, surgical repair of the ventricular septal defect was not considered necessary, and he was discharged and subsequently lost to follow-up.

• • •

Analysis of this patient and 28 reported patients[2-28] with isolated ventricular septal defect caused by blunt chest trauma disclosed the following: 25 (86%) were men; 28 (97%) were young (aged 5 to 38 years [mean, 19 years]), and the remaining patient, a woman, was 75 years old. The trauma in 17 (59%) involved an automobile, and in all but 2 the steering wheel compressed the anterior chest. Other types of trauma included a kick in the chest by a horse, a fall from a moving truck, a crush between a 3-ton bucket and a steam shovel, a fall of a heavy bookcase, a 20-m fall to the roof of a car, a crush under a cattle drop gate, a crush by an auto engine dislodging from its attachments, a forceful throw from a moving sled, a kick in the chest, a crush by the fall of a heavy tree limb, and a fall from 9 floors.

A precordial murmur, systolic in time and loud in intensity, occurred in 25 (86%) of 29 patients, but it was not always present immediately. The time of appearance of the precordial murmur following the accident varied considerably: in 15 the murmur was audible immediately; in the others the murmur was absent initially but appeared anywhere from 6 to 10 days later; and in 1, it appeared 4 months later. When the murmur is delayed, it may be that the ventricular septum is initially only contused; the contused myocardium then becomes necrotic, sloughs, and finally ruptures. The presence of shock also may account for the absence of a precordial murmur immediately.

Abrasions or lacerations of the skin of the chest wall or fractures of the thoracic bones occurred in 17 (61%) of 28 patients in whom associated injuries were described. Rib fractures occurred in only 6 patients (21%), and 11 patients were completely free of injuries to the external chest. An electrocardiogram recorded in the immediate postinjury period in 24 patients was normal in 1 patient and abnormal in 23 (96%), showing changes of acute myocardial ischemia or infarction in 15 patients, nonspecific ST-segment and/or T-wave changes in 4 patients, and conduction disturbances (bundle branch block [5 patients] or complete heart block [2 patients]) in 7 patients. Cardiac catheterization in 19 patients showed left-to-right shunts at the ventricular level in each and pulmonary hypertension (pulmonary systolic pressures, 37–70 mm Hg) in 9 patients.

The ventricular septal defect in each of the patients who underwent operation (15 patients) or autopsy (9 patients [2 died postoperatively]) was muscular in type in all but one and usually linear in shape, varying from 1.0 to 5.5 cm in longest diameter. Multiple defects in the ventricular septum occurred in 2 patients. The patients who died tended to have larger defects than those who underwent operative closure of the ventricular septal defect. Most patients having operative closure of the defect were asymptomatic months after the procedure.

Since the traumatic septal perforations are nearly always of the muscular type, it is possible that these defects may close spontaneously. Eddying of the blood adjacent to the defects tends to produce local endocardial proliferation ("jet lesions"), and this fibrous thickening in itself may at times close defects of the muscular type. Of the 5 patients who survived nonpenetrating rupture of the ventricular septum as proved by cardiac catheterization and did not undergo operation, 4 were asymptomatic >8 months following the accident and the other one had only mild congestive cardiac failure 18 months later.

Since many of these patients do well with temporary medical assistance alone, operative closure of the defect appears to be warranted only in the acutely or progressively deteriorating patient. Even when operation is indicated, it would seem reasonable to delay the procedure for several weeks following the accident if possible to allow healing of the edges of the defect so that sutures can be well secured. These ventricular septal defects often can be closed directly without the aid of a patch.

REFERENCES

1. Corvisart JN. An essay on the organic diseases and lesions of the heart and great vessels. Gates J Trans. Boston: Bradford and Read 1812:344.
2. Pollock BE, Markelz RA, Shuey HE. Isolated traumatic rupture of the interventricular septum due to blunt force. Am Heart J 1952;43:273.
3. Guilfoil PH, Doyle JT. Traumatic cardiac septal defect. Report of a case in which the diagnosis is established by cardiac catheterization. J Thoracic Surg 1953;25:510.
4. Leonard JJ, Harvey WP, Hufnagel CA. Rupture of the aortic valve. A therapeutic approach. N Engl J Med 1955;252:208.
5. Paulin C, Rubin IL. Complete heart block with perforated interventricular septum following contusion of the chest. Am Heart J 1956;52:940.
6. DeWitte PE, Van Der Hauwoaert LG, Joossens JV. Traumatic rupture of the interventricular septum. Am Heart J 1957;54:628.

7. Pierce EC, Dabbs CH, Rawson FL. Isolated rupture of the ventricular septum due to nonpenetrating trauma. Report of a case treated by open cardiotomy under simple hypothermia. *AMA Arch Surg* 1958;77:87.
8. Inkley SR, Barry FM. Traumatic rupture of interventricular septum proved by cardiac catherization. *Circulation* 1958;18:916.
9. Cary FH, Hurst JW, Arentzen WR. Acquired interventricular septal defect secondary to trauma. Report of four cases. *N Engl J Med* 1958;258:355.
10. Campbell GS, Vernier R, Varco RL, Lillehei CW. Traumatic ventricular septal defect. Report of two cases. *J Thoracic Surg* 1959;37:496.
11. Coe JI, Maslansky RA, Woodson RD. Traumatic interventricular septal defect. *Minn Med* 1959;42:1798.
12. Feruglio GA, Bayley A, Greenwood WF. Non-penetrating chest injury resulting in isolated rupture of the ventricular septum and angina pectoris. *Can Med Assoc J* 1960;82:261.
13. Kay JH, Tolentino P, Anderson RM, Bloomer WE, Meihaus JE, Lewis RR. Surgical correction of traumatic partial separation of ventricular septum. *Calif Med* 1960;93:104.
14. Miller DR, Crockett JE, Potter CA. Traumatic interventricular septal defect: A review and report of two cases. *Ann Surg* 1962;155:72.
15. Stern WR, Stoddard LD. Traumatic interventricular septal defect of heart. A case report. *Am Heart J* 1962;63:821.
16. Scheinman JI, Kelminson LL, Vogel JH, Rosenkrantz JG. Early repair of ventricular septal defect due to nonpenetrating trauma. *J Pediatr* 1969;74:406–412.
17. Rotman M, Peter RH, Sealy WC, Morris JJ Jr. Traumatic ventricular septal defect secondary to nonpenetrating chest trauma. *Am J Med* 1970;48:127–131.
18. Rosenthal A, Parisi LF, Nadas AS. Isolated interventricular septal defect due to nonpenetrating trauma. *N Engl J Med* 1970;283:338–341.
19. Moraes CR, Victor E, Arruda M, Cavalcanti I, Raposo L, Lagreca JR, Gomes JM. Ventricular septal defect following nonpenetrating trauma. Case report and review of the surgical literature. *Angiology* 1973;24:222–229.
20. Rees A, Symons J, Joseph M, Lincoln C. Ventricular septal defect in a battered child. *Br Med J* 1975;1:20–21.
21. Stephenson LW, MacVaugh H III, Kastor JA. Tricuspid valvular incompetence and rupture of the ventricular septum caused by nonpenetrating trauma. *J Thorac Cardiovasc Surg* 1979;77:768–772.
22. Merzel DI, Stirling MC, Custer JR. Massive fatal ventricular septal defect due to nonpenetrating chest trauma in a six-year-old boy: the role of early invasive monitoring in an evolving lesion. *Pediatr Emerg Care* 1985;1:138–142.
23. Knapp JF, Sharma V, Wasserman G, Hoover CJ, Walsh I. Ventricular septal defect following blunt chest trauma in childhood: a case report. *Pediatr Emerg Care* 1986;2:242–243.
24. Salvatore L, Chella PS, Di Bello V, Magagnini E, Pozzolini A, Giusti C. Cardiac damage due to nonpenetrating trauma. Report of four cases. *G Ital Cardiol* 1987;17:246–251.
25. Genoni M, Jenni R, Turina M. Traumatic ventricular septal defect. *Heart* 1997;78: 316–318.
26. Harel Y, Szeinberg A, Scott WA, Frand M, Vered Z, Smolinski A, Barzilay Z. Ruptured interventricular septum after blunt chest trauma: ultrasonographic diagnosis. *Pediatr Cardiol* 1995;16:127–130.
27. Tsikaderis D, Dardas P, Hristoforidis H. Incomplete ventricular septal rupture following blunt chest trauma. *Clin Cardiol* 2000;23:131–132.
28. Ansari MZ, Chaudhry MA, Singal A, Joshi R. Unusual cardiac injury following blunt chest trauma. *Eur J Emerg Med* 2001;8:229–231.

Case 1590 Massive Bloody Pericardial Effusion as an Initial Manifestation of Chronic Kidney Disease

Poorya Fazel, MD, Ravi C. Vallabhan, MD, and William C. Roberts, MD

We describe a 35-year-old man with a massive bloody pericardial effusion, which was his initial manifestation of chronic kidney disease. Pericardiocentesis and hemodialysis restored cardiac function and relieved the associated massive anasarca.

A 35-year-old Latin American immigrant man, a known alcohol, cocaine, and tobacco abuser, presented with a 2-week history of progressive dyspnea, dark stools, and epigastric discomfort. He was anasarcous and oliguric. On precordial examination, the cardiac sounds were faint and no murmurs were noted. There was evidence of a large quantity of fluid in the abdominal, pericardial, and pleural cavities. Chest radiograph confirmed the large pleural effusions and the enlarged cardiac silhouette (Figure 1). Electrocardiogram showed low voltage and an ectopic atrial tachycardia (Figure 2). An echocardiogram confirmed the massive pericardial effusion (Figure 3). Results of pertinent laboratory values are shown in the *Table*.

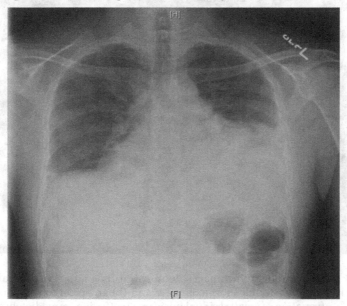

Figure 1   Chest radiograph revealing a large pleural effusion and a large "cardiac" silhouette.

From the Division of Cardiology, Department of Internal Medicine, Baylor University Medical Center at Dallas and the Baylor Heart and Vascular Institute.

Corresponding author: Poorya Fazel, MD, Division of Cardiology, Department of Internal Medicine, Baylor University Medical Center at Dallas, 3500 Gaston Avenue, Dallas, TX 75246 (e-mail: poorya.fazel@gmail.com).

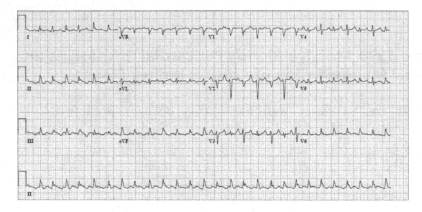

Figure 2 Electrocardiogram demonstrating low voltage and an ectopic atrial tachycardia with a nonspecific intraventricular conduction delay.

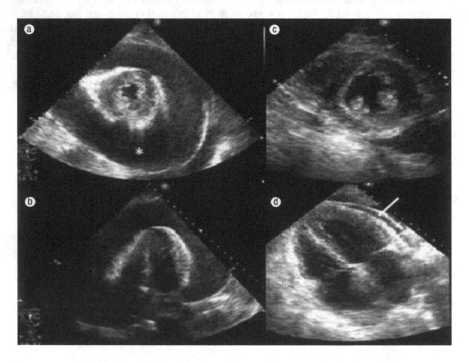

Figure 3 Echocardiographic images demonstrating a large pericardial effusion (asterisk) in **(a)** a parasternal short-axis view and **(b)** an apical four-chamber view. **(c and d)** Confirmation of small residual pericardial effusion immediately after pericardiocentesis (arrow) in the same echocardiographic views.

Pericardiocentesis yielded 1300 mL of bloody fluid having a hematocrit of 11%. Cultures for bacteria, fungi, and acid-fast organisms were negative. No neoplastic cells were identified by cytology examination. Another 525 mL was drained from the pericardial sac over the next 48 hours. Renal sonogram confirmed small echogenic kidneys with kidney length equal to 6.3 cm and 6.8 cm (normal 10–12 cm),

Table 1: Laboratory values

Variable	Hospital day		
	1	5	10
Blood hematocrit (%)	20	26.6	30.4
Aspartate aminotransferase (U/L)	156	41	21
Alanine aminotransferase (U/L)	245	152	33
Sodium (mEq/L)	129	139	137
Potassium (mEq/L)	5.6	3.6	4.6
Chloride (mEq/L)	86	106	101
Bicarbonate (mEq/L)	15	24	27
Blood urea nitrogen (mg/dL)	229	51	42
Creatinine (mg/dL)	25.8	7.5	6.6
Anion gap (mEq/dL)	28	9	9
Body weight (kg)	82.1	74.3	71.2

respectively. This finding was consistent with chronic kidney disease. The patient received hemodialysis, and repeat echocardiogram afterwards showed only a small residual pericardial effusion (Figure 3c, 3d). He was discharged in stable condition to return to Mexico and establish outpatient care.

Pericardial effusion is a known clinical manifestation of chronic kidney disease. With the advent of advanced renal replacement therapy, the incidence of hemodynamically significant effusions has decreased.[1-3] The above described patient presented with symptoms related to a massive pericardial effusion (with pretamponade) as the initial indication of chronic renal failure. The presentation of an effusion as the initial indication of underlying undiagnosed chronic kidney disease is unique. By volume, his pericardial effusion is one of the largest reported and probably the largest of recent memory at Baylor University Medical Center at Dallas.

REFERENCES

1. Alpert MA, Ravenscraft MD. Pericardial involvement in end-stage renal disease. *Am J Med Sci* 2003;325(4):228–236.
2. Colombo A, Olson HG, Egan J, Gardin JM. Etiology and prognostic implications of a large pericardial effusion in men. *Clin Cardiol* 1988;11(6):389–394.
3. Kabukcu M, Demircioglu F, Yanik E, Basarici I, Ersel F. Pericardial tamponade and large pericardial effusions: causal factors and efficacy of percutaneous catheter drainage in 50 patients. *Tex Heart Inst J* 2004;31(4):398–403.

Case 1618 Cardiac Restriction Secondary to Massive Calcific Deposits in the Left Ventricular Cavity

William C. Roberts, MD[a,b,c]*, Randall L. Rosenblatt, MD[d], Jong Mi Ko, BA[a], Paul A. Grayburn, MD[a,c], Johannes J. Kuiper, MD[c], and Joseph M. Guileyardo, MD[b]

Described herein are clinical and necropsy findings in a 61-year-old woman with fatal left ventricular diastolic failure secondary to massive calcific deposits primarily within the left ventricular cavity. At age 3, an isthmic aortic coarctation was resected, and at age 44, a stenotic congenitally bicuspid aortic valve was replaced. The cause of the intracavitary calcific deposits remains unclear, but surgical resection of the deposits has been an effective form of therapy. © 2014 Elsevier Inc. All rights reserved. (Am J Cardiol 2014;113:1442–1446)

Calcific deposits are common in the heart particularly in older individuals and especially in atherosclerotic plaques in coronary arteries, in aortic valve cusps, and in the mitral annulus.[1] These deposits may also occur but far less commonly in other areas of the heart. In 1984, Silver et al[2] described clinical and necropsy findings in a 56-year-old woman with numerous calcific deposits in the left ventricular cavity causing severe impairment to left ventricular filling. This report describes clinical and necropsy findings in a similar patient and reviews other reported cases of large, mainly intracavitary, left ventricular calcific deposits.

CASE REPORT

This 61-year-old white woman had resection of an aortic isthmic coarctation at age 3. At age 44, she underwent an aortic valve replacement with a bileaflet mechanical prosthesis for a stenotic congenitally bicuspid aortic valve. At age 54 (2006), she experienced her first episode of acute pulmonary edema requiring mechanical ventilator. Coronary angiography showed significant narrowing of the left circumflex coronary artery and a stent was inserted. A year later (age 55), another acute episode of heart failure occurred. Repeat angiography disclosed that the lumen of the stent in the left circumflex coronary artery was partially thrombosed, the clot was extracted, and angioplasty was performed. Echocardiogram disclosed a left ventricular ejection fraction of about 30%, but the prosthesis in the aortic valve position was functioning well. She had another episode of acute pulmonary edema 1 year later.

Because of increasing fatigue and periodic evidence of worsening heart failure, she was admitted to the Baylor University Medical Center, Dallas, for the first time at age 59 (February 2011). An echocardiogram, at that time, disclosed severe left ventricular endocardial thickening with numerous intracavitary calcific deposits,

[a]Baylor Heart and Vascular Institute, [b]Department of Pathology, and Divisions of [c]Cardiology and [d]Pulmonology, Department of Internal Medicine, Baylor University Medical Center, Dallas, Texas. Manuscript received December 19, 2013; revised manuscript received and accepted December 26, 2013.

The study was funded by the Baylor Health Care System Foundation, Dallas, Texas.

* Corresponding author: Tel: (214) 820–7911; fax: (214) 820–7533.

E-mail address: wc.roberts@baylorhealth.edu or ajc@baylorhealth.edu (W.C. Roberts).

DOI: 10.1201/9781003408321-23

a restrictive left ventricular filling pattern without respiratory variation, normal-sized right and left ventricular cavities, and a normally functioning aortic valve prosthesis. The cavitary calcific deposits were also seen by chest radiographs and by chest computed tomography. Right-sided cardiac catheterization showed the following pressures in mm Hg: pulmonary arterial wedge mean 20, a wave 26, v-wave 40, pulmonary artery 72/24, and right ventricle 78/15. The cardiac index was 2.25 L/min/m².

Over the next 2 years, the heart failure gradually worsened. Her body mass index was 17 kg/m². The pulmonary arterial pressure rose to 99/29, the right ventricular pressure to 99/0, and the pulmonary arterial wedge pressure to mean 30, a wave 38, and v wave 33 mm Hg. Echocardiogram (Figure 1) revealed findings similar to the one performed 2 years earlier. Repeat chest radiograph showed more left ventricular intracavitary calcific deposits (Figure 2) than had been seen 5 years earlier. Computed tomography (Figure 3) showed the calcific deposits filling the left ventricular cavity. An electrocardiogram a month before death is shown in Figure 4. Cardiopulmonary transplantation was deemed inappropriate and she died of heart failure in August 2013 at age 61.

Numerous serum calcium levels were available between June 2007 and August 2013 and ranged from 8.1 to 9.5 mg/dl. Several serum phosphorous levels in February 2008 ranged from 2.4 to 3.6 mg/dl.

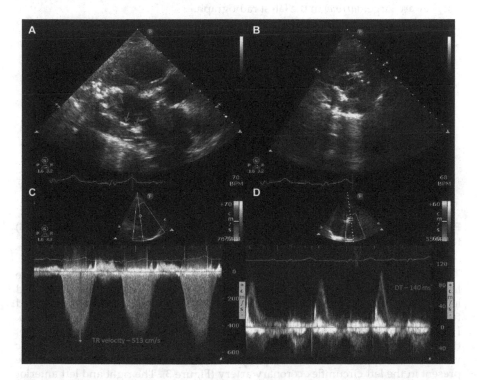

Figure 1 End-systolic frames (*A*) from parasternal long-axis view and (*B*) from short-axis view. *Arrows* point to dense endocardial calcium, which is bright white. (*C*) Continuous-wave Doppler profile from tricuspid regurgitation shows a peak velocity of 513 m/s, consistent with systemic pulmonary artery pressure. (*D*) Mitral inflow pattern exhibits a short deceleration time of 140 ms, consistent with restrictive filling.

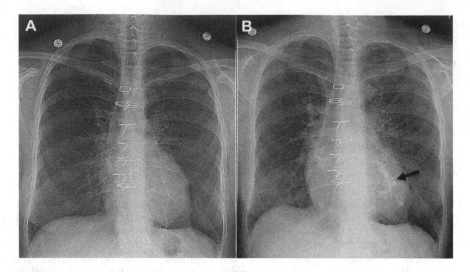

Figure 2 Chest radiographs. (*A*) Taken 5 years before death and (*B*) taken 4 months before death. The left ventricular intracavitary calcific deposits are visible in both, but they are larger (*arrow*) in the latest radiograph.

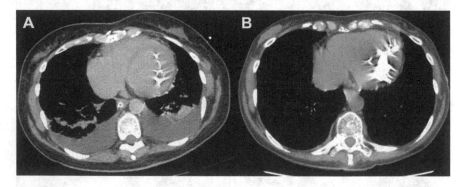

Figure 3 Computed tomographic studies. (A) Taken 6 years before death and (B) taken 4 months before death.

At necropsy, the heart weighed 440 g. Huge calcific deposits were present in the left ventricular cavity from apex to base (Figures 5 and 6). The right ventricular and left ventricular walls and the ventricular septum were of similar thicknesses and free of grossly visible myocardial lesions, and neither ventricular cavity was dilated. Histologically, sections of the myocardium were normal except for enlargement of the myofibers. The discs of the mechanical prosthesis (St. Jude Medical) in the aortic valve position appeared to move properly without interference. Metallic stents were present in the left circumflex coronary artery (Figure 3). The right and left anterior descending coronary arteries were virtually free of atherosclerotic plaques. The right atrium was larger than the left atrium. A saccular aneurysm with a very thin wall was present at the aortic anastomotic site where the isthmic aortic coarctation had been resected.

The right pleural space contained 750 ml and the left 950 ml of serous fluid. Sections of the lungs stained by the Movat method showed that the media of the

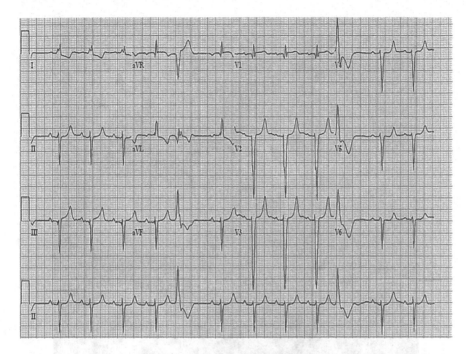

Figure 4 Electrocardiogram, recorded 3 months before death, showing changes of marked right ventricular hypertrophy and frequent ventricular premature complexes.

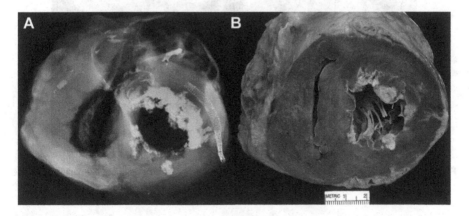

Figure 5 (A) Radiograph and (B) photograph of transverse section of the heart at the base showing extensive left ventricular endocardial calcific deposits and severe thickening of the right ventricular free wall.

pulmonary arteries were thickened, and many had mild thickening of the intima, but no plexiform lesions were present. The intrapulmonary pulmonary veins were dilated, the interlobular septa were thickened (Kerley B lines), and extravasated erythrocytes and hemosiderin-laden macrophages were present in some alveolar spaces. Although most were of normal thickness, some alveolar septa were thickened by fibrous tissue.

117

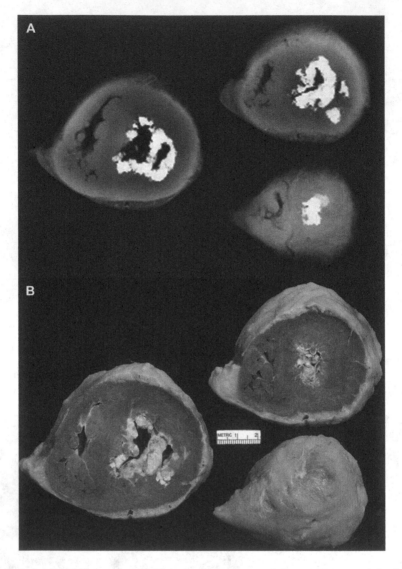

Figure 6 (*A*) Radiograph and (*B*) transverse views of the cardiac ventricles in the apical half again show the extent of the calcific deposits.

DISCUSSION

The patient described herein is virtually identical to the one described in 1984 by Silver et al[2] with huge intracavitary left ventricular calcific deposits leading to extreme difficulty in filling the left ventricular cavity with resulting severe secondary pulmonary hypertension.

In recent years, a number of reports have appeared describing calcific deposits in 1 or more cardiac chambers.[3–20] Reynolds et al[5] in 1997 coined the phrase "calcified amorphous tumor of the heart" to characterize the cardiac calcific deposits because the individual calcific deposits are held together by an "amorphous material," mainly fibrous tissue. In our patient, the intracavitary calcific deposits were essentially

Table 1: Previously reported patients with large left ventricular intracavitary calcific deposits

	First Author	Publication Year	Reference Number	Age (yrs)	Sex	Method of Diagnosis	ESRD	DM
1	Silver	1984	2	56	F	Necropsy	0	0
2	Reynolds	1997	5	30	M	Operation	0	0
3	Tom	2006	6	36	F	CT	+*	+
4	Ho	2008	9	44	M	CT	0	0
5	Kubota	2010	12	64	F	E	+	+
				44	M	CT†	+‡	0
6	Habib	2010	14	58	F	E	0	0
7	van Kruijsdijk	2011	15	56	M	CT	0	0
8	Segura	2011	18	20	M	CT§	0	0
9	Mana	2012	18	55	F	E	0	0
10	Nasli*	2013	19	54	F	CT†	0	0

CT = computed tomography; DM = diabetes mellitus; E = echocardiogram; ESRD = end-stage renal disease; F = female; M = male.
* Secondary hyperparathyroidism.
† The calcific deposits were successfully excised at operation.
‡ Patient had systemic lupus erythematosus.
§ Patient underwent successful cardiac transplantation.

"glued" together and to the mural endocardium by the "amorphous" material that prevented the left ventricular cavity from expanding much during ventricular diastole. Similar huge calcific deposits within the left ventricular and ventricular septal walls unassociated with similar intracavitary calcific deposits can result in similar restriction of left ventricular diastolic filling. A list of reported cases of left ventricular wall and/or intracavitary huge calcific deposits is listed in Table 1. The calcific deposits in each of these patients were clearly visible by echocardiographic and/or computed tomographic studies. Cases in which the calcific deposits involved cardiac valves were excluded from the list.

The cause of "calcified amorphous tumor of the heart" unassociated with heavy calcific deposits involving 1 or more cardiac valves is unclear. At least 4 of the 10 patients listed in Table 1 had chronic renal disease with chronic hemodialysis and at least 1 had secondary hyperparathyroidism. The serum calcium levels in these patients were nearly always normal.

What is the proper management of patients with left ventricular diastolic heart failure secondary to huge intracavitary calcific deposits? The answer appears to be operative excision of the calcific deposits. Both Reynolds et al[5] and Kubota et al[12] have reported operative success by this procedure leading to complete resolution of the left ventricular diastolic heart failure. Cardiac transplantation has been also successful.[18]

DISCLOSURES

The authors have no conflicts of interest to disclose.

REFERENCES

1. Roberts WC. The senile cardiac calcification syndrome. *Am J Cardiol* 1986; 58:572–574.
2. Silver MA, Bonow RO, Deglin SM, Maron BJ, Cannon RO III, Roberts WC. Acquired left ventricular endocardial constriction from massive mural calcific deposits: a newly recognized cause of impairment to left ventricular filling. *Am J Cardiol* 1984;53:1468–1470.

119

3. Dean DC, Pamukcoglu T, Roberts WC. Rocks in the right ventricle. A complication of congenital right ventricular infundibular obstruction associated with chronic pulmonary parenchymal disease. *Am J Cardiol* 1969;23:744–747.
4. Waller BF, Maron BJ, Morrow AG, Roberts WC. Hypertrophic cardiomyopathy mimicking pericardial constriction or myocardial restriction. *Am J Cardiol* 1981;102:790–792.
5. Reynolds C, Tazelaar HD, Edwards WD. Calcified amorphous tumor of the heart (cardiac CAT). *Hum Pathol* 1997;28:601–606.
6. Tom CW, Talreja DR. Heart of stone. *Mayo Clin Proc* 2006;81:335.
7. Lewin M, Nazarian S, Marine JE, Yuh DD, Argani P, Halushka MK. Fatal outcome of a calcified amorphous tumor of the heart (cardiac CAT). *Cardiovasc Pathol* 2006;15:299–302.
8. Fealey ME, Edwards WD, Reynolds CA, Pellikka PA, Dearani JA. Recurrent cardiac calcific amorphous tumor: the CAT had a kitten. *Cardiovasc Pathol* 2007;16:115–118.
9. Ho HH, Min JK, Lin F, Wong SC, Bergman G. Images in cardiovascular medicine. Calcified amorphous tumor of the heart. *Circulation* 2008;117:e171–e172.
10. Gutiérrez-Barrios A, Muriel-Cueto P, Lancho-Novillo C, Sancho-Jaldón M. Calcified amorphous tumor of the heart. *Rev Esp Cardiol* 2008;61:892–893.
11. Vaideeswar P, Karunamurthy A, Patwardhan AM, Hira P, Raut AR. Cardiac calcified amorphous tumor. *J Card Surg* 2010;25:32–35.
12. Kubota H, Fujioka Y, Yoshino H, Koji H, Yoshihara K, Tonari K, Endo H, Tsuchiya H, Mera H, Soga Y, Taniai S, Sakata K, Sudo K. Cardiac swinging calcified amorphous tumors in end-stage renal failure patients. *Ann Thorac Surg* 2010;90:1692–1694.
13. Gupta R, Hote M, Ray R. Calcified amorphous tumor of the heart in an adult female: a case report. *J Med Case Rep* 2010;4:278.
14. Habib A, Friedman PA, Cooper LT, Suleiman M, Asirvatham SJ. Cardiac calcified amorphous tumor in a patient presenting for ventricular tachycardia ablation: intracardiac echocardiogram diagnosis and management. *J Interv Card Electrophysiol* 2010;29:175–178.
15. van Kruijsdijk RC, van der Heijden JJ, Uijlings R, Otterspoor LC. Sepsis-related myocardial calcification. *Circ Heart Fail* 2011;4:e16–e18.
16. Greaney L, Chaubey S, Pomplun S, St Joseph E, Monaghan M, Wendler O. Calcified amorphous tumour of the heart: presentation of a rare case operated using minimal access cardiac surgery. *BMJ Case Rep* 2011. http://dx.doi.org/10.1136/bcr.02.2011.3882.
17. Vlasseros I, Katsi V, Tousoulis D, Tsiachris D, Bousiotou A, Souretis G, Stefanadis C, Kallikazaros I. Visual loss due to cardiac calcified amorphous tumor: a case report and brief review of the literature. *Int J Cardiol* 2011;152:e56–e57.
18. Segura AM, Radovancevic R, Connelly JH, Loyalka P, Gregoric ID, Buja LM. Endomyocardial nodular calcification as a cause of heart failure. *Cardiovasc Pathol* 2011;20:e185–e188.
19. Mana M, Sanguineti F, Unterseeh T, Bouvier E, Garot J. Petrified myocardium: the age of stone? *Circulation* 2012;126:1139–1142.
20. Nazli Y, Colak N, Atar IA, Alpay MF, Haltas H, Eryonucu B, Cakir O. Sudden unilateral vision loss arising from calcified amorphous tumor of the left ventricle. *Tex Heart Inst J* 2013;40:453–458.

Case 1746 Thrombotic Thrombocytopenic Purpura with Graves' Disease During Pregnancy

Junlin Zhang, MD, PhD[a], Laura Baugh, DO, PhD[a], Joseph Guileyardo, MD[a], and William C. Roberts, MD[a,b]

ABSTRACT Thrombotic thrombocytopenic purpura may be seen with several autoimmune disorders such as immune thrombocytopenia purpura, immune hemolytic anemia, and systemic lupus erythematosus, but it is rarely associated with Graves' disease. We report a patient with thrombotic thrombocytopenic purpura associated with Graves' disease.

Thrombotic thrombocytopenic purpura (TTP) is an uncommon disease with a high mortality. Most TTP cases are associated with autoantibodies to ADAMTS13, which normally degrades large, thrombogenic von Willebrand factor multimers. The loss of functional ADAMTS13 results in intravascular platelet aggregation and microangiopathic hemolytic anemia with associated hemorrhage. Plasma exchange is considered the mainstay of treatment; however, immunosuppressive therapies such as corticosteroids and rituximab are also used.[1] Graves' disease (GD) is another autoimmune disorder characterized by hyperthyroidism and diffuse hyperplasia associated with thyroid-stimulating hormone receptor autoantibodies. Management generally involves antithyroid medications, beta-blockers, radioiodine ablation, and surgery, but plasma exchange may also be effective.[2] We describe herein a pregnant woman with combined TTP and GD.

CASE DESCRIPTION

A 39-year-old morbidly obese woman (body mass index 42 kg/m²), who had had two previous full-term pregnancies, developed TTP while pregnant (ADAMTS13 activity <3 units with reference range of 68–163 units). Her mother had immune thrombocytopenic purpura (ITP) and her grandmother had systemic lupus erythematosus. Her platelet level on admission was 6000/µL, and her total 12-lead QRS voltage was 79 mm (standard 10 mm tracing). Her TTP initially responded to plasma exchange but quickly relapsed, prompting a therapeutic abortion at 17 weeks' gestation. Unfortunately, TTP recurred weeks later despite the abortion, and it remained refractory to additional plasma exchanges. Terminally, she developed gastrointestinal hemorrhage and cardiac arrest.

The autopsy disclosed myocardial hemorrhage, most pronounced within the dilated right ventricular wall, the ventricular septum, and the right and left atrial walls (Figure 1a). The heart weighed 495 g. Occlusive platelet-rich microthrombi were present in the small arteries and arterioles of the myocardium (Figure 1b), the lungs, and the intestines. The thyroid gland was diffusely enlarged (weight 95 g). Histologically, the gland was composed of uniform admixtures of mainly

[a]Department of Pathology, Baylor University Medical Center, Dallas, Texas; [b]Division of Cardiology, Department of Internal Medicine, Baylor University Medical Center, Dallas, Texas
Corresponding author: Junlin Zhang, MD, PhD, Department of Pathology, Baylor University Medical Center, 3500 Gaston Avenue, Dallas, TX 75246 (e-mail: junlin.zhang@bswhealth.org)
Received October 10, 2019; Revised December 31, 2019; Accepted January 6, 2020.

DOI: 10.1201/9781003408321-24　　　　　　　　　　　　　　　　**121**

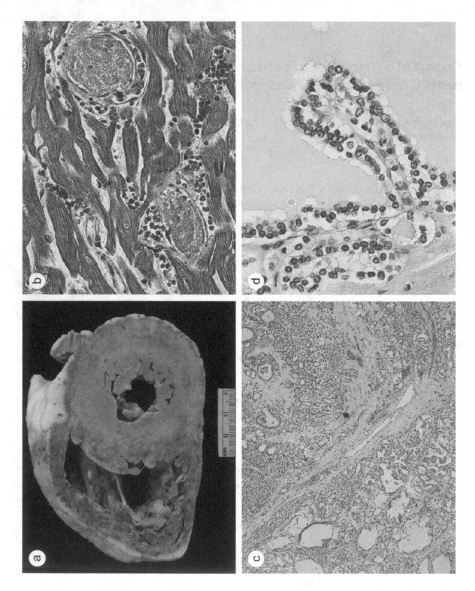

Figure 1 **(a)** Multifocal myocardial hemorrhage. **(b)** Occlusive platelet-rich fibrin thrombi within small intramyocardial vessels (trichrome stain). **(c)** Uniform admixture of hyperplastic follicles and quiescent colloid-filled follicles with no normal parenchyma. **(d)** Follicular hyperplasia with papillary in-folding and colloid scalloping.

hyperplastic follicles and scattered quiescent colloid-filled follicles with no normal parenchyma (Figure 1c, 1d).

DISCUSSION

Patients with an autoimmune disorder are at risk for additional autoimmune diseases, resulting in various combinations including immune-hemolytic anemia,[3] systemic lupus erythematosus,[4] Sjögren syndrome,[5] systemic sclerosis,[6] and others. However, we found only six reported cases of concomitant TTP and GD (Table 1),[7–12]

Table 1: Previous cases of concomitant thrombotic thrombocytopenic purpura and graves' disease (all women)

Variable	Reference number						
	7	8	9	10	11	12 (case 1)	12 (case 2)
Age (years)	49	51	66	51	37	40	25
Pregnant	No*	No*	No*	No*	No*	No*	Relapsed**
TTP duration (days)	7	10	365	120	1	2190	1460
GD duration (days)	7	730	–	120	–	1	730

GD indicates Graves' disease; TTP, thrombotic thrombocytopenic purpura; —, no information available.
* Pregnancy not noted in case report.
** TTP relapsed after uneventful pregnancy.

although several mechanisms have been proposed in which GD may be causally related to TTP.[10,12]

The differential diagnosis for thrombocytopenia in pregnancy is broad and includes ITP, HELLP syndrome (hemolysis, elevated liver enzymes, and low platelets), gestational thrombocytopenia, hemolytic-uremic syndrome, congenital TTP (Upshaw-Schulman syndrome), acquired TTP, and heparin-induced thrombocytopenia.[13] Furthermore, the occurrence of ITP and TTP is greatly increased during pregnancy. ITP complicates 1 in every 1000 to 10,000 pregnancies, accounting for 3% of all thrombocytopenic pregnancies, and pregnancy- or postpartum-related TTP accounts for 10% to 25% of all TTP cases. In addition, preexisting ITP is a known risk factor for developing TTP during pregnancy.[14]

Our patient had recurrent thrombocytopenia, and her ADAMTS13 level met the diagnostic criteria for TTP. However, the TTP subtype (congenital vs acquired) remains unknown since anti-ADAMTS13 IgG levels and genetic analysis were not performed.

The uniform microscopic finding of hyperplastic follicles with scattered quiescent colloid follicles in a diffusely abnormal and enlarged thyroid is highly characteristic of partially treated GD (as opposed to nodular goiter, which exhibits areas of normal parenchyma). However, reliable postmortem serum tests for GD were not possible due to extensive plasma exchange therapy, and no thyroid function tests were available in the medical records. In addition, the plasma exchange therapy for TTP resulted in inadvertent treatment of the GD, altering the histological appearance of the thyroid gland and probably masking other clinical features of GD.

Although combined TTP and GD is uncommon, patients diagnosed with GD who develop thrombocytopenia should be screened for TTP, due to the high mortality associated with delayed treatment of TTP. Conversely, clinical and laboratory evaluation for GD should be considered in patients with relapsed or refractory TTP, and obviously if they develop thyrotoxicosis.

Extremely low platelet levels, as seen in this patient, are known to cause intramyocardial hemorrhage,[15] and myocardial ischemia due to platelet thrombi was contributory to this death. Also, pregnancy is clearly a trigger for the development of ITP and TTP,[12,14,16,17] warranting a high index of suspicion in pregnant patients who develop thrombocytopenia.

ACKNOWLEDGMENTS
The authors acknowledge the support of Carol F. Adair, MD, Department of Pathology at Baylor University Medical Center, for assisting in this study.

ORCID
Junlin Zhang ID http://orcid.org/0000-0003-0371-3113

REFERENCES

1. Scully M, Hunt BJ, Benjamin S, et al. British Committee for Standards in Haematology. Guidelines on the diagnosis and management of thrombotic thrombocytopenic purpura and other thrombotic microangiopathies. *Br J Haematol.* 2012;158(3):323–335. doi:10.1111/j.1365-2141.2012.09167.x.

2. Piskinpasa H, Mert M, Dural AC, et al. Therapeutic plasma exchange in the treatment of hyperthyroidism. *Endocrine Abstracts.* 2017;49:EP1235. doi:10.1530/endoabs.49.EP1235.

3. Morgensztern D, Kharfan-Dabaja MA, Tsai HM, Lian EC. Warm-antibody auto-immune hemolytic anemia developing after thrombotic thrombocytopenic purpura. *Acta Haematol.* 2002;108(3):154–156. doi:10.1159/000064706.

4. Musio F, Bohen EM, Yuan CM, Welch PG. Review of thrombotic thrombocytopenic purpura in the setting of systemic lupus erythematosus. *Semin Arthritis Rheum.* 1998;28(1):1–19. doi:10.1016/S0049-0172(98)80023-1.

5. Yamashita H, Takahashi Y, Kaneko H, Kano T, Mimori A. Thrombotic thrombocytopenic purpura with an autoantibody to ADAMTS13 complicating Sjogren's syndrome: two cases and a literature review. *Mod Rheumatol.* 2013;23(2):365–373. doi:10.3109/s10165-012-0644-7.

6. Towheed TE, Anastassiades TP, Ford SE, Ford PM, Lee P. Thrombotic thrombocytopenic purpura as an initial presentation of limited systemic sclerosis. *J Rheumatol.* 1999;26(7):1613–1616.

7. Chaar BT, Kudva GC, Olsen TJ, Silverberg AB, Grossman BJ. Thrombotic thrombocytopenic purpura and Graves disease. *Am J Med Sci.* 2007;334(2):133–135. doi:10.1097/MAJ.0b013e31812e9735.

8. Zheng WL, Zhang GS, Deng MY. Thrombotic thrombocytopenic purpura complicating Graves disease: dramatic response to plasma exchange and infusion. *Transfus Med.* 2011;21(5):354–355. doi:10.1111/j.1365-3148.2011.01092.x.

9. Chhabra S, Tenorio G. Thrombotic thrombocytopenic purpura precipitated by thyrotoxicosis. *J Clin Apheresis.* 2012;27(5):265–266. doi:10.1002/jca.21210.

10. Bellante F, Redondo Saez P, Springael C, Dethy S. Stroke in thrombotic thrombocytopenic purpura induced by thyrotoxicosis: a case report. *J Stroke Cerebrovasc Dis.* 2014;23(6):1744–1746. doi:10.1016/j.jstrokecerebrovasdis.2014.01.003.

11. Chitnis SD, Mene-Afejuku TO, Aujla A, et al. Thrombotic thrombocytopenic purpura possibly triggered by Graves' disease. *Oxf Med Case Rep.* 2017;10:199–201. doi:10.1093/omcr/omx057.

12. Lhotta K, Zitt E, Sprenger-Mähr H, Loacker L, Becherer A. Treatment of concurrent thrombotic thrombocytopenic purpura and Graves' disease: a report on two cases. *Case Rep Endocrinol.* 2018;2018:5747969. doi:10.1155/2018/5747969.

13. Faridi A, Rath W. Differential diagnosis of thrombocytopenia in pregnancy. *Zentralbl Gynakol.* 2001;123(2):80–90. doi:10.1055/s-2001-12410.

14. Ai-Husban N, Al-Kuran O. Post-partum thrombotic thrombocytopenic purpura (TTP) in a patient with known idiopathic (immune) thrombocytopenic purpura: a case report and review of the literature. *J Med Case Rep.* 2018;12(1):147. doi:10.1186/s13256-018-1692-1.

15. Joly BS, Coppo P, Veyradier A. Thrombotic thrombocytopenic purpura. *Blood.* 2017;129(21):2836–2846. doi:10.1182/blood-2016-10-709857.

16. Roberts WC, Kale IP, Guileyardo JM. Potential cardiac consequences of thrombocytopenia and thrombocytosis. *Cardiovasc Pathol.* 2018;37:34–38. doi:10.1016/j.carpath.2018.08.002.

17. Neave L, Scully M. Microangiopathic hemolytic anemia in pregnancy. *Transfus Med Rev.* 2018;32(4):230–236. doi:10.1016/j.tmrv.2018.08.002.

DISEASES OF
THE AORTA

Case 44 Idiopathic Panaortitis, Supra-Aortic Arteritis, Granulomatous Myocarditis and Pericarditis*

A Cause of Pulseless Disease and Possibly Left Ventricular Aneurysm in the African

William C. Roberts, M.D. and Ernest A. Wibin, M.D.

DURING the past fifteen years numerous reports have appeared describing patients with absent or markedly diminished subclavian and carotid arterial pulses. Approximately twenty-five names have been used to describe this abnormality, but "pulseless disease" and "aortic arch syndrome" appear most appropriate. It has become apparent that there is no single etiology, since syphilis, arteriosclerosis, trauma, dissecting aneurysm, emboli and thrombi, and congenital anatomic variation all have been shown at times to cause absent or markedly diminished subclavian and carotid arterial pulsations.[1] A large group of patients with pulseless disease, however, do not fit into any of these etiologic categories. This *idiopathic* form of pulseless disease is far more common in the Orient than in the United States or Europe,[2-4] and most frequently involves young women ("young female arteritis" or "Takayasu's disease").[3-5] Few reports of idiopathic pulseless disease have appeared from Africa.[6] This paper describes the pathologic conditions which led to absent neck and arm pulsations in an African boy. In addition, this child had diffuse panaortitis with generalized ectasia, focal aneurysms of the aorta and right subclavian artery, and focal granulomatous myocarditis and pericarditis.

CASE REPORT

R.M., a fifteen year old Negro boy living in the Republic of Congo, was well until December 1962 when weakness, paresthesia and numbness of the right arm appeared, and a few weeks later also pain in the right arm and shoulder. In April 1963, a pulsatile mass the size of a nut was noted in the right supraclavicular region. Dyspnea, dysphagia, hoarseness and a cardiac arrhythmia appeared two months later, and in August 1963 he was admitted to the Lovanium University Hospital.

On examination, he appeared thin but well developed. No pulses were palpable in the arms, in the left side of the neck or in either temporal area, and the right carotid pulse was weak. Blood pressures were unobtainable in the arms, but were 190/110 mm. Hg in the legs. A pulsatile, expansive mass was present in the right supraclavicular area, and this was further delineated by chest roentgenogram and angiocardiogram. (Figure 1.) The electrocardiogram disclosed sinus rhythm and occasional premature ventricular contractions. (Figure 2.)

The blood hemoglobin was 11.3 gm. per 100 ml., white blood cell count 12,600 per cu. mm. and erythrocyte sedimentation rate 57 mm. in 1 hour. The serologic tests for syphilis were negative. The serum electrolytes and blood urea nitrogen were normal, but the serum total proteins were 8.8 gm. with albumin 1.6 gm. and globulins 7.2

* From the Laboratory of Pathology, Clinic of Surgery, National Heart Institute, National Institutes of Health, Bethesda, Maryland, and the Department of Surgery, University of Lovanium, Leopoldville, Republic of Congo. Manuscript received November 22, 1965.
Bethesda, Maryland Leopoldville, Republic of Congo

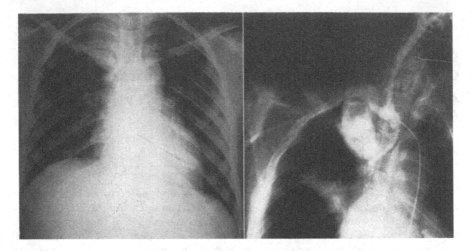

Figure 1 Chest roentgenogram (*left*) and arteriogram (*right*) of the patient described. The ascending aorta is considerably dilated. The mass in the right supra-clavicular area communicates with the right subclavian artery as demonstrated by injection of contrast material into the innominate artery. The right subclavian artery thereafter is totally occluded. The right common carotid artery is narrowed, and neither the left common carotid nor the left subclavian artery is demonstrated.

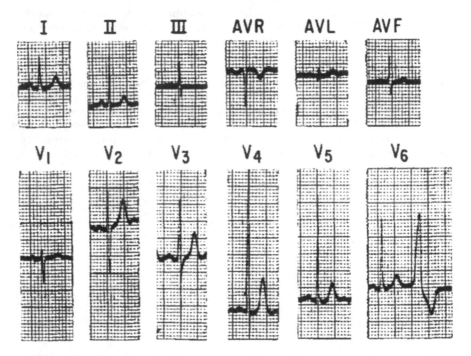

Figure 2 Electrocardiogram of patient obtained on August 19, 1963. An occasional ventricular premature contraction is present. The voltage of the QRS complexes in leads V_4 and V_5 is considerable.

gm. per 100 ml. Urine tests for protein and glucose gave negative results, but a few erythrocytes and leukocytes were found in the urine sediment.

The aneurysm was resected on September 11, 1963. A right femoral to right common carotid arterial bypass was installed via a Tygon® tube in order to clamp the innominate artery. Following this procedure the right subclavian arterial aneurysm, which was surrounded by thick fibrous tissue and many collateral vessels, was resected. The aneurysm had extended behind the right common carotid artery and had compressed the walls of the trachea and esophagus to the left, causing some luminal narrowing of the structures. The child lived 5 hours postoperatively, during which time he had hypotension, fever (40°C) and convulsions.

The autopsy was performed at the Lovanium University Hospital by Dr. David Fluck, who subsequently submitted the heart to Dr. Gregory T. O'Conor and to one of us (W.C.R.). The findings at necropsy are summarized in Figure 3, and described in detail in Figures 4 through 12. The multiple sections of aorta, supra-aortic arteries and myocardium were stained for acid-fast and pyogenic organisms, spirochetes and fungi; none were found. The cause of this widespread disease thus was never determined. The renal, iliac, mesenteric and celiac arteries were normal. Lesions consistent with acute severe hypoxia were present in the brain.

COMMENTS

It has become apparent in recent years that idiopathic pulseless disease is simply one clinical variety of an anatomically relatively widespread arterial disease.[3,6–16] Autopsy and angiographic studies in patients with clinical evidence of isolated subclavian and carotid arterial involvement have demonstrated that the disease process may involve the entire aorta and many of its branches, including the coronary, intercostal, renal, mesenteric, iliac, femoral, popliteal and tibial as well as the pulmonary arteries. Histologic study of these involved arteries has shown that all three layers of the wall are involved (panarteritis), but that the actual obstruction of the vessel results mainly from intimal fibrous proliferation.[14] Giant cells may or may not be present in the involved vessels, but when they are the histologic picture may be identical with that seen in temporal or giant cell arteritis.[1,8,14,15] As in patients with idiopathic pulseless disease, autopsy studies in patients with temporal arteritis have shown that the arteritis is widespread, and may involve the aorta and many of its branches as well as the pulmonary artery.[17–20]

Idiopathic aortitis is another condition in which the histology and distribution of the lesions are similar to those seen in idiopathic pulseless disease and in temporal arteritis.[6,21–28] Despite the anatomic similarities among these three conditions, however, the clinical pictures are different. Patients with temporal arteritis are usually older men (more than sixty-five years old), and their signs and symptoms are related to the temporal arteries.[29] Patients with idiopathic pulseless disease are usually young women (aged fifteen to forty years), and their clinical manifestations are related to inadequate perfusion of the subclavian and carotid arteries.[2–5,30] Patients with idiopathic aortitis are most often children (aged five to fifteen years), and their symptoms are usually related to systemic hypertension resulting from extension of the arteritis to the renal arteries or ostia.[20–22,31] Although patients with temporal arteritis and idiopathic aortitis anatomically may have panarteritis of the subclavian or common carotid arteries, occlusions of these vessels in these two entities are most unusual. Likewise, although aortitis is very common in idiopathic pulseless disease and in temporal arteritis, aortic aneurysms and coarctations, renal arterial stenoses and aortic regurgitation are uncommon.

The patient described herein represents an unusual example of idiopathic pulseless disease. First, he was a boy. Second, he had a large aneurysm of one of the supra-aortic arteries (subclavian) in addition to complete occlusion of this

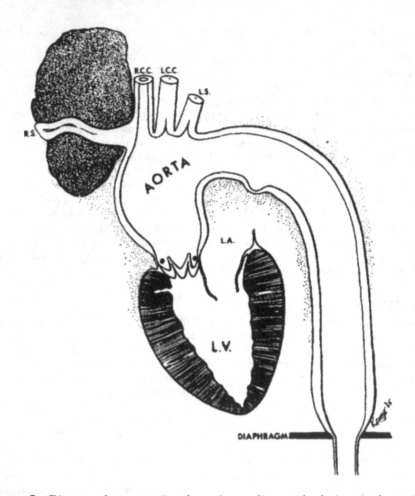

Figure 3 Diagram demonstrating the major cardiovascular lesions in the patient described. The entire thoracic aorta is diffusely dilated, and its wall, uniformly thickened. At the level of the diaphragm the aorta suddenly becomes normal. A small saccular aneurysm is present in the descending aorta. The walls of the vessels arising from the aortic arch are thickened, and the lumens of the right subclavian (R.S.), left common carotid (L.C.C.) and left subclavian (L.S.) arteries are obliterated, and the lumen of the right common carotid artery (R.C.C.) is narrowed. A huge aneurysm filled with a loose fibrin thrombus is present in the first portion of the right subclavian artery. In the ventricular septum and adjacent left ventricular (L.V.) free wall just below the aortic valve there is an invagination into the myocardium from the endocardium. Surrounding this invagination and extending into the adjacent subepicardial tissue are inflammatory and giant cells. The remaining myocardium, cardiac valves and extramural coronary arteries are normal. The pericardial space contained many fibrous adhesions. L.A. = left atrium.

vessel. Third, he had extensive aortitis involving the entire thoracic aorta, leading to generalized ectasia and focal aneurysmal formation. Fourth, he had striking focal granulomatous myocarditis and pericarditis.

Idiopathic pulseless disease appears to be less common in Africa than idiopathic aortitis.[6,21] Isaacson in 1961 reported from Johannesburg "an idiopathic aortitis"

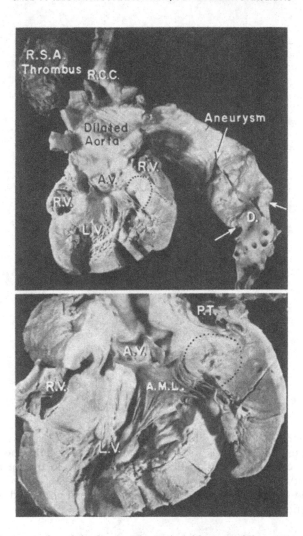

Figure 4 Photographs of the heart. The intimal lining of the entire thoracic aorta is corrugated in contrast to the smooth lining of the abdominal aorta. Neither ventricle is enlarged. The 1.5 by 1.2 cm. sized area of necrosis and inflammation in the ventricular septum is enclosed by the black dots. R.S.A. = right subclavian artery; R.C.C. = right common artery; D. = level of diaphragm; A.V. = aortic valve; R.V. = right ventricle; L.V. = left ventricle; P.T. = pulmonary trunk; A.M.L. = anterior mitral leaflet.

in six children aged seven to sixteen years, each dying of complications of severe systemic hypertension.[21] At autopsy each had widespread aortitis with extension into the renal arteries. In two patients the supra-aortic arteries were involved: a common carotid artery was occluded in one and a common carotid and a subclavian artery was narrowed in another. In 1964 Schrire and Asherson from Cape Town, South Africa, described nineteen patients with idiopathic "arteritis of the aorta and its major branches".[6] Each of the nineteen patients, who ranged in age from four to forty-one years, had extensive aortitis. Only two had clinical evidence of narrowing or obstruction of the carotid arteries, but fifteen showed clinical manifestations of

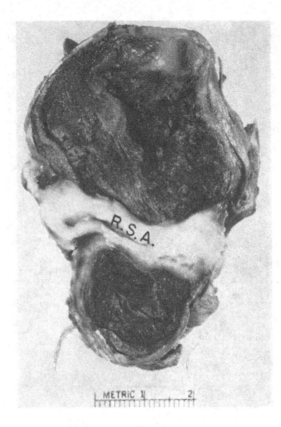

Figure 5 Hemisection of right subclavian artery (R.S.A.) aneurysm filled with fibrin thrombus. The artery is totally occluded. Histologically, the outer wall of the aneurysm consists entirely of fibrous tissue similar to that of the adventitia of the adjacent artery. This aneurysm appears to have resulted from dissection of the intima and media, and rupture appears to have been prevented by the marked fibrous thickening of the adventitia.

narrowing or obstruction of the subclavian arteries. Reports of isolated panarteritis of the supra-aortic arteritis from Africa are most unusual, however, in contrast to the frequency of such reports from the Orient or Europe.[1-4]

In our patient it appears that the large aneurysm of the right subclavian artery and the focal aneurysm of the aortic isthmus are consequences of the panaortitis. Aneurysm formation is not uncommon in association with granulomatous arteritis. Gelfand described a two year old South Rhodesian boy who had extensive panaortitis and a huge fusiform aneurysm of the aorta.[20] Interestingly, this child also had an organized thrombus of the right subclavian artery. One of the patients (Case 2) with "giant cell chronic arteritis" described by Gilmour died from rupture of an aneurysm of the right subclavian artery.[17] This twenty-three year old woman had extensive idiopathic panarteritis of the aorta and the branches of the aortic arch. Schrire and Asherson[6] and others[13,23,28,29] have described similar patients.

An intriguing aspect of the present patient is the associated focal granulomatous myocarditis of the left ventricle and its possible relationship to formation of an aneurysm in the left ventricle. Several reports from Africa in recent years have described an unusual cardiac aneurysm of unknown etiology located in the basal

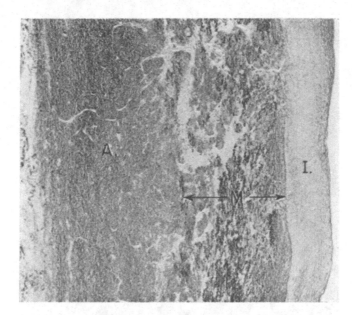

Figure 6 Photomicrograph of section of ascending aorta disclosing severe involvement of all three layers—adventitia (A.), media (M.), and intima (I.)—by the disease process. The adventitia is greatly thickened due to proliferation of fibrous tissue. This scarring process extends into the media causing disruption of the elastic fibers (stained black). Many vascular channels surrounded by mononuclear cells, mainly plasmacytes and lymphocytes, are present in the fibrous scars of the media as well as in the adventitia. The intimal thickening possibly represents a reaction to the underlying medial and adventitial involvement. Verhoff-Van Gieson elastic tissue stain, original magnification × 20.

aspect of the left ventricle immediately below the aortic valve or immediately above the mitral valve.[32-34] The location of this aneurysm, which apparently occurs only in Negroes, corresponds to the focal area of granulomatous myocarditis in the heart of our patient. It is conceivable that the necrotizing granulomatous myocarditis, such as was seen in this patient, is simply a forerunner of an aneurysm in the left ventricle. Further support for this belief is the nature of the cardiac lesion in this patient. The endocardium is deeply invaginated into the focus of myocarditis in the septal and left ventricular walls, and the inflammation simply surrounds this "herniated" endocardium. Abrahams and associates, who originally applied the term "annular subvalvular left ventricular aneurysms," believe that the aneurysms originate as "herniations" of endocardium into the wall of the heart.[33] Reports of the histologic appearance of the walls of these aneurysms have indicated that they consist most commonly of only fibrous tissue.[33,34] Miliary tubercules, however, were found in the myocardium of one patient studied by Abrahams et al., and in each of three patients with this type of left ventricular aneurysm studied by Beheyt and Vandeputte.[32] No reports have appeared describing the "pre-aneurysm" histology of the affected myocardium in patients in whom these unusual cardiac aneurysms subsequently develop. Probably, the myocardium, which becomes the aneurysm wall, heals, and at autopsy only fibrous tissue remains.

133

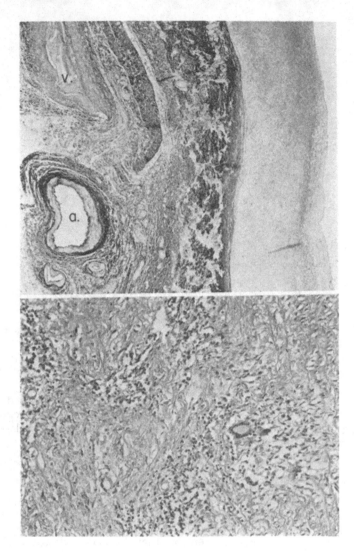

Figure 7 Thoracic aorta. *Top,* section similar to the one shown in Figure 6, but here several adventitial vessels are shown. Both arteries (a.) and veins (v.) are thick-walled. The lumen of the vein is narrowed by intimal fibrous proliferation. The lumens of the adventitial arteries are often severely narrowed also, and generally are surrounded by mononuclear cells. *Bottom,* close-up of media disclosing irregular scars containing vascular channels, lymphocytes, plasma cells, and occasionally Langhans and foreign-body type giant cells. A few remaining elastic fibrils are seen in the right portion of the field. Elastic tissue stain (top) and hematoxylin and eosin stain (bottom); original magnification × 16 (top), × 185 (bottom).

The relationship between the aortitis and the myocarditis is not known, but it would appear reasonable to believe that the two processes are etiologically related. The patients with the annular left ventricular aneurysms usually are several years older than the patients described with idiopathic aortitis. Schrire and Asherson found valvular, coronary or hypertensive disease commonly in

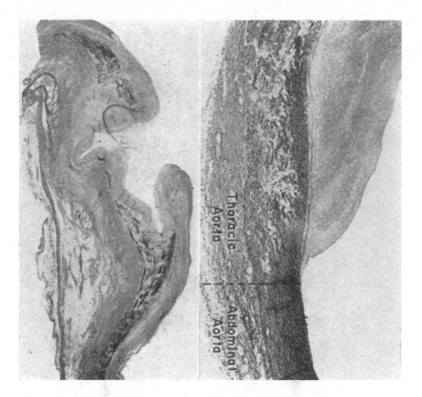

Figure 8 Descending thoracic aorta. *Left*, saccular aneurysm. The media has been disrupted completely, and the base of the aneurysm consists of intima and adventitia. The media is disected for a short distance. *Right*, junction of thoracic and abdominal aorta at the level of the diaphragm. There is an abrupt change to normal at this point. Elastic tissue stains; original magnification × 4 (*left*), × 16 (*right*).

their patients with "arteritis of the aorta and its major branches".[6] Cardiac failure occurred in some patients independently of these conditions, and consequently the heart was believed to be involved directly by the disease process. Several of their patients had aortic or mitral regurgitation, and these lesions together with myocardial ischemia or infarction are the usual findings in patients with "annular subvalvular left ventricular aneurysms".[33,34] None of their patients with clinical cardiac disease, however, had been studied at autopsy. Palmer and Michael recently described extensive giant cell myocarditis of unknown etiology in a patient who also had granulomas in the adventitia of the aorta, liver and thyroid gland.[35]

SUMMARY
The pathologic findings in a fifteen year old Congolese boy, who had idiopathic thoracic aortitis, supra-aortic arteritis with "pulseless disease," aneurysms of the right subclavian artery and aorta, and focal granulomatous myocarditis and pericarditis, are described. Previous reports have indicated that idiopathic aortitis is fairly frequent in African children, but that pulseless disease is unusual in that continent. The etiology of the arteritis and carditis, although unknown, is believed

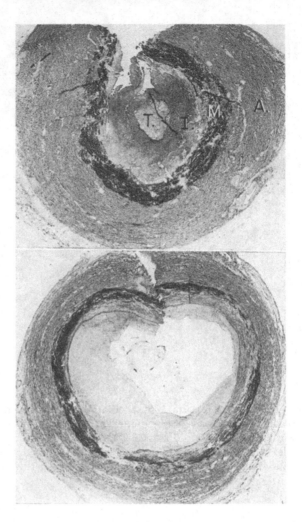

Figure 9 Supra-aortic arteries. *Top*, left subclavian artery 1 cm. from its origin. The left common carotid and left subclavian arteries also were totally occluded and histologically identical to this vessel. The final occlusion is produced by a thrombus (T.) which has organized. I. = intima; M. = media; A. = adventitia. *Bottom*, right common carotid artery which is not completely occluded. Elastic tissue stains; original magnification of each × 13.

to be similar. The location and nature of the myocarditis in this patient suggests that it may be a precursor of an unusual type of left ventricular aneurysm (annular, subvalvular) which occurs in Africa.

Acknowledgment: We wish to thank Dr. Gregory T. O'Conor for his assistance in the preparation of this manuscript. The photomicrographs were taken by Mr. Gebhard Gsell.

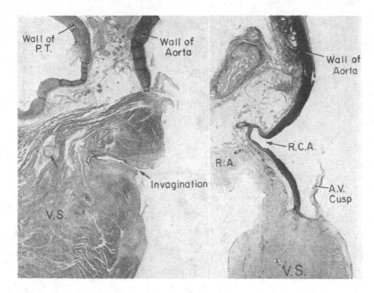

Figure 10 Sections of left ventricular outflow tract and aortic root. *Left*, this section demonstrates the invagination into the ventricular septum (V.S.) just below the aortic valve. The endocardium adjacent to the invagination is considerably thickened, and the adjacent myocardium is inflamed, degenerated, and edematous. In addition, the intramural coronary vessels (arrow), both arteries and veins, in this area show severe luminal narrowing and perivascular inflammation. P.T. = pulmonary trunk. *Right*, in this section the origin of the right coronary artery (R.C.A.) is shown. The panaortitis starts a few millimeters above the coronary ostia as seen here. A.V. = aortic valve; R.A. = right atrial wall. Elastic tissue stains; original magnification × 32 (left), × 135 (right).

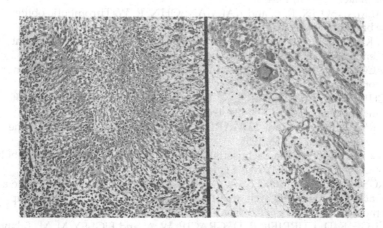

Figure 11 Close-up of ventricular septum adjacent to the invagination. *Left*, numerous inflammatory cells are present, sometimes having a spoke-wheel type of arrangement about bands of necrosis. Plasma cells and lymphocytes predominate, but some histiocytes and polymorphonuclear leukocytes also are present. *Right*, in addition, occasional giant cells are seen in the inflamed, vascular, and edematous cardiac muscle. Hematoxylin and eosin stains; original magnification X 150 (left), X 135 (right).

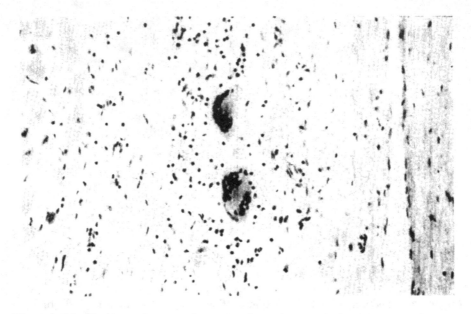

Figure 12 Section of pericardium. In the subepicardial adipose tissue some inflammatory cells and giant cells are present. Hematoxylin and eosin stain; original magnification × 119.

REFERENCES

1. ROSS, R. S. and MCKUSICK, V. A. Aortic arch syndromes. Diminished or absent pulses in arteries arising from arch of aorta. *Arch. Int. Med.*, 92: 701, 1953.
2. ASK-UPMARK, E. On the "pulseless disease" outside of Japan. *Acta Med. Scandinav.*, 149: 161, 1954.
3. KALMANSOHN, R. B. and KALMANSOHN, R. W. Thrombotic obliteration of the branches of the aortic arch. *Circulation*, 15: 237, 1957.
4. MCKUSICK, V. A. A form of vascular disease relatively frequent in the Orient. *Am. Heart J.*, 63: 57, 1962.
5. CACCAMISE, W. C. and WHITMAN, J. F. Pulseless disease. A preliminary case report. *Am. Heart J.*, 44: 629, 1952.
6. SCHRIRE, V. and ASHERSON, R. A. Arteritis of the aorta and its major branches. *Quart. J. Med.*, 33: 439, 1964.
7. BARKER, N. W. and EDWARDS, J. E. Primary arteritis of the aortic arch. *Circulation*, 11: 486, 1955.
8. Case records of the Massachusetts General Hospital: Weekly clinicopathological exercises (Case 23–1961). *New England J. Med.*, 264: 664, 1961.
9. FRÖVIG, A. G. and LÖKEN, A. C. The syndrome of obliteration of the arterial branches of the aortic arch, due to arteritis. A postmortem angiographic and pathological study. *Acta Psychiat. et Neurol. Scandinav.*, 26: 313, 1951.
10. JUDGE, R. D., CURRIER, R. D., GRACIE, W. A. and FIGLEY, M. M. Takayashu's arteritis and the aortic arch syndrome. *Am. J. Med.*, 32: 379, 1962.
11. COPPING, G. A. Pulseless syndrome. *Canad. M.A.J.*, 83: 892, 1960.
12. ASK-UPMARK, E. and FAJERS, C. M. Further observations on Takayashu's syndrome. *Acta Med. Scandinav.*, 155: 275, 1956.
13. CORREA, P. and ARAUJO, J. Arteritis of the aorta in young women. Report of a case. *Am. J. Clin. Path.*, 29: 560, 1958.

14. WARSHAW, J. B. and SPACH, M. S. Takayasu's disease (primary aortitis) in childhood. Case report with review of literature. *Pediatrics*, 35: 620, 1965.
15. NASU, T. Pathology of pulseless disease. A systematic study and critical review of twenty-one autopsy cases reported in Japan. *Angiology*, 14: 225, 1963.
16. RIEHL, J. L. and BROWN, W. J. Takayasu's arteritis. An autoimmune disease. *Arch. Neurol.*, 12: 92, 1965.
17. STRACHAN, R. W. The natural history of Takayasu's arteriopathy. *Quart. J. Med.*, 33: 57, 1964.
18. GILMOUR, J. R. Giant-cell chronic arteritis. *J. Path. & Bact.*, 53: 263, 1941.
19. CARDELL, B. S. and HANLEY, T. A fatal case of giant-cell or temporal arteritis. *J. Path. & Bact.*, 63: 587, 1951.
20. HEPTINSTALL, R. H., PORTER, K. A. and BARKLEY, H. Giant-cell (temporal) arteritis. *J. Path. & Bact.*, 67: 519, 1954.
21. GELFAND, W. Giant-cell arteritis with aneurysmal formation in an infant. *Brit. Heart J.*, 17: 264, 1955.
22. ISAACSON, C. An idiopathic aortitis in young Africans. *J. Path. & Bact.*, 81: 69, 1961.
23. MCMILLAN, G. C. Diffuse granulomatous aortitis with giant cells associated with partial rupture and dissection of the aorta. *Arch. Path.*, 49: 63, 1950.
24. LOMAS, R. W., BOLANDE, R. P. and GIBSON, W. M. Primary arteritis of the aorta in a child. *J. Dis. Child.*, 97: 87, 1959.
25. AUSTEN, W. G. and BLENNERHASSETT, J. B. Giant-cell aortitis causing an aneurysm of the ascending aorta and aortic regurgitation. *New England J. Med.*, 27 (2): 80, 1965.
26. MCGUIRE, J., SCOTT, R. C. and GALL, E. A. Chronic aortitis of undetermined cause with severe and fatal aortic insufficiency. *Am. J. M. Sc.*, 235: 349, 1958.
27. MAGAREY, F. R. Dissecting aneurysm due to giant-cell aortitis. *J. Path. & Bact.*, 62: 445, 1950.
28. DANARAJ, T. J., WONG, H. O. and THOMAS, M. A. Primary arteritis of aorta causing renal artery stenosis and hypertension. *Brit. Heart J.*, 25: 153, 1963.
29. WAGENVOORT, C. A., HARRIS, L. E., BROWN, A. L. and VEENEKLAAS, G. M. H. Giant-cell arteritis with aneurysm formation in children. *Pediatrics*, 32: 861, 1963.
30. HARRISON, C. V. Giant-cell or temporal arteritis; a review. *J. Clin. Path.*, 1: 197, 1948.
31. PATON, B. C., CHARTIKAVANIJ, K., BURI, P., PRACHUABMOH, K. and JUMBALA, M. R. B. Obliterative aortic disease in children in the tropics. *Circulation*, 31 (supp. 1): 197, 1965.
32. BEHEYT, P. and VANDEPUTTE, M. L'anevrisme ventriculaire, d'origine tuberculeuse, chez de jeunes Africains. Etude de 3 cas. *Acta Cardiol.*, 13: 419, 1958.
33. ABRAHAMS, D. G., BARTON, C. J., COCKSHOTT, W. P., EDINGTON, G. M. and WEAVER, E. J. M. Annular subvalvular left ventricular aneurysms. *Quart. J. Med.*, 31: 345, 1962.
34. CHESLER, E., JOFFE, N., SCHAMROTH, L. and MEYERS, A. Annular subvalvular left ventricular aneurysms in the South African Bantu. *Circulation*, 32: 43, 1965.
35. PALMER, H. P. and MICHAEL, I. E. Giant-cell myocarditis with multiple organ involvement. *Arch. Int. Med.*, 116: 444, 1965.

Case 87 The Prepulseless Phase of Pulseless Disease, or Pulseless Disease with Pulses*

A Newly Recognized Cause of Cardiac Disease, Monoclonal Gammopathy and "Fever of Unknown Origin"

William C. Roberts, M.D., Rob Roy MacGregor, M.D., Harold J. DeBlanc, Jr., M.D., G. David Beiser, M.D. and Sheldon M. Wolff, M.D.
Bethesda, Maryland

The clinical and pathologic findings are described in a forty-six year old woman with arteritis involving the aorta and all vessels arising from it. The unusual features of her illness were "fever of unknown origin," atypical bacterial septicemia, monoclonal gammopathy and changing precordial murmurs. Necropsy disclosed widespread aortitis and large vessel arteritis including severe involvement of the coronary arteries and a hitherto undescribed diffuse valvular and focal mural endocardial disease.

DURING recent years numerous reports have appeared describing occlusive disease of arteries arising from the aortic arch. Most patients with the "aortic arch syndrome" (Takayasu's arteritis, disease or syndrome) have been women between fifteen and forty-five years of age, and clinical features have been related to occlusions of the subclavian and common carotid arteries. Autopsies in patients with "pulseless disease" have shown that the arterial involvement is not limited to the supra-aortic arteries but may also involve the aorta and other vessels arising from it.[1] The cause of the arterial involvement is unknown, and few patients with "pulseless disease" or other forms of large vessel panarteritis have been studied during the "preocclusive phase." Recently, this opportunity was presented to us by a middle-aged woman who demonstrated features of a systemic disease of unknown type for fourteen months; at necropsy she was found to have panaortitis with narrowing of all arteries arising from the aorta. A description of the multiple clinical manifestations of her illness and the findings at necropsy constitute this report.

CASE REPORT

This forty-six year old white woman (D.M., 06–91–79), who died on December 17, 1966, had been well until October 1965 (fourteen months before death) when she had the first of many episodes of fever (104°F.), shaking chills, nausea and vomiting, and swelling and tenderness of the tips of her fingers. These episodes lasted from five to seven days and in between she was symptom free until anorexia with weight loss appeared about two months after the onset of her illness. The episodes recurred every seven to fourteen days and were unresponsive to the administration of penicillin or other antibiotics. In January 1966 she had a profuse nose bleed which lasted several hours and required packing at a local hospital.

* From the Section of Pathology and Cardiology Branch, National Heart Institute, Laboratory of Clinical Investigations, National Institute of Allergy and Infectious Diseases and Department of Anatomic Pathology, Clinical Center, National Institutes of Health, Bethesda, Maryland 20014. Requests for reprints should be addressed to William C. Roberts, M.D., Section of Pathology, National Heart Institute, Bethesda, Maryland 20014. Manuscript received February 6, 1968.

DOI: 10.1201/9781003408321-27

On February 28, 1966, because of another episode of high fever, nausea and vomiting "similar to pregnancy sickness," and swelling and tenderness of the tips of her fingers and toes, the patient was admitted to a private hospital. The hemoglobin was 9 gm. per cent and the white blood cell count 20,000 per cu. mm. Serum protein electrophoresis disclosed a "myeloma-type" globulin spike. A bone marrow aspirate showed 8 per cent plasma cells. Fifteen blood cultures yielded no growth. Urinalysis and urine cultures were unremarkable. From April 25 until June 1, 1966, she was hospitalized and again, despite extensive workup, including hepatic biopsy, lymphangiogram and intravenous pyelograms which were normal, a diagnosis was never made. On May 10, while she was hospitalized, a systolic murmur over the lower left sternal border was heard for the first time, and persisted thereafter. Six blood cultures were positive for an atypical bacterial form which reverted to a streptococcus (performed by Dr. P. Charache, Johns Hopkins University School of Medicine), and antibiotic therapy was recommended.

On June 18, the patient was readmitted to the local hospital and examination disclosed a grade 2/6 rough holosystolic murmur, located over the apex and lower left sternal border. The fingernails were slightly clubbed. The hemoglobin was 9.1 gm. per cent, hematocrit 30 per cent and white blood cell count 7,600 cu. mm., with 13 per cent eosinophils on differential smear. The erythrocyte sedimentation rate was 127 mm. per hour and blood urea nitrogen 13 mg. percent. The electrocardiogram was within normal limits and phonocardiograms suggested mitral regurgitation. Chest roentgenograms revealed no abnormalities. As suggested, the patient was treated with penicillin (20,000,000 units daily, intravenously) and streptomycin (1 gm. daily, intramuscularly) for eighteen days at which time this therapy was discontinued because of the possibility of an allergic reaction to the drugs. Following two days of no therapy she was given tetracycline (500 mg. every five hours, orally) and erythromycin (500 mg. every four hours, orally) and finally sulfadiazine (2 gm. orally every four hours) for nine days. Despite the antibiotic therapy, the episodes of fever persisted.

The patient was admitted to the National Institute of Allergy and Infectious Diseases on August 7, 1966. At the time she weighed 107 pounds compared to a weight of 143 pounds one year previously. The patient revealed that she had had intermittent sharp acute pain in the right lower quadrant for the past ten months without obvious provocation or easy relief. Despite the nausea and vomiting there was no history of postprandial abdominal pain, jaundice, melena, diarrhea or tenesmus. Also, during the previous ten months the patient had noted that her toes would "curl up" and "become kinked" and this spasm was relieved by walking. There had been no similar problems with her fingers nor was there any history of Raynaud's phenomenon, skin rashes, splinter hemorrhages or muscular pain. The patient stated that she was markedly dyspneic when walking upstairs. She denied a history of acute rheumatic fever or chorea and had not been aware of a precordial murmur until the present illness. Also, during recent weeks when exercising or upset she noted "a squeezing feeling" in the lower anterior mediastinum as though she was having difficulty breathing. She had never had palpitations or pedal edema.

Initial examination in August 1966 disclosed the patient to be in no distress. No dermal petechiae or nodules were noted. Palpation of the carotid arteries bilaterally showed good pulsations and no thrills. A loud pleural friction rub was heard over the right posterior chest and in the right axilla. A grade 3/6 systolic ejection murmur was heard along the left sternal border with radiation to the back, and a faintly palpable thrill was present over the lower left sternal border. Neither atrial nor ventricular gallops nor a pericardial friction rub were audible. The abdominal aorta was palpable and pulsatile. No abdominal organs were palpable. The fingertips and toes were clubbed but not cyanotic. The radial and dorsalis pedis pulses were brisk bilaterally. The neurologic examination was noncontributory.

The blood hemoglobin was 9.3 gm. per cent, hematocrit 30 per cent and white blood cell count 12,000 cu. mm., with a normal differential. The erythrocyte sedimentation rate was 124 mm. in one hour (Westergren method) and the platelet count was 400,000 per cu. mm. Serum iron was 17 μg. per cent and the total iron-binding capacity was 180 gm. per cent. No Bence Jones protein or casts were present in the urine, but a few erythrocytes and an occasional leukocyte was seen. The serum total protein was 7.5 units with albumin 2.8 gm. per 100 ml. The results of the serum electrophoresis (Figure 1) were albumin 2.2 gm., alpha$_1$ globulin 0.5, alpha$_2$ globulin 1.2, beta globulin 1.3 and gamma globulin 2.1 gm. per cent. Immunoglobulin determinations, as measured by radial diffusion on agar gel, on two separate occasions revealed grossly elevated IgG levels of 31 and 29.6 mg. per cent whereas IgA levels of 1.4 and 1.3 mg. per cent and IgM levels of 0.84 and 0.66 mg. per cent were normal. Immunoelectrophoresis of the monoclonal gammopathy revealed it to be IgG with only lambda chain determinants. Serum vitamin B$_{12}$ level was 100 μg. per cent. The serologic test for syphilis was negative. The following tests were either within normal limits or negative: direct and indirect Coombs' tests, antistreptolysin O titer, lupus erythematosus preparations, cryoglobulins, pyroglobulin, ear lobe histiocyte count, blood fibrinogen, latex fixation, Bentonite® flocculation for rheumatoid factor, blood urea nitrogen (11 mg. per cent), creatinine, fasting blood sugar, total bilirubin, serum glutamic oxalacetic transaminase, uric acid, electrolytes, blood calcium and phosphorus, stool for blood, ova and parasites, and cultures of urine, sputum and feces. Electrocardiograms revealed no abnormalities. Roentgenograms of the hands, wrists, feet, ribs, skull and chest (Figure 2) were within normal limits. The heart was always of normal size. The kidneys were of normal size on abdominal roentgenogram. Bone marrow biopsy disclosed 20 per cent plasma cells, focal erythroid hyperplasia, no stainable iron, amyloid or granulomas. No abnormal plasma cells were seen in any of the bone marrow sections.

During hospitalization, intermittent episodes of fever (to 39°C., rectally) associated with anorexia, vomiting, swelling and redness of the fingers and toes, and occasional splinter hemorrhages under the nail beds, occurred. Weekly electrophoretic determinations of serum proteins showed the albumin to vary between 1.9 and 3.0, and gamma globulin, from 1.7 to 2.5 gm. per 100 ml. The anemia

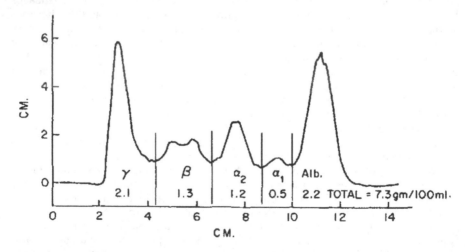

Figure 1 Serum electrophoretic pattern showing the high peak in the gamma globulin fraction.

142

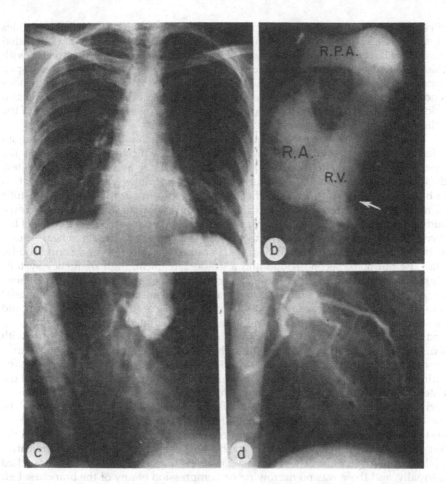

Figure 2 Posteroanterior roentgenogram (*a*) right-sided angiocardiogram (*b*) and aortogram (*c* and *d*). *a*, the heart is of normal size. *b*, following injection of contrast material into the superior vena cava, the right atrium (R.A.), right ventricle (R.V.) and major pulmonary arteries are visualized. (R.P.A. = right main pulmonary artery.) The arrow points toward the ventricular septal wall which was believed to be impinging on the right ventricular cavity. *c*, and *d*, following injection of contrast material into the aortic root all three major coronary arteries are visualized and no filling defects are seen in them.

was normocytic, normochromic and unimproved by iron therapy. Each of six blood cultures grew an aberrant, possibly an atypical form, of bacteria (performed by Dr. Viola May Young). Repeated attempts to subculture these unusual forms of microorganisms yielded a Staphylococcus epidermidis from two cultures and beta hemolytic streptococcus from another. It was impossible to determine whether these bacteria were true reversions to normal, or merely contaminants.

The patient was treated with large doses of penicillin and streptomycin for six weeks because of reported success elsewhere with such a regimen in some patients with atypical bacterial septicemias.[2] A total of sixteen blood cultures drawn during and after this therapy failed to show any forms similar to those originally isolated at The Johns Hopkins Hospital or seen at the National Institutes of Health, or other bacteria, fungi or mycoplasma. Nevertheless, the febrile episodes persisted. In addition to penicillin and streptomycin, erythromycin was added during the last two weeks of therapy. In November 1966 the patient was treated with chloramphenicol because of possible persistence of atypical bacterial forms despite negative cultures, but still the febrile episodes persisted. During one of the episodes tenderness and redness of the right elbow and left knee developed, but there was no evidence of swelling or fluid in the joints. At one point right-sided tenderness of the deltoid bursa region also developed.

Throughout the four month period of hospitalization the patient had an intermittent and fleeting right pleural friction rub which increased during the febrile episodes, despite negative chest roentgenograms, and at times completely disappeared. The precordial murmur changed several times, varying from ejection to blowing quality and increased during inspiration. In addition, a faint diastolic rumble at the cardiac apex and atrial and ventricular diastolic gallops became audible. In late November an atrial myxoma was suggested as a possible cause of the fever[3] and changing murmurs. Phonocardiograms recorded a loud first heart sound at the apex, a normally split second heart sound, the aortic second sound louder than the pulmonic second sound and a grade 2/6 apical, high frequency systolic murmur with an initial low frequency component. Since a myxoma had been suggested, angiocardiography was performed with injection of contrast material into the superior vena cava on December 5, 1966 (Figure 2). The right atrium and venae cavae were normal, but the right ventricle expanded poorly during diastole and "appeared to have a mass either in or immediately adjacent to the septum, with a distinctly convex surface toward the right ventricular cavity, reducing its volume by approximately 25 per cent." No intraluminal filling defect was seen and the pulmonary arteries and veins and left atrium appeared normal. Compression of the anterolateral wall of the left ventricle was suggested by levocardiogram. The thoracic aorta and its branches were "normal." An injection into the aortic root, while the patient was performing a Valsalva maneuver, showed that the aortic valve opened and closed normally, and that there was minimal reflux of contrast material in the left ventricle, presumably secondary to the Valsalva maneuver and not indicative of aortic regurgitation. The coronary arteries (Figure 2) arose and branched normally, and there was no narrowing or compression of any of the branches. Left ventricular injection (Figure 3) disclosed regurgitation of contrast material into the left atrium during ventricular systole; the left ventricle contracted and expanded normally and was of normal size. The mitral valvular leaflets moved normally. The coronary arteries again appeared normal. Following retrograde catheterization of the right brachial artery thrombosis of this vessel developed and embolectomy was performed.

Upon wakening on December 16, 1966, the patient felt "sore and tired" and had a dry cough. The chest was normal on physical and roentgenographic examinations. Nine hours later dyspnea appeared and expiratory wheezes were audible, but the electrocardiogram revealed no abnormalities. Early left ventricular failure was believed to be present; consequently, the patient was given digoxin and morphine intravenously and nasal oxygen. On this therapy her condition improved for an hour, but then she again became dyspneic. Shortly thereafter the blood pressure began to fall and the electrocardiogram showed progressive elevation of the S-T segments. The blood pressure subsequently became unobtainable and cardiac resuscitation was unsuccessful.

At necropsy (A66–237) the entire aorta was thick (Figure 4) and there was mild narrowing of the proximal portions of the innominate and left common carotid arteries and severe narrowing of the left subclavian artery. In addition, the celiac, superior mesenteric, renal, ovarian and common iliac arteries were severely

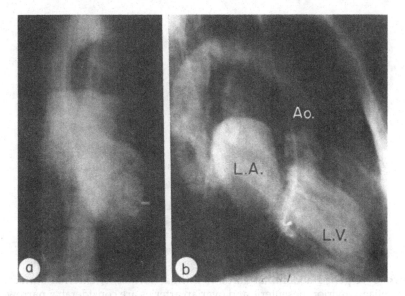

Figure 3 Left ventriculogram. Contrast material refluxes into the left atrium (L.A.) during ventricular systole. *a*, anteroposterior projection, *b*, lateral view. L.V. = left ventricular cavity; Ao. = aorta.

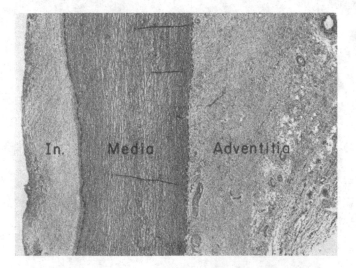

Figure 4 Ascending aortic wall. The intima (In.) and adventitia are thickened by fibrous tissue. Hematoxylin and eosin stain, original magnification × 20.

narrowed at and just proximal to their origins (Figure 5 and 6). The narrowing of these vessels and the thickening of the aorta was secondary to fibrous proliferation of the intima and adventitia. No giant cells were present, but occasionally foci of mononuclear cells were seen in the adventitia. Special stains for bacteria and fungi of these vessels were negative. The coronary arteries were severely narrowed (Figure 7

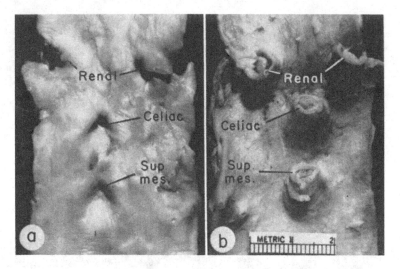

Figure 5 Opened abdominal aorta. *a*, intimal surface, *b*, external surface. The renal, celiac, superior mesenteric and ovarian arteries are considerably narrowed.

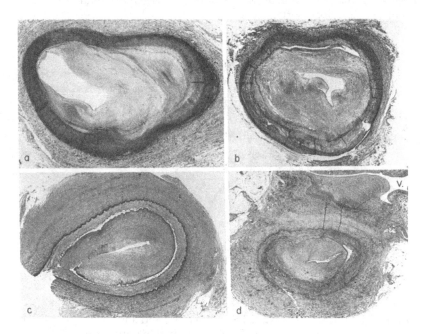

Figure 6 Arteries arising from the aorta. *a*, left subclavian artery just following its origin from the aorta. The innominate and left common carotid arteries were only mildly narrowed in contrast to the severe narrowing of this vessel. *b*, celiac artery. *c*, left renal artery. *d*, artery arising from right common iliac artery. Not only is there severe intimal proliferation in these arteries, but also the adventitia is thickened by more dense fibrous tissue. There is focal intimal and adventitial fibrous proliferation in the vein (v.) draining the right common iliac adjacent to the artery (*d*.). Movat stains; original magnifications × 11 (*a*) and × 14 (*b, c* and *d*).

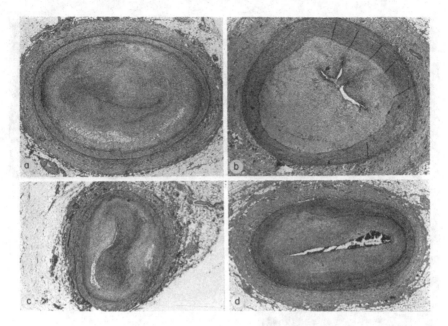

Figure 7 Extreme narrowing of the coronary arteries. *a*, right coronary artery 3 cm. from its origin from the aorta. The lumen of the first 4.5 cm. of the right coronary artery was narrowed between 80 to 100 per cent. Thereafter, it was wide open. *b*, left main coronary artery. *c*, left circumflex coronary artery. The lumen of the entire vessel was severely narrowed. *d*, anterior descending branch 1.5 cm. from its origin from the left main coronary artery. There is both intimal and adventitial fibrous proliferation. Movat stain (*a*), hematoxylin and eosin stains (*b, c* and *d*); original magnification of each × 22.

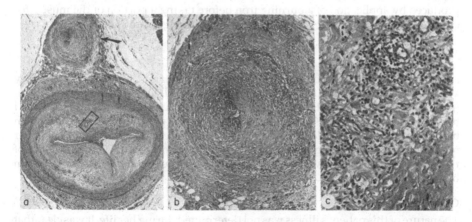

Figure 8 Coronary panarteritis. *a*, right coronary artery 2.5 cm. from its origin from the aorta. *b*, close-up of the small branch (arrow) shown in *a*. This vessel contains numerous inflammatory cells, including eosinophils and other polymorphonuclear leukocytes, lymphocytes, plasma cells and epitheloid cells, as well as many vascular channels. *c*, close-up of the area shown in brackets in *a*. Hematoxylin and eosin stains, original magnifications × 20 (*a*), × 70 (*b*) and × 210 (*c*).

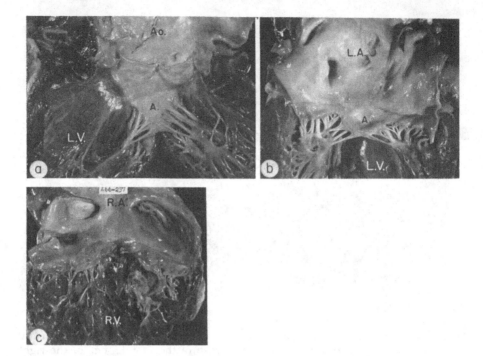

Figure 9   Interior of heart. *a*, opened left ventricle (L.V.) aortic valve, and ascending aorta (Ao.). Each of the three aortic valve cusps is diffusely although mildly thickened. The ostia of the coronary arteries are narrowed, and the aorta is thick. The left ventricle is normal. *b*, opened mitral valve showing mild but diffuse thickening of its leaflets and chordae tendineae. L.A. = left atrium. *c*, opened right atrium (R.A.) tricuspid valve, and right ventricle (R.V.). There is minimal diffuse thickening of the leaflets. The discolored area on the septal wall of the right ventricle is an artefact produced by application of a burning iron before taking a portion of the muscle for culture. No tumor or other lesions are present in the right ventricle.

and 8) but there were no old or recent myocardial infarcts. Some of the coronary arteries contained numerous mononuclear cells in all three layers of their wall (panarteritis) (Figure 8). All cardiac valves were diffusely and uniformly thickened by fibrous tissue which was devoid of elastic fibers and which was superimposed on both surfaces of the valve leaflets (Figure 9 and 10). There was no evidence of either recent or past vegetative endocarditis. The heart was enlarged (350 gm.) and free of tumor. The lungs, brain, liver, spleen, kidneys and skeletal muscles were normal on histologic examination.

COMMENTS

The nature of this patient's illness was not determined during her life. It was clear that she had a systemic illness which involved several organ systems. She was originally admitted to the National Institutes of Allergy and Infectious Disease because of "fever of unknown origin." Blood cultures suggested the presence of what appeared to be atypical bacterial forms but the source of this infection was never determined; antibiotic therapy resulted in disappearance of these organisms from the blood (sixteen cultures negative), but had no effect on her clinical syndrome, myeloma

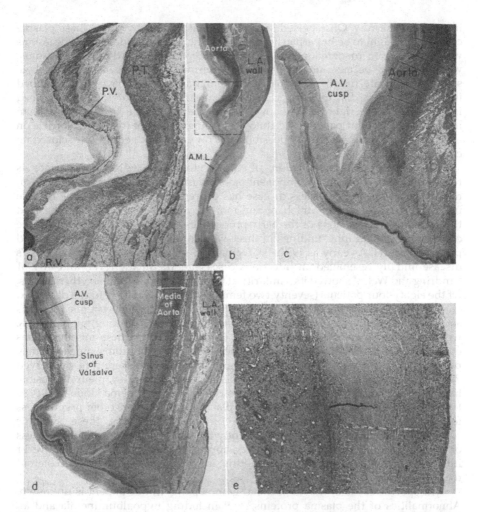

Figure 10 Histologic sections of cardiac valves. *a*, pulmonic valve (P.V.) cusp is well delineated by the black-staining elastic membrane. Superimposed on this membrane is fibrous tissue which is devoid of elastic fibers. P.T. = pulmonary trunk; R.V. = right ventricle. *b*, section includes anterior mitral leaflet (A.M.L.), aortic valve cusp (in brackets) and walls of the aorta and left atrium (L.A.). Both mitral and aortic leaflets are diffusely thickened as is the wall of the aorta. *c*, close-up of aortic valve shown in brackets in *b*. The cusp *per se* is normal but fibrous tissue devoid of elastic fibers is superimposed on it. *d*, this section includes another aortic valve cusp. Both the cusp and the aortic wall is thick. *e*, close-up of the area in solid brackets shown in *d*. The cusp contains numerous mononuclear cells, vascular channels, and small areas which are necrotic. Elastic van Gieson stains (*a*, *b*, *c*, *d*), hematoxylin and eosin stain (*e*); original magnification × 15 (*a*), × 3 (*b*), × 11 (*c* and *d*) and × 50 (*e*).

protein or sedimentation rate. Infective endocarditis was considered because of the bacteremia, fever, changing precordial murmurs, splinter hemorrhages and anemia, but at necropsy there was no localized endocardial damage which could have been attributed to the site of a previous vegetation. Multiple myeloma was considered because of the monoclonal gammopathy and the increased numbers of plasma cells in the bone marrow. On repeated study by hematologists, however, these plasma cells were thought to be hyperplastic, not neoplastic, and no evidence of lytic lesions was ever seen on roentgenograms. An intracardiac tumor, particularly myxoma, was considered because of the precordial murmur, fever, elevated erythrocyte sedimentation rate, mild leukocytosis and anemia, all of which have been described in patients with cardiac myxoma.[3] Elevations in serum gamma globulin described in myxomas of the right atrium, however, have always been diffuse, rather than monoclonal, as in our patient. The abnormal configuration of the right ventricle on angiocardiogram supported the possibility of myxoma, but necropsy disclosed no cardiac tumor.

Although persistent elevation of the erythrocyte sedimentation rate is recognized to be a common component of Takayasu's arteritis,[4-6] overemphasis on the advanced form of pulseless disease has prevented recognition of the disease in the prepulseless phase. Strachan[5] and more recently, Nakao et al.[6] emphasized the protean manifestations of the early prepulseless stage. Strachan described the clinical and angiographic findings in three women with the disease and reviewed previous reports. As early as 1954 Ask-Upmark[7] pointed out how often Takayasu's disease initially resembled an infectious disease or rheumatic fever, and in 1961 Sandring and Welin[8] showed its similarity at times to systemic lupus erythematosus. Of the eighty-four patients (seventy-two female) with Takayasu's arteritis described clinically by Nakao and associates[6] about two-thirds manifested systemic reactions such as malaise, fever, stiffness of the shoulders, nausea, vomiting, night sweats, weight loss and menstrual irregularities. "In most patients, these manifestations occurred a few weeks or more before the local signs and symptoms appeared; they persisted for a few weeks after the local signs appeared and were rarely observed during the later stages of the disease".[6] Anemia, cough, pleurisy, pleural effusion, hemoptysis, pericarditis, polyarthralgia, ulceration or erythema nodosum type lesions of the legs and abnormalities of the plasma proteins were other prepulseless features emphasized by Strachan who further stated "that these systemic manifestations may be present intermittently for many years before pulselessness or symptoms of circulatory insufficiency appear".[5] Recognition of the active or inflammatory stage of Takayasu's arteritis is important because corticosteroid therapy may induce clinical remission.[6]

The specific cause of the monoclonal gammopathy in our patient is unknown. Abnormalities of the plasma proteins,[5,6,9-11] including hypoalbuminemia and an increase in the fibrinogen, gamma or alpha$_2$ globulin fractions, have been reported in patients with Takayasu's arteriopathy, but monoclonal gammopathy has not been described previously. An increase in the IgG globulin is the rule, and occasionally the IgM globulin is increased as well. Monoclonal gammopathy is classically described in myeloma, macroglobulinemia and neoplasms of the reticuloendothelial system, but there are reports[11-14] of such monoclonal elevations in patients with myopathy, neuropathy, pernicious anemia and rheumatoid arthritis. In light of these reports it seems reasonable to ascribe the monoclonal gammopathy in our patient to her underlying inflammatory disease producing the arteriopathy.

Although it is fairly common in patients with Takayasu's arteriopathy,[5,6] fever has not been emphasized as a component of this disease. The patient described demonstrates that large vessel arteritis and aortitis should be added to the diagnostic list of causes of fever, particularly "fever of unknown origin." It is not surprising that fever as well as some of the other manifestations of a systemic illness should accompany the prepulseless stage of the illness since the primary lesion is a panarteritis. The inflammatory infiltrate initially contains polymorphonuclear leukocytes, and later, only mononuclear cells.[15] The final occlusion of the arteries arising from the aorta is the result of intra-arterial thrombosis, and when this stage (pulseless phase) is reached the inflammatory infiltrate has generally disappeared. Thus, the active process is essentially over by the time vascular obstruction occurs.

The significance of the atypical bacteria isolated from the blood in our patient is speculative. The possibility must be considered that a bacterium may have been the cause of the large vessel panarteritis and aortitis despite the fact that its eradication had no effect on the patient's clinical syndrome. Similar isolations have not been described to our knowledge in previously reported cases of Takayasu's arteritis, although it requires specialized culture procedures to grow these forms.

Another intriguing aspect of our patient is the unusual cardiac disease. Aortic regurgitation has been described in at least fourteen patients with Takayasu's arteriopathy,[5,8,10,15-21] but in only four of them[10,18-20] have the anatomic features of the aortic valve and ascending aorta been described at necropsy and then only briefly. Mitral and/or tricuspid regurgitation has been mentioned in the reports of five patients with pulseless disease and in only one[18] were these valves described at necropsy. In a thirty-nine year old woman with Takayasu's arteritis and murmurs typical of aortic regurgitation, aortic stenosis and mitral regurgitation, described by Judge et al. (Case 4[10]), the aortic valve cusps at necropsy were "contracted." A forty-nine year old woman with Takayasu's arteritis described by Castleman[19] had "obvious" aortic regurgitation, probable mitral regurgitation as well, and at necropsy each of the three aortic valve cusps were diffusely although mildly thickened, their edges rolled and the commissural spaces slightly widened. The mitral valve "seemed normal." It seems reasonable to believe that the valvular lesion in this patient was related to the arterial lesion. Yamada and associates[18] described thickening and hardening of the aortic valve cusps and a "hard, thick, contracted" mitral valve in a twenty-eight year old man with the aortic arch syndrome (Case 3[18]). Aortic regurgitation was his most significant hemodynamic lesion, but it is uncertain whether the valvular lesions were a part of the arteritis or secondary to another disease (rheumatic). In a fourteen year old girl with "arteritis of the aorta and its major branches" described by Schrire et al. (Case 3[20]) the aortic valve was described as normal at necropsy although during life murmurs typical of aortic regurgitation and of mitral regurgitation and stenosis had been heard. The mitral valve was not described at necropsy. Nakao et al.[6] described "aortic and mitral valvular disease" in one of six patients who died with Takayasu's arteritis. None of the reports mentioning valvular cardiac disease in patients with Takayasu's arteritis have described the valves histologically, and in none of the previous reports have anatomic abnormalities of the tricuspid or pulmonic valves been described. In our patient all four cardiac valves were slightly but uniformly thickened, and both atrioventricular valves were mildly incompetent. On histologic study the valvular thickening was found to be secondary to deposits of fibrous tissue which contained mononuclear cells, mainly lymphocytes, small vascular channels and no elastic fibers. This mildly inflamed fibrous tissue did not extend into the valvular cusps *per se* but was superimposed on their lining membranes, reminiscent of the type of endocardial disease observed in the carcinoid syndrome.[22] It differed from that found in the carcinoid syndrome, however, in one important feature. In our patient the superimposed fibrous tissue was deposited on *all* surfaces of the cardiac valves, whereas in the carcinoid syndrome the fibrous tissue, which is devoid of elastic fibers, is present only on the under or ventricular surfaces of the atrioventricular valves and only on the arterial surfaces of the semilunar valves. Fibrous tissue similar to that which was located on the valvular endocardium of our patient also involved mural endocardium, although focally. The type endocardial involvement in this patient is unique in our experience, and we have not found reported descriptions or illustrations of this type of cardiac lesion. The cause of the diffuse valvular and focal mural endocardial fibrosis in this patient is unknown, but it is reasonable to believe that its etiology is the same as that causing the arteritis and aortitis.

The other striking anatomic cardiac abnormality in the patient described was the extensive narrowing of the extramural coronary arteries, some of which contained an active inflammatory reaction. Narrowing of coronary arterial ostia has been reported in at least four patients with Takayasu's arteritis,[19,23-25] and involvement of the coronary arteries has been described in this entity in at least six patients.[20,26-29] Six[20,21,24,26,28,29] of the ten subjects had myocardial infarctions as a result of the coronary ostial or arterial narrowing, and two additional patients with Takayasu's arteritis had acute myocardial infarctions but were living when described by Burstein et al.[30] Myers et al.[26] described pulseless disease and old myocardial infarction in a thirty-nine year old man who at necropsy had occluded right and left coronary arteries. Schrire and Asherson[20] described aortitis and arteritis involving all vessels arising from the aorta in an eleven year old girl who died from acute myocardial infarction (Case 19[20]). Both left and right coronary arteries were occluded, the right entirely by fibrous tissue. Hudson[27] described extensive aortitis and large vessel arteritis in an eighteen month old girl who had severely narrowed major coronary arteries at necropsy. Juzi[28] described Takayasu's arteritis in two women, aged fifty-six and fifty-nine years, each of whom died of acute myocardial infarctions secondary to panarteritis with narrowing of the coronary arteries. In one of the patients acute myocardial infarction was the only complication of Takayasu's arteritis. Scully[29] described "severe, diffuse coronary arteritis of a nonspecific (Takayasu's) type" and acute myocardial infarction in a forty-five year old man who had diffuse aortitis and apparently narrowing of all arteries arising from the aorta. Despite the widespread coronary arterial narrowing in our patient there was no myocardial scarring or anatomic evidence of acute myocardial infarction.

Still another unusual aspect of the patient described was the striking discrepancy between the normal appearance of the coronary arteries at aortic root arteriography and their nearly occluded appearance at necropsy. The roentgenologic interpretation was based on aortic root injection and not on selective coronary arterial injection, and angiocardiograms from only two views were performed and not cineangiocardiograms from several projections. Hazards in interpreting nonselective coronary arteriograms have been pointed out by Kemp and associates,[31] who also have shown the diagnostic accuracy of good quality selective coronary cinearteriograms.

REFERENCES

1. ROBERTS, W. C. and WIBIN, E. A. Idiopathic panaortitis, supra-aortic arteritis, granulomatous myocarditis and pericarditis. A cause for pulseless disease and possibly left ventricular aneurysm in the African. *Am. J. Med.*, 41: 453, 1966.
2. CHARACHE, P. Personal communication.
3. GOODWIN, J. F. Diagnosis of left atrial myxoma. *Lancet*, 1: 464, 1963.
4. MCKUSICK, V. A. A form of vascular disease relatively frequent in the Orient. *Am. Heart J.*, 63: 57, 1962.
5. STRACHAN, R. W. The natural history of Takayasu's arteriopathy. *Quart. J. Med.*, 33: 59, 1964.
6. NAKAO, K., IKEDA, M., KIMATA, S.-I., NIITANI, H., MIYAHARA, M., ISHIMI, Z.-I., HASHIBA, K., TAKEDA, Y., OZAWA, T., MATSUSHITI, S. and KURAMOCHI, M. Takayasu's arteritis. Clinical report of eighty-four cases and immunological studies of seven cases. *Circulation*, 35: 1141, 1967.
7. ASK-UPMARK, E. On the "pulseless disease" outside of Japan. *Acta Med. Scandinav.*, 149: 161, 1954.

8. SANDRING. H. and WELIN, G. Aortic arch syndrome with special reference to rheumatoid arthritis. *Acta Med. Scandinav.*, 170: 1, 1961.
9. BIRKE, G., EJRUP, B. and OLHAGEN, B. Pulseless disease. A clinical analysis of ten cases. *Angiology*, 8: 433, 1957.
10. JUDGE, R. D., CURRIER, R. D., GRACIE, W. A. and FIGLEY, M. M. Takayasu's arteritis and the aortic arch syndrome. *Am. J. Med.*, 32: 379, 1962.
11. IKEDA. M. Immunologic studies on Takayasu's arteritis. *Japan Circulation J.*, 30: 87, 1966.
12. WALDENSTROM, J. The occurrence of benign, essential, monoclonal, non-macromolecular hyperglobulinemia and its differential diagnosis. *Acta Med. Scandinav.*, 176: 345, 1964,
13. BACHMANN, R. The diagnostic significance of the serum concentration of pathological proteins (M-components). *Acta Med. Scandinav.*, 178: 801, 1965.
14. ZAWADZKI, Z, and EDWARDS, G. Dysimmunoglobulinemia in the absence of clinical features of multiple myeloma and macroglobulinemia. *Am. J. Med.*, 42: 67, 1967.
15. NASU, T. Pathology of pulseless disease. A systematic study and critical review of twenty-one autopsy cases reported in Japan. *Angiology*, 14: 225, 1963.
16. JERVELI., A. Pulseless disease. *Am. Heart J.*, 47: 780, 1954.
17. LESSOF, M. H. and GLYNN, L. E. The pulseless syndrome. *Lancet*, 1: 799, 1959.
18. YAMADA, H., HARUMI, K., OHTA, A., NOMURA, T. and OKADA, R. Aortic arch syndrome with cardiomegaly and aortic calcification. *Jap. Heart J.*, 2: 538, 1961.
19. Case records of the Massachusetts General Hospital: Weekly clinicopathological exercises (Case 23–1961). *New England J. Med.*, 264: 664, 1961.
20. SCHRIRE, V. and ASHERSON, R. A. Arteritis of aorta and its major branches. *Quart. J. Med.*, 33: 439, 1964.
21. CHEITLIN, M. D. and CARTER, P. B. Takayashu's disease. Unusual manifestations. *Arch. Int. Med.*, 116: 283, 1965.
22. ROBERTS, W. C. and SJOERDSMA, A. The cardiac disease associated with the carcinoid syndrome (carcinoid heart disease). *Am. J. Med.*, 36: 5, 1964.
23. FRÖVIG, A. G. and LÖKEN, A. C. The syndrome of obliteration of the arterial branches of the aortic arch, due to arteritis. A post-mortem angiographic and pathological study. *Acta Psychiat. et Neurol. Scandinav.*, 26: 313, 1951.
24. BARKER, N. W. and EDWARDS, J. E. Primary arteritis of the aortic arch. *Circulation*, 11: 486, 1955.
25. DANARAJ, T. J., WONG, H. O. and THOMAS, M. A. Primary arteritis of aorta causing renal artery stenosis and hypertension, *Brit. Heart J.*, 25: 153, 1963.
26. MYERS, J. D., MURDAUGH, H. V., MCINTOSH, H. D. and BLAISDELL, R. K. Observations on continuous murmurs over partially obstructed arteries. An explanation for the continuous murmur found in the aortic arch syndrome. *Arch. Int. Med.*, 97: 726, 1956.
27. HUDSON, R. E. B. *Cardiovascular Pathology*, vol. 1, p. 532. Baltimore, 1965. Williams & Wilkins Co.
28. JUZI, U. Takayasuche Arteriitis mit Herzinfarkt. *Schweiz, Med. Wehnschr.*, 97: 397, 1967.
29. DESANCTIS, R. W., and SCULLY, R. E. Case records of the Massachusetts General Hospital: Weekly clinicopathological exercises (Case 46–1967). *New England J. Med.*, 277: 1025, 1967.
30. BURSTEIN, J., LINDSTRÖM, B, and WASASTJERNA, C. Aortic arch syndromes A survey of five cases. *Acta Med. Scandinav.*, 157: 365, 1957.
31. KEMP, H. G., EVANS, H., ELLIOTT, W. C. and GORLIN, R. Diagnostic accuracy of selective coronary cinearteriography. *Circulation*, 36: 526, 1967.

Case 127 Late Vascular Manifestations of the Rubella Syndrome

A Roentgenographic-Pathologic Study

*Nicholas J. Fortuin, M.D., Andrew G. Morrow, M.D. and
William C. Roberts, M.D.*
Bethesda, Maryland

Attention is called to the late development of complete aortic luminal occlusion with severe systemic hypertension in a seven year old boy with clinical features of the rubella syndrome. Necropsy showed that the aorta was occluded by fibrocalcific material, probably the result of organization of thrombus. The distal abdominal aorta and the branches arising from it were severely hypoplastic, as were the renal arteries. Aortic thrombosis and systemic arterial hypoplasia have not been described previously as complications of the rubella syndrome.

Many new features of the rubella syndrome emerged after the 1964 epidemic,[1, 2] in particular, a better understanding of the effects of the in utero infection on the cardiovascular system of the fetus. Before 1964, patent ductus arteriosus was believed to be the most common cardiac malformation associated with the rubella syndrome.[3] Subsequently, stenosis or hypoplasia of the pulmonic valve, pulmonary trunk or its branches have been shown to be as frequent or possibly more frequent manifestations.[4–6] In addition, lesions of systemic arteries have been recognized recently as consequences of fetal rubella infection.[7–9] Such lesions have been responsible for the development of renal arterial stenosis with systemic hypertension[9, 10] and supravalvular aortic stenosis.[11] These effects have been described in infants. This report describes the rubella syndrome in an older child in whom severe hypertension and total occlusion of the abdominal aorta developed as a consequence of systemic arterial lesions attributable to in utero rubella infection.

CASE REPORT

This seven year old white boy (M.M., 02–52–30) died on February 17, 1966. He was the product of a pregnancy complicated by rubella in the first trimester. At age six weeks he became dyspneic, and on examination a grade 3/6 systolic precordial murmur and a ventricular gallop were heard, and cardiomegaly and hepatomegaly were found. He was given digitalis, diuretics and a sodium-restricted diet with subsequent improvement in symptoms; at age six months he was admitted to the National Heart and Lung Institute for further study. At this time no precordial murmur was audible, but the heart was still enlarged. Electrocardiograms revealed sinus tachycardia and biventricular hypertrophy. At cardiac catheterization, the pulmonary arterial pressure was 65/30 mm Hg (mean 44) and right ventricular pressure 70/0 mm Hg. A large left to right shunt at the level of the pulmonary trunk was demonstrated by oximetry. A catheter passed from the pulmonary trunk to the ascending aorta via

From the Section of Pathology and the Clinic of Surgery, National Heart and Lung Institute, National Institutes of Health, Bethesda, Maryland 20014. Requests for reprints should be addressed to Dr. William C. Roberts, Section of Pathology, National Heart and Lung Institute, National Institutes of Health, Bethesda, Maryland 20014. Manuscript received April 28, 1970.

DOI: 10.1201/9781003408321-28

a patent ductus arteriosus. Pressure in the thoracic aorta was 82/38 mm Hg (mean 54) and in the abdominal aorta 75/40 mm Hg (mean 52). A thoracotomy performed on June 26, 1959, disclosed a large ductus and a hypoplastic aortic arch. The ductus was divided.

When examined in 1960 and 1961 the patient was asymptomatic and had no precordial murmur, but he was deaf, spastic in the lower extremities, and his growth and development were retarded.

The patient was lost to follow-up until 1966 (age seven) when acute pneumonia developed and he was again admitted to the National Heart and Lung Institute. The lungs were clear, and the heart was enlarged. A grade 3/6 harsh systolic murmur was heard along the left sternal border. No murmur was heard over the back or abdomen. The femoral, dorsalis pedis and posterior tibial arterial pulsations were absent. The chest and abdominal wall showed evidence of collateral circulation. The blood pressure was 210/170 mm Hg in the left arm, 230/180 mm Hg in the right arm and only 90 mm Hg systolic in the left leg. No retinal hemorrhages or exudates were observed, and the optic discs were flat. A serologic test for syphilis was negative. The urine was normal except for 10 leukocytes/ high power field, and the blood urea nitrogen was 12 mg/100 ml. The electrocardiogram (Figure 1) showed sinus tachycardia, left axis deviation, right ventricular conduction delay and left ventricular hypertrophy with associated ST-T wave changes. Chest roentgenograms revealed generalized cardiomegaly. Abdominal roentgenograms demonstrated calcific deposits in the wall of the aorta overlying vertebral bodies from the eleventh thoracic through the fourth lumbar vertebrae.

Asystole occurred on the third hospital day, but resuscitation was successful. Aortograms (Figure 2) were obtained the next day with injections into both

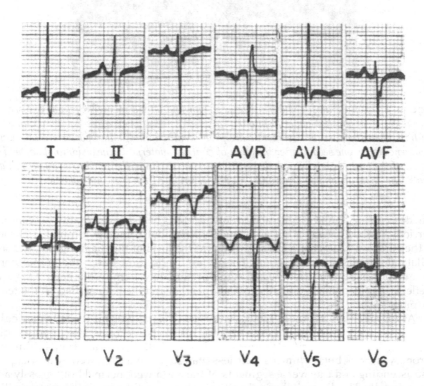

Figure 1 *Electrocardiogram taken February 8, 1966.*

155

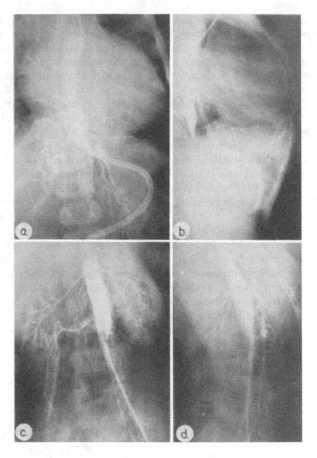

Figure 2 *Aortograms. a and b, anteroposterior and lateral roentgenographs one second after injection of contrast material into the transverse aorta. The aorta is totally occluded at the level of the diaphragm. Collaterals are prominent, c and d, anteroposterior and lateral roentgenographs one second after injection of contrast material in the abdominal aorta. The lumen of the aorta is totally occluded just above the origin of the renal arteries, which are small. The distal abdominal aorta and the arteries arising from it are hypoplastic.*

the descending thoracic and abdominal aorta. The transverse and descending portions of the thoracic aorta appeared normal, but complete luminal occlusion of the aorta was demonstrated, beginning at the level of the diaphragm. Extensive collateral circulation was present. The renal arteries and lower abdominal aorta were hypoplastic, the latter measuring approximately 1 cm in diameter. Oliguria, areflexia, papilledema and finally coma appeared, and the patient died on the tenth hospital day.

At autopsy (A66–24), the heart was enlarged (weight, 190 gm), the left ventricular wall was hypertrophied (Figure 3), and histologic sections disclosed medial hypertrophy and focal intimal fibrous proliferation in the extramural and intramural coronary arteries, but the lumens were less than 25 per cent narrowed by the plaques. The ascending and transverse segments of the aorta were normal both grossly and histologically. The distal abdominal aorta was hypoplastic, as were the common iliac and renal arteries (Figure 4). The intima of the descending thoracic aorta was focally

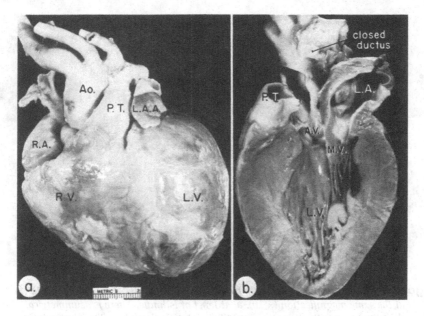

Figure 3 *Heart, a, exterior anteriorly. The left ventricle is very hypertrophied. Note the relatively large soldier's plaques (milk spots) in the epicardium of both right (R.V.) and left (L.V.) ventricles. R.A. = right atrium; L.A.A. = left atrial appendage; Ao. = aorta; and P.T. = pulmonary trunk. b, longitudinal section of left ventricle showing thickening of its wall and dilatation of its cavity. A.V. = aortic valve; M.V. = mitral valve; and L.A. = left atrium.*

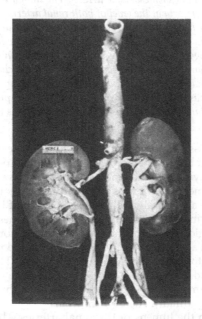

Figure 4 *Descending thoracic and abdominal aorta, renal arteries, hemisections of kidneys and ureters. The aorta here begins at the isthmus. Note the varying size of the aorta exteriorly and that the distal portion is hypoplastic. The pelves and proximal ureters are dilated.*

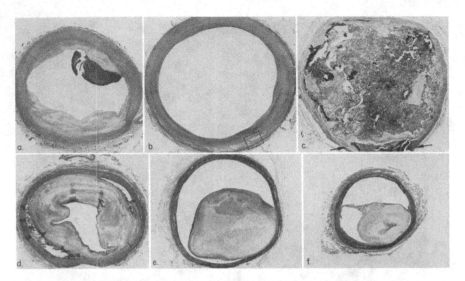

Figure 5 *Cross sections of the aorta from isthmus (**a**) to distal abdominal aorta (**f**), each taken at the same magnification (× 10). **a**, at level of isthmus. There is asymmetrical fibrous intimal proliferation with a superimposed fibrin-platelet thrombus. The fibrous intimal proliferation is probably the result of organization of thrombus. **b**, at level of mid-descending thoracic aorta. At this level there is no intimal proliferation, but the media is thickened and elastic fibers are focally degenerated. A close-up view of focally destroyed elastic fibers in this vessel is shown in Figure 6d. **c**, at level of celiac axis. At this point the lumen is occluded by masses of fibrous tissue and calcific deposits. The origin of the celiac axis is designated by the arrows. **d**, at level of superior mesenteric artery. The lumen is narrowed but not totally occluded. A cross section of aorta at the level of both renal arteries is shown in Figure 6a. **e**, at level 1.5 cm below origin of renal arteries, a fibrous nodule attached to the intima wall on about 20 per cent of its circumference is present in the aortic lumen. The nodule is bordered by elastic fibers suggesting that they split off from the aortic media. Note that the media is much thinner than that of the aorta proximal to the occlusion (**a** and **b**). **f**, at level 3.3 cm below origin of renal arteries. The diameters of the aorta at this point and distally are much smaller. Still a fibrous nodule, bordered by elastic fibers, is present in the aortic lumen. Hematoxylin and eosin stains (**a** and **c**); elastic van Gieson stains (**b**, **d**, **e**, **f**).*

thickened by fibrous tissue and an occasional fibrin-platelet thrombus (Figure 5). At the level of the diaphragm the aorta was completely occluded by fibrocalcific material which partially occluded the aortic lumen for several centimeters distally (Figure 5). There was moderate fibrous intimal proliferation of the proximal renal arteries (Figure 6). The aortic wall at all levels was free of inflammatory cells, and the adventitia was normal. The internal elastic membranes appeared intact at all sites examined histologically, but the media of the aorta showed disruption of a few elastic fibers in several areas (Figure 6). At the level of the renal arteries, the inner aortic media had split to form a false channel (Figure 6). The aortic media at most sites, however, appeared normal.

The renal parenchyma appeared grossly normal, but the left pelvis was dilated, as were both ureters proximally. Histologically, the kidneys were normal except for rare calcific deposits in the lumens of the renal arteries. The elastic and muscular pulmonary arteries and arterioles were normal. Focal alveolar edema and acute

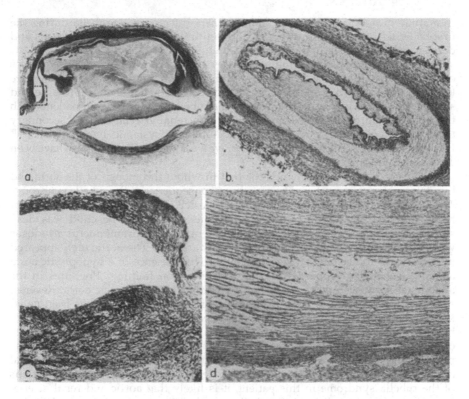

Figure 6 *Cross sections of aorta at level of renal arteries (**a**), one renal artery (**b**) and close-up views of media of aorta (**c** and **d**). **a**, the aorta is partially obstructed at this level. The ostia of both renal arteries are visible. The media of the aorta is split at two sites and one (enclosed in the brackets) is shown in high power in **c**. The cause of the disruption of the aortic intima is uncertain. **b**, renal artery showing intimal proliferation. The internal elastic membrane is well preserved but the intimal fibrous tissue is also covered by another elastic membrane. **d**, closeup of media of aorta at level of mid-descending thoracic aorta (see Figure 5b). Some elastic fibers are disrupted. Elastic van Gieson stains, original magnifications × 10 (**a**), × 60 (**b**) and × 95 (**c** and **d**).*

pneumonia were present. The liver, adrenal glands and pancreas were normal. Sections of brain disclosed foci of acute encephalomalacia.

COMMENTS

The characteristic vascular lesion in neonates with the rubella syndrome is fibrous intimal proliferation in various arteries.[7,9,12,13] This lesion was first described by Campbell[7] in a four month old infant. Changes were found in the pulmonary arteries and the aorta and its large branches. In addition to intimal thickening, the internal elastic membrane in these vessels was focally fragmented, and the media contained vacuoles. Since Campbell's original description, other investigators[8,9,12,13] have made similar observations. Alterations of the internal elastic membrane or media or both have not been constant features, however, but have been noted in more severe cases. Vascular lesions may be seen soon after in utero infection.

In a study of abortuses obtained from mothers infected with rubella during the first trimester of pregnancy, Tondury and Smith[14] found endothelial necrosis and damage to blood vessels of the chorion and fetus.

Stenosis or hypoplasia of the pulmonary trunk are recognized consequences of rubella virus infection.[4,5] The effects of this virus on the systemic circulation are less well documented. Rorke and Spiro[15] noted endothelial changes in large and small cerebral arteries of nine infants with the rubella syndrome. Four patients with the rubella syndrome have been described with renal arterial stenosis secondary to intimal hyperplasia, and two had documented systemic hypertension.[8,10,16] Hypoplasia of the aortic isthmus[17] and supravalvular aortic stenosis[11] also have been attributed to the effects of rubella.

The patient described herein is the first in whom thrombosis of the aorta and hypoplasia of systemic arteries occurred as a consequence of the rubella syndrome. The mother had had rubella in the first trimester of pregnancy, and the patient had many characteristic manifestations of the syndrome. The child was deaf, spastic and retarded in growth and development. A large patent ductus arteriosus was responsible for congestive heart failure in infancy. The aortic arch appeared hypoplastic at thoracotomy at age six months. The presence of a hypoplastic aorta at this time is also supported by the catheterization findings. Pressures in the abdominal aorta were lower than those recorded in the thoracic aorta. Reversal of the normal increase in pressure from proximal to distal aorta has been noted in other patients with aortic hypoplasia.[18,19] Six years later the aortic arch was not hypoplastic by aortography or at autopsy. The explanation for the increase in size of the proximal aorta between age six months and seven years is uncertain but was probably the result of severe hypertension. At death, however, the distal abdominal aorta and renal arteries were hypoplastic. In light of the many other manifestations of the rubella syndrome in this patient, it is likely that aortic and renal arterial hypoplasia also are attributable to rubella infection. The marked intimal thickening of the aorta, renal and other systemic arteries in our patient is similar to the arterial lesions described in younger children with the rubella syndrome.[8–12] Also consistent is the absence of inflammatory changes within the aortic wall and the absence of involvement of adventitia or vasa vasorum.

Our patient presented as a case of acquired coarctation of the aorta, a condition which is seen frequently in children in the Orient and Africa.[20–22] In those patients, however, aortic occlusion or stenosis is related to panaortitis, histologically similar to Takayusu's aortitis.[23,24] The roentgenologic finding of a smooth-walled aorta up to the point of occlusion, the absence of inflammatory cells in the aortic wall and the lack of adventitial involvement distinguish our patient from those described in the Orient and in Africa. Thrombosis of the aorta, however, has been described in this country and in Europe[25,26] in newborns, but inflammatory cells have been found in the aortic media. Inflammatory changes in the liver and kidney and the presence of abnormalities of the ductus arteriosus (patency[26] or aneurysm[25]) are changes which occur in rubella, although the presence or absence of this infection was not mentioned in any report.[25,26]

The patient described is unusual in that the clinical manifestations of systemic vascular lesions did not appear until age seven. The progression of systemic arterial disease in our patient, and of pulmonary arterial lesions in patients described by others,[27] is probably not due to persistent viral infection. Wasserman et al.[27] postulated that hemodynamic stress in a vessel weakened by subtle changes in vessel makeup induced by the viral infection in utero is responsible for the pulmonary arterial lesions. This explanation seems reasonable in our patient in whom systemic hypertension probably resulted initially from the combined effects of aortic and renal arterial hypoplasia and intimal proliferation in renal arteries producing renal ischemia. Hypertension may have augmented intimal hyperplasia in the aorta and renal arteries with subsequent narrowing of the aortic lumen, eventual complete occlusion by thrombus, further increase in blood pressure and ultimately death.

Manifestations of a fetal viral infection, as illustrated by our patient, may be absent early in life but appear later. Had aortic thrombosis not occurred, the patient may have remained well and perhaps presented in adulthood with systemic hypertension. The association between rubella infection and the vascular lesions would be less clear at a later age or if other manifestations of the rubella syndrome had not been present. Congenital rubella infection thus might be considered in other patients, especially younger ones, with occlusive vascular disease.

It is interesting to speculate upon the possibility of in utero rubella infection as the hitherto unsuspected cause of other malformations of vessels present from birth. Diffuse tortuosity of the aorta and its branches has been described recently in two young patients.[28, 29] In addition to having truly spectacular tortuosity of the aorta and all of its branches, the ten year old living girl described by Ertugrul[28] also had a small atrial septal defect (without a shunt), mild right ventricular systolic hypertension of undetermined etiology, mild aortic regurgitation and fragmented internal elastic membranes in a biopsied artery. In addition to having tortuous and abnormally long systemic and pulmonary arteries, the seventeen month old boy described by Beuren et al.[29] who underwent autopsy, also had severe supravalvular and peripheral pulmonic stenosis, fragmentation of internal elastic membranes and intimal thickening of most arteries including the coronaries. The six week old infant with total occlusive fibroelastosis of both coronary arteries described by MacMahon and Dickinson[30] also had pulmonic valve stenosis and a "patent" foramen ovale. In none of these three patients was the possibility of in utero rubella mentioned, but each had lesions well recognized as consequences of this infection, which obviously can be overlooked in the pregnant mother.

ADDENDUM

Since submitting this manuscript, Witzleben[31] described widespread "intimal fibrous proliferation in elastic and muscular arteries, elastic tissue degeneration and scant calcification" in an infant. No mention of rubella is made. It is likely, however, that the lesions described at necropsy in his patient are also the result of rubella.

REFERENCES

1. Plotkin SA, Oski FA, Hartnett EM, Hervada AR, Friedman S, Gowing J: Some recently recognized manifestations of the rubella syndrome. *J Pediat* 67: 182, 1965.
2. Cooper LZ, Ziring PR, Ockerse AB, Fedun BA, Kiely B, Krugman S: Rubella: Clinical manifestations and management. *Amer J Dis Child* 118: 18, 1969.
3. Campbell M: The place of maternal rubella in the aetiology of congenital heart disease. *Brit Med J* 1: 691, 1961.
4. Rowe RD: Maternal rubella and pulmonary artery stenosis. *Pediatrics* 32: 180, 1963.
5. Venables AW: The syndrome of pulmonary stenosis complicating maternal rubella. *Brit Heart J* 27: 49, 1965.
6. Rowe RD: Cardiovascular lesions in rubella (letter to the editor). *J Pediat* 68: 147, 1966.
7. Campbell PE: Vascular abnormalities following maternal rubella. *Brit Heart J* 27: 134, 1965.
8. Esterly JR, Oppenheimer EH: Vascular lesions in infants with congenital rubella. *Circulation* 36: 544, 1967.

9. Esterly JR, Oppenheimer EH: Pathologic lesions due to congenital rubella. *Arch Path (Chicago)* 87: 380, 1969.

10. Menser MA, Dorman DC, Reye RDK, Reid RR: Renal artery stenosis in the rubella syndrome. *Lancet* 1: 790, 1966.

11. Varghese PJ, Izukawa I, Rowe RD: Supravalvular aortic stenosis as part of the rubella syndrome, with discussion of pathogenesis. *Brit Heart J* 31: 59, 1969.

12. Singer DB, Rudolph AJ, Rosenberg HS, Rawls WE, Boniuk M: Pathology of the congenital rubella syndrome. *J Pediat* 71: 665, 1967.

13. Forrest JM, Menser MA, Reye RDK: Obstructive arterial lesions in rubella. *Lancet* 1: 1263, 1969.

14. Tondury G, Smith DW: Fetal rubella pathology. *J Pediat* 68: 867, 1966.

15. Rorke LB, Spiro AJ: Cerebral lesions in congenital rubella. *J Pediat* 70: 243, 1967.

16. Menser MA, Dorman DC, Reye RDK, Reid RR: Renal artery stenosis in rubella. *Lancet* 1: 571, 1967.

17. Hastreiter AR, Joorabchi B, Pujatti G, vander Horst RL, Patalsil G, Sever JL: Cardiovascular lesions associated with congenital rubella. *J Pediat* 71: 59, 1967.

18. Eklof O, Ilha DO, Zetterquist P: Aortic hypoplasia. *Acta Paediatrica* 53: 377, 1964.

19. Pyörälä K, Heikel P, Halonen, PI: Hypoplasia of the aorta. *Amer Heart J* 57: 289, 1959.

20. McKusick VA: A form of vascular disease relatively frequent in the Orient. *Amer Heart J* 63: 57, 1962.

21. Sen PK, Kinare SG, Engineer SD, Parulkai GB: The middle aortic arch syndrome. *Brit Heart J* 25: 610, 1963.

22. Isaacson C: An idiopathic aortitis in young Africans. *J Path Bact* 81: 69, 1961.

23. Roberts WC, Wibin EA: Idiopathic panaortitis, supraaortic arteritis, granulomatous myocarditis and pericarditis. A cause of pulseless disease and possibly left ventricular aneurysm in the African. *Amer J Med* 41: 453, 1966.

24. Roberts WC, MacGregor RR, De Blanc HJ Jr, Beiser GD, Wolff SM: The prepulseless phase of pulseless disease, or pulseless disease with pulses. A newly recognized cause of cardiac disease, monoclonal gammopathy and "fever of unknown origin." *Amer J Med* 46: 313, 1969.

25. Morison JE: Thrombosis of the aorta in the newborn: three cases, one with infarction of the liver. *J Path Bact* 57: 221, 1945.

26. Heggtveit HA, Hill DP: Thromboaortitis in the newborn. *Arch Path (Chicago)* 76: 578, 1963.

27. Wasserman MP, Varshese PJ, Rowe RD: The evolution of pulmonary arterial stenosis. *Amer Heart J* 76: 638, 1968.

28. Ertugrul A: Diffuse tortuosity and lengthening of the arteries. *Circulation* 37: 400, 1967.

29. Beuren AJ, Hort W, Kalbfleisch H, Müller H, Stoermer J: Dysplasia of the systemic and pulmonary arterial system with tortuosity and lengthening of the arteries. A new entity, diagnosed during life, and leading to coronary death in early childhood. *Circulation* 39: 109, 1969.

30. MacMahon HE, Dickinson PCT: Occlusive fibroelastosis of coronary arteries in the newborn. *Circulation* 35: 3, 1967.

31. Witzleben CL: Idiopathic infantile arterial calcification—a misnomer? *Amer J Cardiol* 26: 305, 1970.

Case 135 Stenosis of the Right Pulmonary Artery

A Complication of Acute Dissecting Aneurysm of the Ascending Aorta

L. Maximilian Buja, M.D., Nayab Ali, M.D., Ross D. Fletcher, M.D., William C. Roberts, M.D., Washington, D. C.

Common complications of acute dissecting aortic aneurysm include external rupture with fatal hemorrhage, dissection and occlusion of major branches of the aorta, and aortic regurgitation.[1-5] Although lesions of the pulmonary vessels may complicate nondissecting (syphilitic, arteriosclerotic, Marian's) thoracic aneurysms,[6-10] pulmonary vascular lesions caused by acute dissecting aortic aneurysm have not been described. This has recently been observed by us and is the subject of this report.

CASE REPORT

A. W., a 57-year-old man, who had a history of systemic hypertension, developed severe persistent precordial chest pain 17 hours before death. When hospitalized 9 hours before death, the patient's blood pressure was 180/120 mm. Hg, and an atrial diastolic gallop was audible. No precordial murmur was heard. An anteroposterior chest roentgenogram showed minimal cardiomegaly and a widened mediastinum. The electrocardiogram (ECG) disclosed sinus tachycardia (120 beats per minute), left ventricular hypertrophy, left atrial enlargement, S-T segment elevation in Leads V_{1-3}, and S-T segment depression with T wave inversion in Leads I, aV_L, and V_{5-6}. Two hours before death, the chest pain worsened and hypotension (100/70 mm. Hg) and ventricular tachycardia appeared. Sinus rhythm and hypertension (170/130 mm. Hg) returned after an intravenous injection of lidocaine. The ECG was unchanged except for the presence of small Q waves in Leads II, III, and aV_f. One hour before death, complete heart block appeared and the patient lost consciousness. Resuscitative efforts including attempted transvenous pacing were unsuccessful.

At autopsy an acute medial dissection of the ascending thoracic aorta (Type II of De Bakey and associates[5]) was found (Figures 1 and 2), and it had ruptured into the pericardial cavity. The aneurysm contained a large hematoma which narrowed the aortic lumen. Extravasated blood also was present in the adventitia of the ascending and transverse portions of the aorta, pulmonary trunk, right and left main pulmonary arteries, and left atrium (superior wall). Extravasated blood also surrounded the proximal right and left coronary arteries, and the lumen of the right coronary artery was slightly compressed by the adventitial blood. The lumen of the right main pulmonary artery was narrowed > 75 per cent by the adventitial hematoma (Figure 3). This obstructed artery was located between the left atrium (inferior) and aortic arch (superior). The heart weighed 550 grams. The left ventricle was hypertrophied but not dilated. The lumens of the coronary arteries were

From the Section of Pathology, National Heart and Lung Institute, Bethesda, Md., and the George Washington and Georgetown University Medical Divisions, District of Columbia General Hospital, Washington, D. C.

Received for publication Aug. 2, 1970.

DOI: 10.1201/9781003408321-29

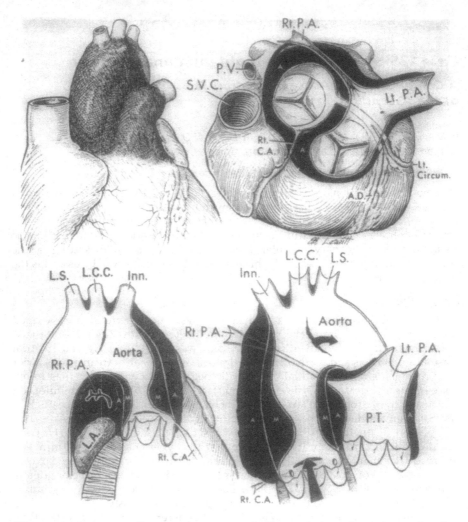

Figure 1 Drawing of heart and great vessels. External view of anterior surface (top left), superior view with cross section of great vessels (top right), and lateral (bottom left) and frontal (bottom right) views of longitudinal sections. Extensive hematoma is present in the adventitia (*A*) of the ascending and transverse aortas, pulmonary trunk (*P.T.*), and right and left main pulmonary arteries (*Rt. P.A.* and *Lt. P.A.*). The lumen of the right main pulmonary artery is severely compressed by the adventitial hematoma (*A*) as the artery passes between aorta and left atrium (*L.A.*). The lumen of the proximal right coronary artery (*Rt. C.A.*) also is narrowed by the adventitial hematoma. The ascending aorta is involved by an acute medial dissection with proximal and distal tears (bottom left and right). Medial hematoma (*M*) in the lumen of the dissecting aneurysm narrows the lumen of the ascending aorta. *A.D.* = left anterior descending coronary artery; *Lt. Circum.* = left circumflex coronary artery; *Inn.* = innominate artery; *L.C.C.* = left common carotid artery; *L.S.* = left subclavian artery; *S.V.C.* = superior vena cava; and *P.V.* = pulmonary vein.

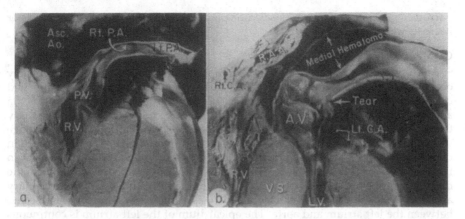

Figure 2 Longitudinal sections through the great vessels (pulmonary trunk, *a*, and ascending aorta, *b*) and the base of the heart. The great vessels show extensive adventitial hemorrhage. The ascending aorta (*Asc. Ao.*) is involved by a medial dissection with hematoma in the lumen of the dissecting aneurysm. A complete tear (arrow) of the aortic wall is present just distal to the left coronary artery (*Lt. C.A.*). *A.V.* = aortic valve; *Rt. C.A.* = right coronary artery; *R.A.A.* = right atrial appendage; *R.V.* = right ventricle; *V.S.* = ventricular septum; *L.V.* = left ventricle; *Rt. P.A.* = right main pulmonary artery; *Lt. P.A.* = left main pulmonary artery.

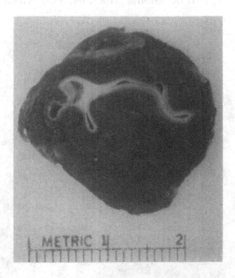

Figure 3 Cross-section of the right main pulmonary artery showing severe luminal compression by adventitial hematoma. Histologic examination showed that the media of this vessel was normal and that the hematoma was entirely in the adventitia.

narrowed < 50 per cent by arteriosclerotic plaques. No foci of myocardial fibrosis or necrosis were present.

COMMENTS

Severe obstruction of the right main pulmonary artery in this patient probably occurred in the following manner. The aortic aneurysm, which originally had dissected through only a part of the media, ruptured through the entire aortic media at a site just above the aortic valve. At this level the ascending aorta and pulmonary trunk share a common investment, visceral pericardium (Figure 4).[11] Hemorrhage was propagated in the adventitia of the aorta and pulmonary trunk, both enclosed in the common visceral pericardium, by systemic pressure transmitted via the tear in the ascending aorta, and the blood extended in this manner into the adventitia of the distal ascending and transverse aortas, and into the right and left main pulmonary arteries. Only the right pulmonary artery was compressed since it was located between the left atrium and aorta. The epicardium of the left atrium is continuous with the adventitia of the right pulmonary artery (Figure 4), and this connection accounts for extravasated blood in the left atrial wall superiorly. The hematoma in the false channel of the aortic dissecting aneurysm probably formed when blood flow slowed severely. This hematoma narrowed the true lumen of the aorta nearly 50 per cent.

SUMMARY

Attention is called to the occurrence of severe obstruction of the right main pulmonary artery as a consequence of acute dissection of the ascending aorta. The pulmonary arterial obstruction appears to have resulted from compression of this artery by an adventitial hematoma which extended from the ascending aorta

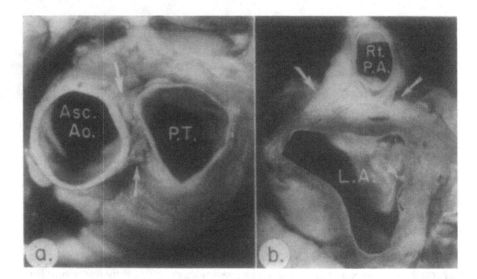

Figure 4 Normal heart. Superior view, *a*, of cross section of pulmonary trunk (*P.T.*) and ascending aorta (*Asc. Ao.*), and lateral view, *b*, of longitudinal section through the right main pulmonary artery (*Rt. P.A.*) and left atrium (*L.A.*). In *a*, the common investment by visceral pericardium (arrows) of the ascending aorta and pulmonary trunk is shown. In *b*, the relationship of the right main pulmonary artery to the left atrium and and continuity of the adventitia of the artery with the visceral pericardium of the atrium are shown.

after medial rupture of the aortic dissecting aneurysm. This complication of acute dissecting aortic aneurysm has not been described previously.

REFERENCES

1. Shennan, T.: *Dissecting aneurysms.* Medical Research Council, Special Report Series No. 193, London, 1934, H. M. Stationary Office.
2. Hirst, A. E., Jr., Johns, V. J., Jr., and Kime, S. W., Jr.: Dissecting aneurysm of the aorta: A review of 505 cases, *Medicine (Balt.)* **37**:217, 1958.
3. Gore, I., and Seiwert, V. J.: Dissecting aneurysm of the aorta, pathological aspects: An analysis of 85 cases, *Arch. Path. (Chicago)* **53**:121, 1952.
4. Lindsay, J., Jr., and Hurst, J. W.: Clinical features and prognosis in dissecting aneurysm of the aorta: A reappraisal, *Circulation* **35**:880, 1967.
5. De Bakey, M. E., Henly, W. S., Cooley, D. A., Morris, G. C., Jr., Crawford, E. S., and Beall, A. C., Jr.: Surgical management of dissecting aneurysms of the aorta, *J. Thorac. Cardiovasc. Surg.* **49**:130, 1965.
6. Nicholson, R. E.: Syndrome of aortic aneurysm rupture into the pulmonary artery: Review of literature with report of two cases, *Ann. Intern. Med.* **19**:286, 1943.
7. Mark, H., Aaron, R. S., Elias, K., Hurwitt, E. S.: Rupture of aortic aneurysm into left pulmonary artery: Attempt at surgical correction, *Amer. J. Cardiol.* **1**:757, 1958.
8. Pearson, J. R., and Nichol, E. S.: The syndrome of compression of the pulmonary artery by a syphilitic aortic aneurysm resulting in chronic cor pulmonale, with report of a case, *Ann. Intern. Med.* **34**:483, 1951.
9. Bevin, A. G., Rojas, R. H., and Stansel, H. C., Jr.: Aneurysm of the ascending aorta causing obstruction of the left pulmonary artery, *J. Thorac. Cardiovasc. Surg.* **52**:245, 1966.
10. Yacoub, M. H., Braimbridge, M. V., and Gold, R. G.: Aneurysm of the ascending aorta presenting with pulmonary stenosis, *Thorax* **21**:236, 1966.
11. Goss, C. M., editor: *Gray's anatomy,* ed. 28, Philadelphia, 1966, Lea & Febiger, Publishers, pp. 545, 574.

Case 386 Death in the Disco

Frank C. Brosius, III, M.D.; Brian D. Blackbourne, M.D.; and William C. Roberts, M.D., F.C.C.P.

Dr. William C. Roberts: Herein we discuss findings in a young man who died while dancing in a disco. Dr. Brosius will present the patient.

Dr. Frank C. Brosius: A 31-year-old white man, who died July 29, 1979, had been healthy until age 25 when he had a transient episode of substernal chest pain with radiation to the left arm. Although not hospitalized, a diagnosis of "pericarditis" was made. An ECG and chest roentgenogram performed at age 26 were normal. The total serum cholesterol level, however, was 360 mg/100 ml. At age 29, transient, substernal chest pain, for which he did not seek medical care, again occurred, and occasional substernal and left arm pain with extreme exertion was noted periodically thereafter. At age 29, an ECG (employment examination) was normal, and the total serum cholesterol level was 380 mg/100 ml. At age 31, a few weeks before death, the total serum cholesterol level was 450 mg/100 ml and the serum triglyceride level, 128 mg/100 ml. The low density lipoprotein (LDL) serum cholesterol level was 356 mg/100 ml, and the very low density lipoprotein (VLDL) level was 26 mg/100 ml. Both his brother and his father had elevated serum cholesterol levels. The patient smoked about 40 cigarettes daily. About two weeks before his sudden death, he began taking phendimetrazine to lose weight. During the afternoon of death, he ate a large picnic meal at which time he told his friends that he "did not feel well," but he expressed no specific complaints. Later that evening, he reportedly inhaled substantial amounts of butyl nitrite, which he had used often in the past year. While dancing in the disco, he collapsed and could not be resuscitated.

Dr. Roberts: Dr. Blackbourne, will you present your findings at necropsy?

Dr. Brian D. Blackbourne: At necropsy, the heart weighed 430 g. A healed transmural infarct was present in the posterior wall of left ventricle and it extended from apex to base. No foci of myocardial necrosis were present. The lumens of the four major coronary arteries were severely narrowed by atherosclerotic plaques. Each of the four major epicardial coronary arteries were divided into 5-mm long segments, and a histologic section was prepared and examined from each segment. Greater than 75 percent cross-sectional area narrowing by atherosclerotic plaque was present in 9 of 14 5-mm segments of the right coronary artery, in 11 of 11 of the left anterior descending, and in 5 of the 5 of the left circumflex (Figure 1). In addition, numerous yellow atherosclerotic plaques were present in the ascending aorta.

Dr. Roberts: Although only 31 years of age, our patient had fatal coronary atherosclerosis ("sudden coronary death"), familial hypercholesterolemia, namely type II hyperlipoproteinemia (hyperbetalipoproteinemia), for which he never received therapy, previous acute myocardial infarction, probably at age 25, as

From the Pathology Branch, National Heart, Lung, and Blood Institute, National Institutes of Health, Bethesda, and The District of Columbia Medical Examiner's Office, Washington, D.C.
Reprint requests: Dr. Roberts, Building 10A, Room 3E30, NIH, Bethesda 20205

DOI: 10.1201/9781003408321-30

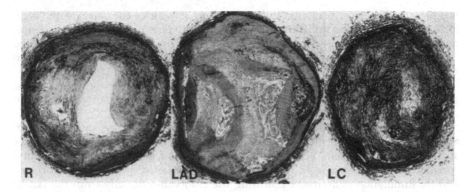

Figure 1 Photomicrographs at sites of maximal narrowing of the right (R), left anterior descending (LAD), and left circumflex (LC) coronary arteries. All three are severely narrowed, (all are Movat stains, original magnification × 16).

evidenced by a transmural left ventricular scar at necropsy, and unrecognized periodic angina pectoris thereafter.

Among the risk factors to premature symptomatic atherosclerosis, hypercholesterolemia is clearly the most important. Of 181 patients with familial hypercholesterolemia reported by Jensen and associates,[1] symptomatic coronary heart disease occurred before age 40 years in 19 percent of the men (25 percent of the women), and before age 50 years in 45 percent of the men (75 percent of the women). Of the patients with familial hypercholesterolemia reported by Slack,[2] 24 percent of the men had evidence of coronary heart disease by age 40 years and 85 percent by age 50 years. The mean age of development of symptomatic coronary heart disease in the men with hypercholesterolemia reported by Harlan and associates[3] was 42 years. Of the male patients with type II hyperlipoproteinemia described by Stone and associates,[4] nearly 10 percent had clinical evidence of coronary heart disease by age 30 years, 16 percent (1 in 6) by age 40 years, and 52 percent by age 50 years. In contrast, among the male patients of similar age but with normal serum lipoprotein patterns, the risk of a fatal or nonfatal coronary event by age 40 was less than 1 percent and by age 50, 13 percent.[4] Thus, type II hyperlipoproteinemia appears to accelerate the development of symptomatic coronary heart disease among American men by more than 20 years.

The amount of coronary arterial narrowing in our 31-year-old patient was extreme. Of 30 5-mm segments of major coronary artery examined histologically, 25 (83 percent) were narrowed greater than 75 percent in cross-sectional area by atherosclerotic plaques. This degree of narrowing is more than is usually observed at necropsy in victims of "sudden coronary death."[5] Among 31 previously reported personally studied necropsy patients with sudden coronary death, examination of histologic sections from each 5-mm segment of the four major (right, left main, left anterior descending and left circumflex) coronary arteries (50 5-mm segments per patient) disclosed that 36 percent were narrowed 76 percent to 100 percent in cross-sectional area by atherosclerotic plaque; 34 percent, 51 percent to 75 percent; 23 percent, 26 percent to 50 percent, and only 7 percent were narrowed 25 percent or less.[5] Thus, the atherosclerotic process in victims of "sudden coronary death" is diffuse and severe, but usually not as severe as in the present patient

Depending on how "sudden coronary death" is defined, histologic evidence of myocardial necrosis may or may not be present. If the definition includes death up to six hours after the sudden change in the symptomatic state, then myocardial necrosis is nearly always absent.[5] If the definition of "sudden coronary death" is up to 24 hours, a definition utilized by the World Health Organization, left ventricular myocardial necrosis may be observed or expected in the victims dying in the time period 12 to 24 hours. Our patient, who died nearly instantaneously, had no myocardial necrosis.

Although never knowingly taking medication for his unrecognized cardiac disease, our patient frequently sniffed butyl nitrite. Dr. Brosius, can you enlighten us about this volatile nitrite?

Dr. Brosius: Butyl nitrite has been popular in the drug culture as an aphrodisiac,[6,7] especially among homosexual men.[8] Amyl nitrite has been used for such purposes for several years, but its availability is legally restricted. The butyl congener, in contrast, is sold over the counter, marketed as a "room odorizer," and its stimulation is derived by sniffing the compound directly from the bottle. Recently, it has been documented that butyl nitrite inhalation can cause subclinical methemoglobinemia in normal persons, and theoretically, if the nitrite exposure were intense or inadequate time were allowed between nitrite inhalations for methemoglobin reduction, obvious clinical manifestations of methemoglobinemia could occur.[9] Increased intraocular pressure and severe hypotension also have been reported as side effects of chronic nitrite use.[6] Although potentially dangerous in the normal individual, butyl nitrite in our patient with extremely narrowed coronary arteries was at least potentially beneficial because of its vasodilator effects. In addition, it may have served to counteract the vasopressor effects of both his antiobesity medication and his cigarette smoking. In contrast to the pleasurable effects described from use of the volatile nitrites in the drug abusers, the giddiness, light headedness, mild disinhibitory action, and "orgasm expander"-effects are virtually never described in patients with angina pectoris. Instead, the coronary patients complain of the odor; the pounding, pulsating headache, or the feeling of fullness behind the eyes. There are no reports of psychological dependence on the volatile nitrites by coronary patients.

REFERENCES

1. Jensen J, Blankenhorn D, Kornerup V: Coronary disease in familial hypercholesterolemia. *Circulation* 1967; 36:77–82.
2. Slack J: Risks of ischaemic heart disease in familial hyperlipoproteinemic states. *Lancet* 1969; 2:1380–1382.
3. Harlan WR, Graham JB, Estes EH: Familial hypercholesterolemia: a genetic and metabolic study. *Medicine* 1966; 45:77–110.
4. Stone NJ, Levy RI, Fredrickson DS, Verter J: Coronary artery disease in 116 kindred with familial type II hyperlipoproteinemia. *Circulation* 1974; 49:476–488.
5. Roberts WC, Jones AA: Quantitation of coronary arterial narrowing at necropsy in sudden coronary death: analysis of 31 patients and comparison with 25 control subjects. *Am J Cardiol* 1979; 44:39–45.
6. Everett GM: Effects of amyl nitrite (Poppers') on sexual experience. *Med Aspects Hum Sexual* 1972; 6:146–151.
7. Cohen S: The volatile nitrites. *JAMA* 1979; 241:20772078.
8. Goode E, Troiden RR: Amyl nitrite use among homosexual men. *Am J Psychiatr* 1979; 136:1067–1069.
9. Horne MK, Waterman MR, Simon LM, et al: Methemoglobinemia from sniffing butyl nitrite. *Ann Intern Med* 1979; 91:416–418.

Case 679 Rupture of the Ascending Aorta During Cocaine Intoxication

Charles W. Barth III, MD, Michael Bray, MD
and William C. Roberts, MD

Cocaine is commonly injected, sniffed and smoked because of its psychotropic effects, but it also has significant cardiovascular effects. Illicit use of cocaine has been associated with ventricular arrhythmias, myocardial infarction, with or without associated significant coronary atherosclerosis, and subarachnoid hemorrhage.[1-4] Herein, we describe rupture of the ascending aorta in a person while smoking cocaine, a complication of cocaine use not previously described.

A healthy 45-year-old man had been smoking "free base" cocaine off and on for several hours. He suddenly collapsed and died while smoking a pipe containing cocaine. Blood cocaine level at necropsy was 9 mg/liter. A circumferential tear through intima and media was present in the ascending aorta about 2 cm above the sinotubular junction (Figure 1). Although there was no dissection distally from the site of aortic rupture, medial dissection extended proximally to the level of the aortic valve cusps. Adventitial hemorrhage extended around the aortic root onto the proximal portion of both the right and left coronary arteries, but it did not cause luminal compression. Hemorrhage also was present in the adventitia of the pulmonary trunk and main right and left pulmonary arteries with partial compression of the lumen of the right pulmonary artery. The heart weighed 500 g. The lumen of the left anterior descending coronary artery was narrowed at one point 76 to 95% in cross-sectional area by atherosclerotic plaque.

Cocaine acts as a sympathomimetic agent by blocking the neuronal re-uptake of catecholamines at adrenergic nerve endings, resulting in dose-dependent increases in heart rate and systemic blood pressure, the latter mainly a result of peripheral vasoconstriction.[5] Additionally, cocaine increases the chronotropic and inotropic effects of catecholamines on the heart.[6] It has been suggested that the previously described cardiovascular complications of cocaine use are a consequence of acute elevation of systemic blood pressure, a marked increase in myocardial oxygen demand and possibly coronary vasoconstriction.

Acute rupture of the ascending aorta in our patient most likely was caused by a large increase in systemic blood pressure due to the extremely high levels of cocaine in his blood in the presence of underlying chronic systemic hypertension.

From the Pathology Branch, National Heart, Lung, and Blood Institute, National Institutes of Health, Bethesda, Maryland 20205, and the Medical Examiner's Office of the District of Columbia, Washington, D.C. Manuscript received and accepted July 15, 1985.

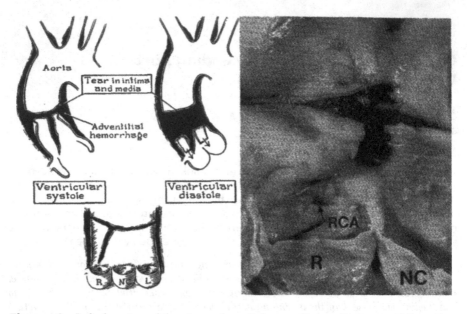

Figure 1 *Left*, drawing of the circumferential ascending aortic tear and the extensive adventitial hemorrhage. *Right*, close-up of the aortic tear. L = left aortic valve cusps; NC = non-coronary; R = right; RCA = ostium of right coronary artery.

REFERENCES

1. Nanji AA, Filipenko JD. Asystole and ventricular fibrillation associated with cocaine intoxication. *Chest* 1984;85:132–133.
2. Lichtenfeld PJ, Rubin DB, Feldman RS. Subarachnoid hemorrhage precipitated by cocaine snorting. *Arch Neurol* 1984;41:223–224.
3. Kossowsky WA, Lyon AF. Cocaine and acute myocardial infarction. A probable connection. *Chest* 1984;86:729–731.
4. Schachne JS, Roberts BH, Thompson PD. Coronary artery spasm and myocardial infarction associated with cocaine use [letter]. *New Engl J Med* 1984;310:1665–1666.
5. Fishman MW, Schuster CR, Resnekov L, Shick JFE, Krasnegor NA, Fennell W, Freedman DX. Cardiovascular and subjective effects of intravenous cocaine administration in humans. *Arch Gen Psychiat* 1976;33:983–989.
6. Masuda Y, Matsuda Y, Levy MN. The effects of cocaine and metanephrine on cardiac responses to norepinephrine infusions. *J Pharmacol Exp Ther* 1980;215:20–27.

Case 837 Hemodynamic Confirmation of Peripheral Pulmonary Stenosis Caused by Aortic Dissection

William C. Roberts, MD, Lowell F. Satler, MD, and Robert B. Wallace, MD

In aortic dissection, the intimal and medial tear most commonly is located in the ascending aorta. The dissecting channel is located in the outer one half or the outer one third of the aortic media.[1] As a consequence, the thickness of the medial wall separating the true and false channels is always greater than the thickness of the medial wall forming the outer wall of the false channel. Because the outer medial wall of the false channel is thin and the thinned wall is subjected to a systemic intra-aortic pressure, additional tearing of the media of the outer wall commonly occurs in the vicinity of the initial intimal-medial aortic tear. The further tearing of the outer aortic wall may lead to extravasation of intra-aortic blood into the adventitia of the aorta. The ascending aorta and pulmonary trunk have a common adventitia, and therefore dissection into the adventitia of the ascending aorta commonly extends into the adventitia of the pulmonary trunk and from there into the right and left main pulmonary arteries and their branches. Because the intraluminal pulmonary arterial pressure is relatively low and the adventitial dissection in both aorta and pulmonary arteries is driven by a systemic pressure, the extravasated blood in the pulmonary arterial adventitia can cause compression and narrowing of the lumens of the major pulmonary arteries. Although peripheral pulmonary stenosis has been observed at necropsy as a consequence of adventitia dissection from initial aortic medial dissection, hemodynamic proof of peripheral pulmonary stenosis from this mechanism has not been reported. Such is the purpose of this report.

W.D., a 45-year-old white male roofer, was well until about 60 hours before death when he developed sub-sternal chest pain that radiated into his neck while sitting drinking a beer. Shortly thereafter he began sweating profusely and when he stood up he fainted. He was taken to a local hospital. On examination, a grade 4/6 systolic ejection murmur was heard over the precordium, loudest in the second right intercostal space, with radiation into the neck. Because of intermittent persistence of the chest pain, he was transferred to Georgetown University Hospital 24 hours before death. The chest pain had worsened, but repeated electrocardiograms did not disclose evidence of myocardial ischemia. Doppler echocardiogram showed a peak systolic pressure gradient across the aortic valve of approximately 80 mm Hg. Cardiac catheterization disclosed a 25-mm Hg peak systolic pressure gradient between right ventricle and an intra-pulmonary pulmonary artery (Figure 1). The mean pulmonary artery wedge pressure was 10 mm Hg. On retrograde aortic catheterization, the stenotic aortic valve could not be crossed by the catheter and neither coronary ostium could be entered. Injection of contrast material into the ascending aorta disclosed true and false aortic lumens. Because of severe hypotension an aortic balloon pump was inserted and the patient was taken to the operating room. After median sternotomy and incision of the parietal pericardium, blood was found in the pericardial sac. The outer wall of the entire ascending aorta, pulmonary trunk

From the Pathology Branch, National Heart, Lung, and Blood Institute, National Institutes of Health, Bethesda, Maryland 20892, and the Division of Cardiology, Department of Medicine, and Department of Surgery, Georgetown University Medical Center, Washington, DC. Manuscript received February 6, 1989; revised manuscript received and accepted March 13, 1989.

DOI: 10.1201/9781003408321-32

173

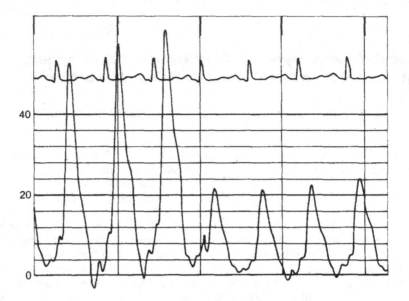

Figure 1 Pressure tracing with catheter tip in right ventricular cavity (*left*) and in pulmonary arterial lumen (*right*) immediately before operation. The peak systolic pressure gradient is approximately 25 mm Hg.

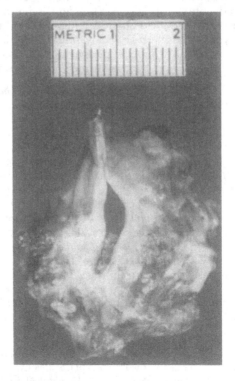

Figure 2 Operatively excised, heavily calcified, severely stenotic, unicuspid aortic valve.

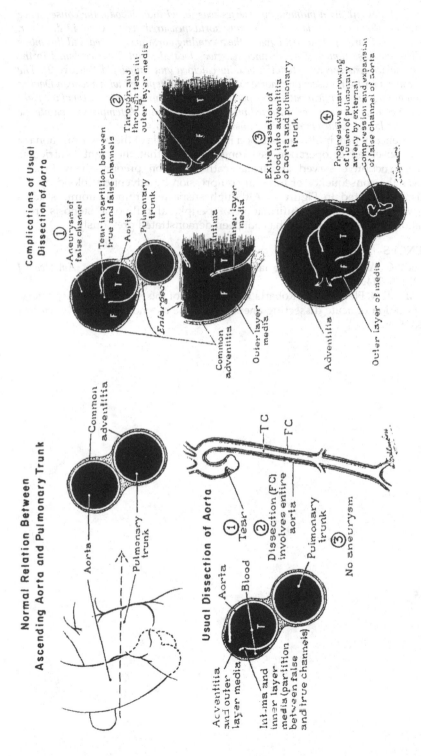

Figure 3   The relation between the adventitia of the ascending aorta and pulmonary trunk, the usual aortic dissection and a major complication of aortic dissection, namely adventitial pulmonary dissection with pulmonary arterial narrowing. Reproduced with permission from Roberts WC.[1]

and main right and left main pulmonary arteries was found to be bloody, the consequence of dissection into their adventitia. The ascending aorta measured about 10 cm in diameter. After institution of cardiopulmonary bypass, the ascending aorta was incised and thrombus was found in the false lumen. The entrance tear was located about 2 cm cephalad to the aortic valve, which was severely stenotic, heavily calcified and unicuspid (Figure 2). *The aortic valve and a portion of ascending aorta were excised and replaced with a woven Dacron conduit containing a mechanical valve. The portions of aorta containing the ostia of the right and left main coronary artery were inserted into the Dacron graft. Attempts to separate the patient from cardiopulmonary bypass were unsuccessful.*

The presence of firm infiltrates of blood in the adventitia of the major pulmonary arteries as observed at operation is strong evidence that the right ventricular outflow obstruction observed at cardiac catheterization preoperatively in this patient was the consequence of luminal compression by adventitial blood by the mechanism illustrated in Figure 3. Although suspected from anatomic studies previously,[1,2] hemodynamic confirmation of peripheral pulmonic stenosis from complications of aortic dissection has not been demonstrated previously.

REFERENCES

1. Roberts WC. Aortic dissection: anatomy, consequences, and causes. *Am Heart J* 1981;101:195–214.
2. Buja LM, Ali N, Fletcher RD, Roberts WC. Stenosis of the right pulmonary artery: a complication of acute dissecting aneurysm of the ascending aorta. *Am Heart J* 1972;83:89–92.

Case 971 Massive Perigraft Aortic Aneurysm Late After Composite Graft Replacement of the Ascending Aorta and Aortic Valve in the Marfan Syndrome

Susanne L. Mautner, MD, Gisela C. Mautner, MD, Charles L. Curry, MD, and William C. Roberts, MD

A major complication of the Marfan syndrome is the development of a fusiform aneurysm of the ascending aorta involving both its sinus and tubular portions. The fusiform aneurysm generally leads to aortic regurgitation, which may become severe, or to aortic rupture, which nearly always is fatal. Treatment of the aneurysm and aortic regurgitation consists of insertion of a composite graft, which involves a substitute aortic valve being sewn into the proximal end of a tube graft. The composite graft is then anastomosed proximally at the aortic valve position and distally to the ascending aorta beyond the aneurysm, and the wall of the aneurysm of the native aorta is wrapped around the composite graft. The coronary arteries are directly anastomosed to small orifices in the tube graft (Bentall operation[1]). This report describes a patient who developed a massive perigraft aortic aneurysm late after operation.

A 30-year-old black man had the Marfan syndrome diagnosed when he was approximately 15 years of age on the basis of ectopia lentis and skeletal features. At the time, the ascending aorta was dilated, and a murmur of aortic regurgitation was audible. Because of progressively worsening aortic regurgitation, the aortic valve and ascending aorta were replaced according to the Bentall operation when he was 23 years old (Figure 1). Within a few months, a mass was observed by echocardiogram surrounding the aortic composite graft, and this mass progressively increased in size to finally reach massive proportions (Figure 2). At age 24 years, retinal detachment occurred that was treated operatively, and also atrial fibrillation appeared. Despite the enlarging periaortic mass, the patient led an active life, including light weight lifting. He weighed 91 kg and was 191 cm in height. A chest radiograph was obtained 7 days before death at a routine follow-up visit (Figure 3). He died suddenly and unexpectedly at home.

Necropsy showed that the large perigraft mass was an aneurysm, the wall of which had been the wall of the previous native aorta (Figure 4). The combined weight of the ascending aorta with the aneurysm and the heart was 1,320 g. The aneurysm surrounded the composite graft, did not compress it and contained a large thrombus. The aneurysm was believed to have resulted from a small detachment of the suture line connecting the left main coronary artery to the composite graft. Both atrial cavities were extremely compressed by the aneurysmal mass (Figure 4). The left ventricular wall was free of foci of necrosis and fibrosis, the left ventricular cavity was moderately dilated, and the leaflets of the mitral and tricuspid valves were focally thickened by fibrous tissue. Histology sections of the wall of the native aorta disclosed massive loss of elastic fibers.

From the Pathology Branch, National Heart, Lung, and Blood Institute, National Institutes of Health, Building 10, Room 2N-258, Bethesda, Maryland 20892, and the Department of Medicine, Howard University Medical Center, Washington, D.C. Manuscript received July 9, 1992; revised manuscript received and accepted August 18, 1992.

DOI: 10.1201/9781003408321-33

177

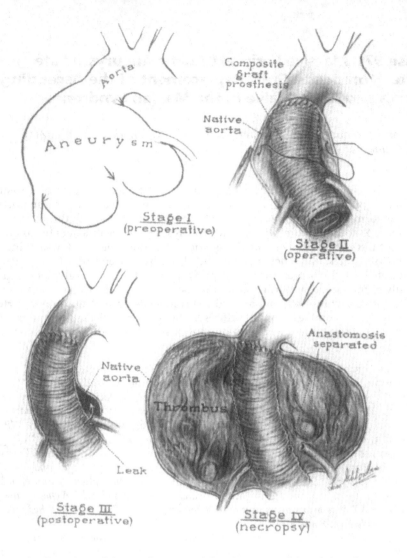

Figure 1 Drawing of the mechanism of development of the perigraft aortic aneurysm. Stage I: preoperative aortic regurgitation due to a dilated ascending aorta. Stage II: Bentall procedure with insertion of a composite graft (i.e., graft for the ascending aorta including a prosthesis [Björk-Shiley] in the aortic position). The coronary arteries are implanted into the tube graft and the wall of the native aorta is wrapped around the graft. Stage III: presumed slow leakage at suture line, most likely at the site of the anastomosis of the left main coronary artery to the graft of the ascending aorta (*arrow*). Stage IV: At necropsy, a massive perigraft aortic aneurysm formed by the wall of the native aorta was present, which was filled with thrombus. The left coronary artery was completely detached from its anastomosis to the composite graft.

The patient described in this report developed a huge (12 X 10 X 9 cm) perigraft aneurysm after replacement of most of the ascending aorta with a graft containing

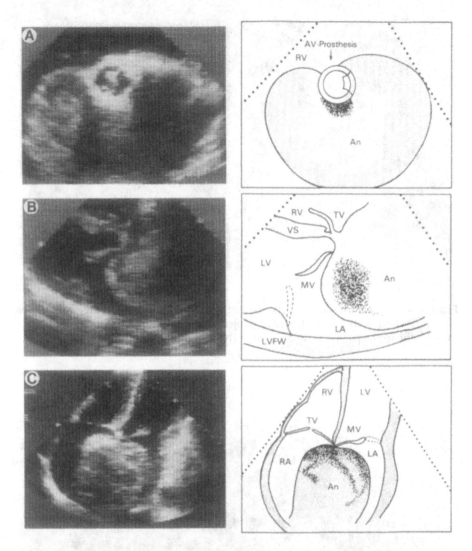

Figure 2 Echocardiogram performed 1 day before death showing the large aortic aneurysm around the graft in the aortic position (*A*), and the compression of the left and right atria (*B and C*). *A*, parasternal short-axis view; *B*, parasternal long-axis view; and *C*, 4-chamber view. An = perigraft aortic aneurysm; AV = aortic valve; LA = left atrium; LV = left ventricle; LVFW = left ventricular free wall; MV = mitral valve; RA = right atrium; RV = right ventricle; TV = tricuspid valve; VS = ventricular septum.

a valve prosthesis, and anastomosis of the coronary arteries directly to the Gortex graft. Detachment of the left main coronary artery to the composite graft appeared to be the cause of the perigraft aortic hematoma and aneurysm.

Several reports mentioned a peri-composite graft aneurysm after replacement of the ascending aorta with a composite graft with anastomosis of the coronary arteries to the graft.[2-9] At least 3 reports have described aortic graft-coronary arterial

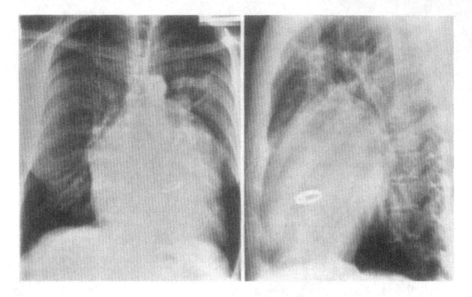

Figure 3 Chest radiograph of the patient obtained 7 days before death. *Left*, posteroanterior projection. *Right*, lateral projection. The enlarged heart silhouette is mainly due to the periaortic aneurysm of the ascending aorta.

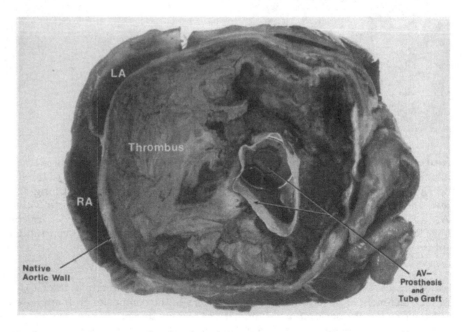

Figure 4 Perigraft aortic aneurysm at necropsy. The left and right atria (LA and RA, respectively) are compressed by the massive aneurysm of the ascending aorta. The mechanical valve prosthesis is in the aortic valve (AV) position.

180

disruption after a similar type of operation. Nath et al[10] reported 4 of 15 patients who late after composite graft replacement of the ascending aorta had leakage into the perigraft, intraaortic space at 1 coronary anastomotic site by angiogram. Gott et al[11] described graft dehiscence of the anastomosis of the left main coronary artery in 1 of 50 patients with the Marfan syndrome undergoing composite graft repair. Marvasti et al[12] described 1 of 30 patients undergoing the composite graft operation with aortic wrapping of the graft who had partial disruption of the anastomosis of the right coronary artery to the graft. Two other patients had "pseudoaneurysms" at the site of the right coronary anastomosis to the graft.

The Bentall procedure performed in this patient has had several technical modifications in recent years, and the dramatic complication described herein will hopefully be less frequent with the newer techniques.[13-17] However, regular follow-up including echocardiography is advisable.

In summary, perigraft aortic aneurysm secondary to coronary artery disruption from a composite graft is an infrequent but potentially fatal complication after replacement of the ascending aorta with a composite graft.

Acknowledgment: We thank Michael W. Spencer for his photographic assistance, and Vivian E. Norman for her secretarial support.

REFERENCES

1. Bentall H, De Bono A. A technique for complete replacement of the ascending aorta. *Thorax* 1968;23:338–339.
2. Nair KK. False aneurysm of the ascending aorta after surgery for Marfan's syndrome. *J Thorac Cardiovasc Surg* 1976;71:765–767.
3. Gallotti R, Ross DN. The Marfan syndrome: surgical technique and follow-up in 50 patients. *Ann Thorac Surg* 1980;29:428–433.
4. Pyeritz RE, Gott VL, McDonald GR, Achuff SC, Brinker JA, Haller JA, Hutchins GM. Surgical repair of the Marfan aorta: technique, indications and complications. *Johns Hopkins Med J* 1982;151:71–82.
5. Probst P, Baur HR, Leupi F, Schüpbach P, Althaus U. Postoperative evaluation of composite aortic grafts: comparison of angiography and CT. *Br J Radiol* 1983;56:797–804.
6. Kitamura S, Onishi K, Nakano S, Kawachi K, Kawashima Y. Early and late results of the Bentall operation for annulo-aortic ectasia. *J Cardiovasc Surg (Torino)* 1983;24:5–12.
7. Kouchoukos NT, Marshall WG Jr, Wedige-Stecher TA. Eleven-year experience with composite graft replacement of the ascending aorta and aortic valve. *J Thorac Cardiovasc Surg* 1986;92:691–705.
8. Josephson RA, Singer I, Levine JH, Maughan L, Pyeritz RE, Gott VL, Weisman HF, Brinker J. Systolic expansion of the aortic root: an echocardiographic and angiographic sign of aortic composite graft dehiscence. *Cathet Cardiovasc Diagn* 1988;14:705–707.
9. Kong B, Ogilby JD, Poynton R. Pseudoaneurysm of a Shiley composite aortic valve and graft prosthesis. *Am Heart J* 1990;120:1002–1004.
10. Nath PH, Zollikofer C, Castaneda-Zuniga WR, Velasquez G, Formanek A, Nicoloff D, Amplatz K. Radiological evaluation of composite aortic grafts. *Radiology* 1979;131:43–51.
11. Gott VL, Pyeritz RE, Magovern GJ Jr, Cameron DE, McKusick VA. Surgical treatment of aneurysms of the ascending aorta in the Marfan syndrome. Results of composite-graft repair in 50 patients. *N Engl J Med* 1986;314:1070–1074.
12. Marvasti MA, Parker FB, Randall PA, Witwer GA. Composite graft replacement of the ascending aorta and aortic valve. Late follow-up with intra-arterial digital subtraction angiography. *J Thorac Cardiovasc Surg* 1988;95:924–928.

13. Cabrol C, Pavie A, Mesnildrey P, Gandjbakhch I, Laughlin L, Bors V, Corcos T. Long-term results with total replacement of the ascending aorta and reimplantation of the coronary arteries. *J Thorac Cardiovasc Surg* 1986;91:17–25.
14. Crawford ES, Svensson LG, Coselli JS, Safi HJ, Hess KR. Surgical treatment of the aneurysm and/or dissection of the ascending aorta, transverse aortic arch, and ascending aorta and transverse aortic arch: factors influencing survival in 717 patients. *J Thorac Cardiovasc Surg* 1989;98:659–674.
15. Belcher P, Ross D. Aortic root replacement—20 years experience of the use of homografts. *Thorac Cardiovasc Surg* 1991;39:117–122.
16. Kouchoukos NT, Wareing TH, Murphy SF, Perrillo JB. Sixteen-year experience with aortic root replacement. Results of 172 operations. *Ann Surg* 1991;214:308–318.
17. Miyamoto AT. Technique for replacing the ascending aorta and aortic valve with a modified Bentall's operation. *Ann Thorac Surg* 1992;53:1125–1126.

Case 1063 Sudden Death While Playing Tennis Due to a Tear in Ascending Aorta (Without Dissection) and Probable Transient Compression of the Left Main Coronary Artery

Susan R. Comfort, MD, * R. Charles Curry, Jr., MD, and William C. Roberts, MD

Although it has many causes,[1] sudden death in an older person is usually the result of atherosclerotic coronary artery disease. Such was not the case in the patient described below, and the cause has not been encountered previously by us or reported previously by others.

• • •

V.M., a 71-year-old white woman, had been asymptomatic all her life until she suddenly collapsed on the tennis court. She was resuscitated, transported to a hospital, where she failed to regain consciousness until her death 8 days later when life support was withdrawn. During a routine examination when she was 64 years old, an electrocardiogram disclosed complete left bundle branch block. Coronary angiogram was recorded at the time and no narrowings were present in the epicardial arteries and no abnormalities in origin or courses of the coronary arteries were noted.

At necropsy, the heart weighed 305 g. The major epicardial coronary arteries had normal origins and courses with a right dominant circulation. The arteries were cut transversely at 5 mm intervals, and although an occasional small plaque was present, the lumen everywhere was wide open. The ventricles were cut at 1 cm intervals transverse to the posterior atrioventricular sulcus; no foci of fibrosis or necrosis were seen in any ventricular wall and histologic sections disclosed no interstitial inflammatory cells. The 4 cardiac valves were normal. None of the 4 cardiac chambers was dilated.

The ascending aorta was of normal size. Small atherosclerotic plaques were present at the sinotubular junction, which overhung both widely patent right and left main coronary ostia. A linear tear measuring 2.5 cm in length was present in the tubular portion of ascending aorta just cephalad to the left and posterior aortic valve cusps (Figure 1). The portion of aorta just caudal to the tear protruded slightly toward the aortic lumen, exposing the intact adventitia of aorta behind the tear. The adventitia at this site contained some blood components and they extended into the aortic wall behind the adjacent sinuses of Valsalva. The tear did not produce any dissection of the aorta.

• • •

From the Division of Cardiology, Department of Medicine, Orlando General Hospital, Orlando, Florida; and the Baylor Cardiovascular Institute, Baylor University Medical Center, Dallas, Texas 75246. Manuscript received and accepted March 15, 1996.
* Present address: Maricopa County Medical Examiner's Office, 120 South 6th Avenue, Phoenix, Arizona 85003.

DOI: 10.1201/9781003408321-34

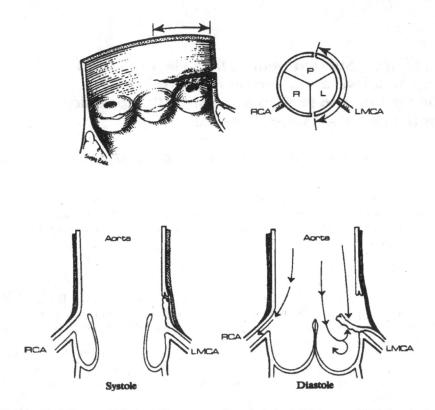

Figure 1 Diagram of ascending aorta showing the tear (upper left), the part of the aortic circumference involved in the tear (upper right), and the presumed location of a part of the aortic wall immediately above the ostium of the left main coronary artery (LMCA) in both ventricular systole and diastole (lower right). L = left; P = posterior; R = right aortic valve sinuses of Valsalva; RCA = right coronary artery.

The heretofore described patient collapsed while playing tennis, was resuscitated, but never regained consciousness. Necropsy disclosed a through-and-through medial tear in the ascending aorta just cephalad to the left and part of the posterior aortic valve cusps. Death could not be attributed directly to the tear because it did not lead to either complete rupture of the aortic wall with hemopericardium or to aortic dissection with its various consequences. We speculate that the tear during ventricular diastole allowed blood to fill the space within the tear, allowing the caudal portion of the wall to compress either the ostium of the left main coronary artery or the left main trunk causing, at least transiently, inadequate perfusion of the left ventricular wall.

REFERENCE

1. Roberts WC. Sudden cardiac death: definitions and causes. *Am J Cardiol* 1986;57:1410–1413.

Case 1178 Aneurysm of the False Channel of Descending Thoracic Aorta Years After Operative Excision of the Initiating Aortic Dissection Tear in Ascending Aorta

Stuart R. Lander, MD; William C. Roberts, MD

Aortic dissection is one of the most dramatic clinical events in cardiovascular disease. The initiating tear is usually in ascending aorta, the dissection proceeds anterograde from the site of the tear, and most commonly involves the entire aorta thereafter. On occasion, the tear is located just distal to the origin of the left subclavian artery (aortic isthmus), and then the dissection proceeds anterograde down the descending thoracic aorta and on occasion retrograde into ascending aorta. In persons who survive the initial ascending aortic tear with dissection, a second tear with dissection is more common than in persons who do not have the first tear followed by dissection. It is important, of course, to diagnose aortic dissection as rapidly as possible because persons with tears in ascending aorta generally die within several days after onset of the event. When the tear is in ascending aorta, about 90% of these individuals die without operation within 30 days of the initial tear. Usually the initial dissection occurs most commonly in persons in their sixth decade of life and less commonly in elderly persons. However, in those persons who have aortic dissection resulting from a tear in ascending aorta and have the tear operatively excised about 75% of these individuals survive the operative repair and, therefore, are at risk for a second aortic tear followed by dissection.

A 70-year-old woman at age 54 had a tear in ascending aorta followed by a dissection of the entire aorta. The tear in ascending aorta was excised and a portion of ascending aorta was replaced with a graft. Five years later she had the sudden appearance of chest pain again and now computed tomography disclosed a second tear most likely at the aortic isthmus and a large aneurysm of the false channel of descending thoracic aorta. She recovered spontaneously from this second event and apparently did well until age 70 when back pain of increasing frequency and intensity prompted her to seek medical care again. Chest radiograph (Figure 1) disclosed marked mediastinal widening and probable aortic aneurysm. Computed tomography (Figure 2) now showed the size of the descending thoracic aorta to be 7 cm, slightly <1 cm larger, since the second aortic tear 11 years earlier. The descending thoracic aorta was operatively excised and a graft was inserted between aortic isthmus and distal descending thoracic aorta. The excised descending thoracic aortic aneurysm was divided transversely to show the large false channel, most of which was filled with thrombus, and the small residual true channel (Figure 3). She did not regain consciousness and died 25 days after this second operation.

The above briefly described the patient 15 years before death. She had a tear in ascending aorta with dissection of the entire aorta and had that tear excised. Five years later she was found to have a large aneurysm of the false channel of the descending thoracic aorta and a new tear at the aortic isthmus. Then at age 70, 15 years after the first aortic tear and 11 years after the second one—each followed by a dissection—a large aneurysm of the false channel of the descending thoracic aorta was excised.

From the Baylor Cardiovascular Institute, Baylor University Medical Center, Dallas, TX

DOI: 10.1201/9781003408321-35

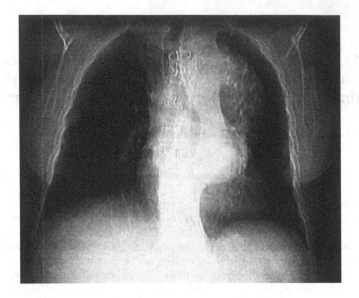

Figure 1 *Radiograph of chest, anteroposterior view, about 30 days before death.*

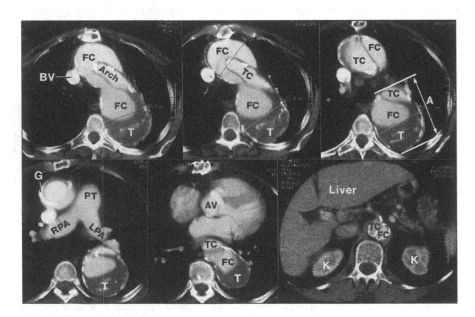

Figure 2 *Tomographic transverse views about 30 days before death through the chest and upper abdomen showing the large aortic dissection with both true channel (TC) and false channel (FC) beginning in the ascending aorta. The false channel in descending thoracic aorta contains a large thrombus (T). A=total aneurysm size (includes both true and false channels); AV=aortic valve; BV=brachiocephalic vein (containing dense contrast material); G=graft (in ascending aorta); K=kidney; LPA=left pulmonary artery; PT=pulmonary trunk; RPA=right pulmonary artery.*

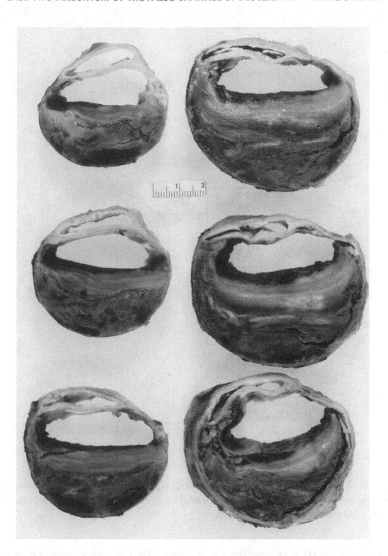

Figure 3 *Cross sections of the operatively excised descending thoracic aortic aneurysm. The lumen of the false channel is much larger than that of the true channel. The lumen of the false channel contains a large thrombus.*

In general, when the tear is excised from ascending aorta the false channel distal to the distal anastomotic site becomes smaller and infrequently becomes aneurysmal. In the present patient, the false channel in descending thoracic aorta became huge and was calcified five years after the initiating tear in ascending aorta. The above described patient illustrates that a large aneurysm of the false channel of descending thoracic aorta may occur in a patient who initially has a tear in ascending aorta and has the tear operatively excised. It is well established that an aneurysm of the false channel of descending thoracic aorta may occur in an occasional patient who survives a tear with dissection of ascending aorta and does not have the tear operatively excised. There will be an increasing number of patients in the elderly group who have survived aortic dissection with tear in ascending aorta and who

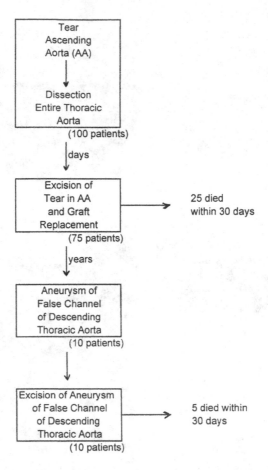

Figure 4 *Diagram of the frequency and consequences of development of an aneurysm of the false channel in descending thoracic aorta after operative resection of the initialing tear and graft replacement of ascending aorta.*[1]

have had the initial tear operatively excised. What the best management of an aneurysm of the false channel of descending thoracic aorta is in someone who has already had partial replacement of ascending aorta is uncertain. Based on a publication by Bachet et al,[1] Figure 4 shows the likely frequency and consequences of the development of an aneurysm of the descending thoracic aorta after operative resection of the ascending aortic entrance tear and graft replacement.

REFERENCE

1. Brachet J, Termignon JL, Dreyfus G, et al. Aortic dissection: Prevalence, cause, and results of late reoperations. *J Thorac Cardiovasc Surg.* 1994;108:199–206.

Case 1381 Abdominal Aortic Aneurysm in Nonagenarians

William C. Roberts, MD;[124] Jong Mi Ko, BA;[4] Gregory J. Pearl, MD[3]

A 92-year-old woman had been healthy all her life until age 88, when dyspnea prompted hospitalization and heart failure secondary to mitral regurgitation was diagnosed. The signs of heart failure vanished after appropriate medical therapy. An asymptomatic abdominal aortic aneurysm (AAA) measuring 6 cm in maximal right-to-left diameter was diagnosed by computed tomography at the time. Operative resection was not recommended then because of her advanced age. Thereafter, she was in her usual active state until age 92 when she was hospitalized again, this time because of abdominal pain, nausea, and vomiting. Her blood pressure was 120/80 mm Hg, a loud precordial murmur consistent with mitral regurgitation was audible, body mass index was 21 kg/m² (body weight, 110 lb; height, 62 in), and hematocrit was 37%. Repeat computed tomography showed that the AAA had increased to 9 cm in diameter and blood was present in the aortic wall of the aneurysm (Figure 1). The patient accepted the high risk of AAA operative resection, which was carried out on May 2, 2006. Her postoperative course was complicated by transient renal and cerebral insufficiency, but both renal and cerebral function gradually returned to normal levels. About a month postoperatively while in the rehabilitation hospital, gastrointestinal blood loss was detected and it, too, has slowly disappeared. She was discharged from the rehabilitation hospital on June 13, 2006, 42 days after the AAA resection.

The operatively excised intraaneurysmal thrombus (Figure 2) weighed 351 g and consisted virtually entirely of fibrin.

COMMENTS

Among patients with AAA, the hitherto described patient is unusual in several respects: (1) her older age, (2) the large size of the AAA and the intraaneurysmal thrombus, (3) her gender, (4) the lack of clinical evidence of myocardial, cerebral, or peripheral arterial insufficiency, and (5) the lack of a history of systemic hypertension or of a recorded elevated systemic arterial pressure.

During the past 6 years (1999–2006), 42 patients have had intraaneurysmal thrombus from AAA operatively excised at Baylor University Medical Center (BUMC) in Dallas, TX.[1] Two of the 42 patients were 90 years of age and older. Bickerstaff and colleagues[2] reviewed records of 616 patients with AAA referred to the Mayo Clinic in 3 separate years in the eighth decade of the 20th century. The oldest of the 616 patients was 91 years of age. How many of the 616 patients were nonagenarians was not stated. The same authors also reviewed records of all patients from the city of Rochester, MN, admitted to the Mayo Clinic during a 30-year period (1951–1980).[2] Of

From the Departments of Internal Medicine, Division of Cardiology;[1] and Pathology;[2] and Surgery;[3] and the Baylor Heart and Vascular Institute,[4] Baylor University Medical Center, Dallas, TX

Address for correspondence: William C. Roberts, MD, Baylor Heart and Vascular Institute, Baylor University Medical Center, 621 North Hall Street, Suite H-030, Dallas, TX 75226

E-mail: wc.roberts@baylorhealth.edu

DOI: 10.1201/9781003408321-36

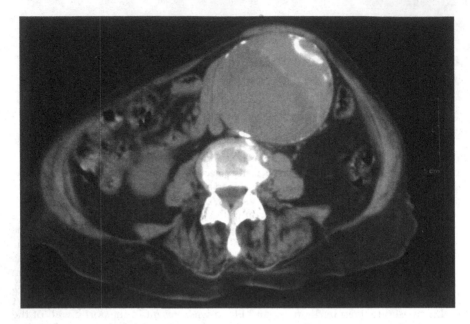

Figure 1 *Computed tomography image of the abdominal aortic aneurysm in the patient presented*

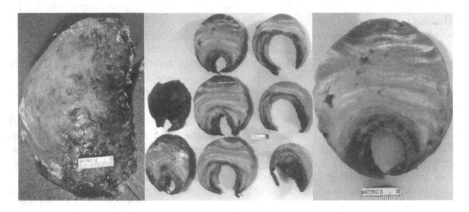

Figure 2 *Operatively excised intra-aneurysmal thrombus in the patient presented. Left, Photo of the intact thrombus. Center, Cross-sections of the thrombus. Right, Close-up of one cross-section. The residual lumen is at the bottom, closest to the ruler.*

296 patients, 27 (14%) were 80 years and older, but the number of those 90 years and older was not stated. Waller and Roberts[3] studied 40 patients 90 years of age and older at necropsy; at least four of them had an AAA.

The large size of the AAA in the patient described is unusual. Of the 42 patients previously mentioned with AAA intraaneurysmal thrombus, 10 were in women; only two weighed >100 g, and the 351 g in the present patient was the largest by far.

AAA is clearly more common in men than in women. Ten (24%) of our 42 patients with AAA and resection of the intraaneurysmal thrombus were women.[1] Of the 616 patients referred to the Mayo Clinic and described by Bickerstaff and associates,[2] 16%

were women. Of the 296 patients with AAA from the city of Rochester, 34% were women.[2] Of the 473 patients with AAA studied at necropsy from 1952–1975 at a single hospital (Massachusetts General) and reported by Darling and associates,[4] 130 (27%) were women.

The present patient had no clinical evidence preoperatively of coronary, cerebral, or peripheral arterial insufficiency, a condition in a minority of patients with AAA. Although this scenario is the case in many patients with AAA, virtually all of them have evidence by angiogram, echocardiogram, computed tomography, and/or anatomic examination of major atherosclerotic involvement of these other vascular systems, and the most common cause of death among patients with AAA is coronary heart disease.[5] Mautner and associates,[6] for example, described coronary arterial findings at necropsy in 27 patients with AAA (>5 cm in widest transverse diameter). During life, 12 (44%) of the 27 patients had symptomatic myocardial ischemia and 10 of the 27 patients died from its consequences. Evidence of acute or healed myocardial infarction was present in 15 patients (56%). Twenty-three (85%) of the 27 patients had narrowing 76%–100% in cross-sectional area of one or more major epicardial coronary artery by atherosclerotic plaque. The mean number of coronary arteries per patient severely (>75%) narrowed was $2.0 \pm 1.3/4.0$. Of the 108 major coronary arteries in the 27 patients, 55 (51%) were narrowed >75% in cross-sectional area by plaque. Of the 1475 5-mm segments of the 4 major coronary arteries in the 27 patients, 18% were narrowed >75% and not a single one was devoid of plaque. Thus, patients with AAA nearly always have diffuse and severe coronary atherosclerosis.

REFERENCES

1. Roberts WC, Ko JM, Pearl GJ. Relation of weights of intraaneurysmal thrombi to maximal right-to-left diameters of abdominal aortic aneurysms. *Am J Cardiol.* In press.
2. Bickerstaff LK, Hollier LH, Van Peenen HJ, et al. Abdominal aortic aneurysm: the changing natural history. *J Vasc Surg.* 1984;1:6–12.
3. Waller BF, Roberts WC. Cardiovascular disease in the very elderly. Analysis of 40 necropsy patients aged 90 years or over. *Am J Cardiol.* 1983;51:403–421.
4. Darling RC, Messina CR, Brewster DC, et al. Autopsy study of unoperated abdominal aortic aneurysms. The case for early resection. *Circulation.* 1977;56(3 suppl):II161–II164.
5. Ernst CB. Current concepts: abdominal aortic aneurysm. *N Engl J Med.* 1993;328:1167–1172.
6. Mautner GC, Berezowski K, Mautner SL, et al. Degrees of coronary arterial narrowing at necropsy in men with large fusiform abdominal aortic aneurysm. *Am J Cardiol.* 1992;70:1143–1146.

Case 1390 Isolated Aortic Valve Replacement Without Coronary Bypass for Aortic Valve Stenosis Involving a Congenitally Bicuspid Aortic Valve in a Nonagenarian

William C. Roberts, MD;[1,2,4] Jong Mi Ko, BA;[4] Gregory John Matter, MD[3]

A 90-year-old man sought care because of rapidly progressing dyspnea and an episode of near syncope. Examination found him to be 71 inches tall and to weigh 180 lb (body mass index, 25 kg/m^2). A grade 5/6 harsh systolic ejection precordial murmur was present, loudest over the right second intercostal space. A murmur of aortic regurgitation was not described. The blood hematocrit was 39%. Cardiac catheterization disclosed the following pressures (mm Hg): left ventricle, 207/15; aorta, 157/60; and peak transvalvular systolic pressure gradient, 50. The left ventricular ejection fraction was 50%, and the calculated aortic valve area was 0.64 cm^2. Angiogram disclosed wide open coronary arteries. The aortic valve was replaced with a 25-mm pericardial bioprosthesis (Baxter, Deerfield, IL). His postoperative course was uncomplicated. The operatively excised aortic valve was congenitally bicuspid, heavily calcified, and rigid, and it weighed 5.73 g. The patient was known to be alive 1507 days after valve replacement.

COMMENTS

The hitherto described patient had congenital heart disease, specifically a bicuspid aortic valve. Symptoms of aortic valve stenosis, namely those of heart failure and near syncope, did not develop until 90 years after birth. By this time, the bicuspid aortic valve was heavily calcified, quite stenotic, and replaced. The operatively excised valve was very heavy (5.73 g [normal, 0.5 g])[1] and immobile[2] (Figure).

Aortic stenosis, of course, is fairly common in older individuals, but it usually manifests itself symptomatically long before the age of 90, particularly when the stenosis involves a congenitally malformed valve. From 1993 to 2006, we studied operatively excised stenotic aortic valves in 9 nonagenarians: 3 had congenitally bicuspid aortic valves, including the present patient, and 6 had 3-cuspid aortic valves.[3] All but 1 patient survived the operative period; 1 died 874 days and 1 died 1011 days after valve replacement; 6 others have survived from 787 to 2324 days postoperatively as of June 29, 2006. The hitherto described patient is doing well 1507 days after valve replacement.

Why some patients with a congenitally bicuspid stenotic valve do not become symptomatic until their 90s and why others become symptomatic in early life is unclear. The stenosis is primarily the result of calcific deposits on the aortic aspects of the cusps. Those with higher serum cholesterol levels may develop calcific deposits on the valve cusps at an earlier age than the patients with lower serum cholesterol numbers. Unfortunately, we were unable to obtain the cholesterol values

From the Departments of Internal Medicine, Division of Cardiology,[1] Pathology,[2] and Cardiothoracic Surgery,[3] and the Baylor Heart and Vascular Institute,[4] Baylor University Medical Center, Dallas, TX

Address for correspondence: William C. Roberts, MD, Baylor Heart and Vascular Institute, Baylor University Medical Center, 621 North Hall Street, Suite H-030, Dallas, TX 75226

E-mail: wc.roberts@baylorhealth.edu

DOI: 10.1201/9781003408321-37

in the above-described patient. The fact that his coronary arteries were virtually free of plaque as determined by angiography suggests that his serum cholesterol levels were relatively low.

In patients with isolated aortic valve stenosis unassociated with mitral valve dysfunction, the absence of coronary narrowing by angiogram suggests that the underlying structure of the aortic valve is bicuspid rather than tricuspid, at least in patients aged 40–70 years.[4] Among 3 patients aged 90–91 years with isolated aortic stenosis and bicuspid aortic valves, 2 by angiogram had 1 or more epicardial coronary arteries narrowed >50% in diameter. In contrast, of 6 patients aged 90–91 years with isolated aortic valve stenosis superimposed on a 3-cusp aortic valve, all had severe narrowing of 1 or more major epicardial coronary arteries by angiogram. Mautner and colleagues[4] examined the structure of stenotic aortic valves in adults and related the valve structure to several variables, including coronary arterial narrowing, useful in predicting that structure. One hundred eighty-eight patients having aortic valve replacement for isolated valvular aortic stenosis were studied. All patients were older than 40 years at the time of aortic valve replacement; all had coronary angiograms preoperatively; 182 (97%) had measurements of serum total cholesterol; and 184 (98%) had body mass index calculated. The structure of the operatively excised valve was classified as unicuspid or bicuspid (congenitally malformed) or as a tricuspid aortic valve. A logistic regression model was developed that found 4 factors (age, serum total cholesterol, angiographic coronary artery disease, and body mass index) to be predictive of aortic valve structure.[1] Patients with at least 3 or all 4 factors high or present (ie, age older than 65 years, serum total cholesterol >200 mg/dL, body mass index >29 kg/m², and coronary artery disease) had a low probability (10%–29%) of having a congenitally malformed valve[2] and patients with at least 3 or all 4 factors low or absent (ie, age 65 years or younger, serum total cholesterol

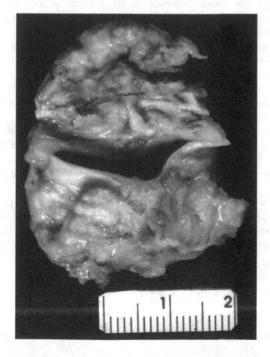

Figure 1 *Congenitally bicuspid aortic valve in the 90-year-old patient described.*

<200 mg/dL, body mass index <29 kg/m^2, and no coronary artery disease) had a high probability (72%–90%) of having a congenitally malformed valve. Thus, the morphology of the operatively excised stenotic aortic valve can be predicted with knowledge of the age, serum total cholesterol, body mass index, and coronary artery status of the patient.

The presence of an elevated systolic systemic arterial pressure in an older person should not be interpreted to mean absent or only minimal or mild aortic valve stenosis. The peak systemic systolic pressure in the present patient at cardiac catheterization was 157 mm Hg and yet the peak left ventricular pressure was 207 mm Hg. We have observed the peak systemic systolic pressure to be as high as 200 mm Hg and yet the degree of aortic stenosis was severe, with a peak left ventricular systolic pressure of 300 mm Hg and a peak transvalvular gradient of 100 mm Hg.[5]

Aortic valve replacement even in nonagenarians is the procedure of choice for severe aortic stenosis. Bacchetta and associates[6] reported 18 patients aged 90 years or older who had aortic valve replacement for aortic stenosis, 13 of whom also had simultaneous coronary bypass grafting. All patients survived the 30-day operative period and, although the data are scant, at least up to 2.5 years postoperatively. Among 9 nonagenarians having aortic valve replacement for aortic stenosis at Baylor University Medical Center (Dallas, TX), all but 1 survived the 30-day postoperative period, 2 died nearly 2+ years later, and the others are alive up to 6+ years postoperatively.

REFERENCES

1. Silver MA, Roberts WC. Detailed anatomy of the normally functioning aortic valve in hearts of normal and increased weight. *Am J Cardiol*. 1985;55:454–461.
2. Roberts WC, Ko JM, Hamilton C. Comparison of valve structure, valve weight, and severity of the valve obstruction in 1849 patients having isolated aortic valve replacement for aortic valve stenosis (with or without associated aortic regurgitation) studied at 3 different medical centers in 2 different time periods. *Circulation*. 2005;112:3919–3929.
3. Roberts WC, Ko JM, Matter GJ. Aortic valve replacement for aortic stenosis in nonagenarians. *Am J Cardiol*. In press.
4. Mautner GC, Mautner SL, Cannon RO III, et al. Clinical factors useful in predicting aortic valve structure in patients > 40 years of age with isolated valvular aortic stenosis. *Am J Cardiol*. 1993;72:194–198.
5. Roberts WC, Perloff JK, Costantino T. Severe valvular aortic stenosis in patients over 65 years of age. A clinicopathologic study. *Am J Cardiol*. 1971;27:497–506.
6. Bacchetta MD, Ko W, Girardi LN, et al. Outcomes of cardiac surgery in nonagenarians: a 10-year experience. *Ann Thorac Surg*. 2003;75:1215–1220.

Case 1501 Full Blown Cardiovascular Syphilis with Aneurysm of the Innominate Artery

William Clifford Roberts, MD[a,b,c,]*, Forrester Dubus Lensing, MD[d],
Harry Kourlis, Jr., MD[e], Jong Mi Ko, BA[c], Jonathan Warren Newberry, MD[b],
Michael John Smerud, MD[d], Elizabeth C. Burton, MD[b], and Robert Frederick
Hebeler, Jr., MD[e]

The investigators report the case of a 44-year-old man who presented acutely and was found to have saccular aneurysm of the innominate artery, narrowed or totally occluded aortic arch arteries, and marked thickening of the thoracic aorta except for the wall behind the sinuses of Valsalva. The abdominal aorta was entirely normal. Results of the serologic test for syphilis were strongly positive. Because cardiovascular syphilis appears to be a disease that affects the vasa vasora and because these channels are limited to the thoracic aorta, the abdominal aorta is uninvolved, as demonstrated so nicely in the patient described in this case report. Because most patients with cardiovascular syphilis are much older than the patient described, it is unusual to see a perfectly normal abdominal aorta, as in the present patient. In conclusion, syphilis producing aneurysm of the innominate artery is unusual but is always associated with syphilitic involvement of the thoracic aorta. © 2009 Elsevier Inc. All rights reserved. (Am J Cardiol 2009;104:1595–1600)

Recently, we studied a young man who presented with evidence of a saccular aneurysm of the innominate artery and narrowing or total occlusions of the arteries from the aortic arch. Operative resection of the aneurysm and bypassing of the 2 obstructed arteries, although initially successful, proved to be unsuccessful, and the entire thoracic aorta and its major branches were found to be affected by cardiovascular syphilis. Because of the unusual opportunity to study the morphologic features of full-blown cardiovascular syphilis in a relatively young patient, and because of the presence of a saccular aneurysm of an arch artery, the present case is described.

CASE DESCRIPTION

A 44-year-old white man born in February 1963 had been in his usual health except for right-hand claudication when doing hard labor until September 2007, when he developed substernal chest pain and fainted. He was brought to his local hospital and found to have marked differences in the pulses in the arms, and because of the possibility of aortic dissection, he was transferred to Baylor University Medical Center.

Computed tomographic angiographic examination (Figure 1) on admission showed a 5.6-cm saccular aneurysm of the innominate artery, severe narrowing of the right common carotid and vertebral arteries and the celiac axis at their origins,

[a]Department of Internal Medicine, Division of Cardiology, and [b]Department of Pathology, [c]Baylor Heart and Vascular Institute; and [d]Departments of Radiology and [e]Cardiothoracic Surgery, Baylor University Medical Center, Dallas, Texas. Manuscript received June 16, 2009; revised manuscript received and accepted June 17, 2009.
* Corresponding author: Tel: 214–820–7911; fax: 214–820–7533.
E-mail address: wc.roberts@baylorhealth.edu (W.C. Roberts).

DOI: 10.1201/9781003408321-38

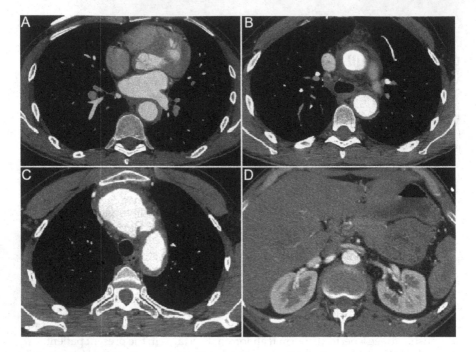

Figure 1 Computed tomographic angiographic images in the patient described. (A) Axial image depicting the normal appearance of the aortic root with normal wall thickness. Note also wall thickening of the descending aorta. (B) Axial image demonstrating severe thickening of the wall of ascending aorta with extensive inflammatory stranding in the prevascular space anterior to the ascending aorta. (C) Axial image of the large saccular aneurysm of the innominate artery. This image does not depict the fusiform dilatation of the more distal innominate artery. This image does not demonstrate fusiform dilatation of the distal innominate artery, from which the right subclavian and right common carotid arteries arose. (D) Axial demonstrating normal wall thickness of the abdominal aorta.

and totally occluded left common carotid and left subclavian arteries. The right subclavian and left vertebral arteries were patent. The wall of the entire thoracic aorta, except for the wall behind the aortic sinuses, was thickened. A 3-dimensional reconstruction best demonstrated the saccular aneurysm of the innominate artery (Figure 2). Gadolinium-enhanced magnetic resonance angiography (Figure 3) better showed the intracerebral and extracerebral blow flow.

Although the results of the Venereal Disease Research Laboratory test for syphilis were nonreactive, the results of rapid plasma reagin were positive (>1:512), and the treponema palladium particle agglutination was also reactive. Antinuclear antibodies were present, and in titer 1 they were 1:2,560, and strong cytoplasmic speckling was noted. The C-reactive protein level was 8.9 mg/dl, and the erythrocyte sedimentation rate was 105 mm/hour. The results of cerebrospinal fluid test for syphilis (rapid plasma reagin) were negative.

At operation in September 2007, the aneurysm was excised, Dacron grafts were placed from the aorta to the right and left common carotid arteries, and a saphenous vein graft was placed from the Dacron graft to the right vertebral artery. The 7-day postoperative course initially was smooth, but the patient's last 2 days of life were characterized by very poor perfusion to essentially all body organs and tissues.

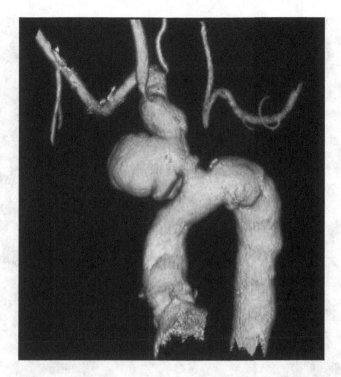

Figure 2 Computed tomographic 3-dimensional reconstruction image demonstrating the large saccular aneurysm of the proximal innominate artery, the fusiform aneurysmal dilatation of the distal innominate artery, and severe stenosis of the right common carotid artery and the origin of the right vertebral artery. This image also demonstrates complete occlusion of the left common carotid and left vertebral artery origins, with back filling of the proximal left vertebral artery. This pattern of obstruction resulted in a left-sided left subclavian steal phenomenon.

At necropsy, there were large bilateral pleural and abdominal effusions, severe centrilobular hepatic necrosis, renal tubular necrosis, focal left ventricular necrosis, and occluding thrombi in the brachiocephalic and subclavian veins and in the left internal carotid artery.

The aortic findings at necropsy are summarized partially in Figure 4.

The wall of the innominate artery aneurysm (excised at operation) was greatly thickened. The wall of the ascending aorta behind the sinuses of Valsalva was not thickened, but beginning at the sinotubular junction and extending to the origin of the celiac axis, the wall of the aorta was severely thickened (Figures 5 and 6). The lumen of the celiac axis just as it arose from the aorta was severely narrowed by the same process affecting the aorta. The wall of the abdominal aorta was normal. Histologic study of the wall of the innominate artery aneurysm showed its wall to be similar to that of the thoracic aorta and typical of cardiovascular syphilis (Figure 7).

COMMENTS
The unusual features of this case are the extent of involvement of the aorta and the severe involvement of the arteries arising from the aortic arch, including a large saccular aneurysm of the innominate artery. The morphologic features of the aorta

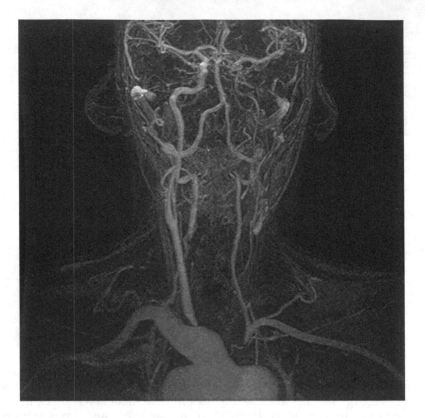

Figure 3 Maximum-intensity projection image from intracranial and extracranial gadolinium-enhanced magnetic resonance angiography demonstrating the fusiform dilatation of the distal innominate artery with severe stenosis of the right common carotid and right vertebral arteries at their origins. The left vertebral artery received backflow from the collaterals from the circle of Willis, resulting in left-sided subclavian steal. The left common carotid and left internal carotid arteries were occluded. Cerebral blood flow essentially was maintained via the right common carotid and right vertebral arteries and by perfusion to the left cerebral hemisphere via circle of Willis collaterals (anterior and posterior communicating arteries), not well visualized in this image.

and arch arteries and celiac axis are typical of cardiovascular syphilis and confirmed by the strongly reactive serologic test for syphilis.

Aneurysm of the innominate artery has been described previously in cardiovascular syphilis. Warfield[1] described x-ray changes in 20 patients, and the aneurysms measured 2.4 to 9.0 cm in diameter and each contained thrombus. Neither the right nor the left subclavian or internal carotid arteries were involved in the "destructive process." The patients ranged in age from 35 to 72 years. The Wassermann reaction was positive in 15 (75%). All had severe involvement of the thoracic aorta. Twelve were studied at necropsy. Gay and Walker[2] described x-ray features of 18 patients, all men, aged 35 to 63 years, with innominate artery aneurysms. Fourteen (78%) had positive serologic results for syphilis, and 7 (39%) had histories of chancres. Tadavarthy et al[3] reported 4 patients with syphilis involving the thoracic aorta, including a saccular aneurysm of the innominate artery. All 4

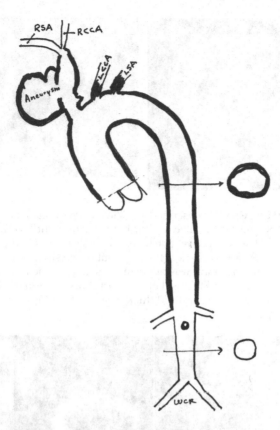

Figure 4 Diagram of aorta and aortic arch branches demonstrating the distribution of syphilitic involvement. Syphilitic involvement started at the sinotubular junction of the aorta and extended just beyond the origin of the renal arteries. The aneurysm of the innominate artery was of the saccular type, and its wall was as thick as the wall of the entire thoracic aorta distal to the sinuses of Valsalva. The origin of the right common carotid artery (RCCA) was severely narrowed, and the proximal portions of the left common carotid artery (LCCA) and left subclavian artery (LSA) were totally occluded. The celiac axis located just caudal to the origins of the renal arteries was also severely narrowed. The wall of the abdominal aorta was entirely normal, in contrast to the marked thickening of the wall of the thoracic aorta. RSA = right subclavian artery.

patients had positive Venereal Disease Research Laboratory test results for syphilis. Goei et al[4] described a 66-year-old man with an aneurysm of the innominate artery, a very dilated ascending aorta, and a history of having been treated for syphilis 20 years earlier.

Characteristically in cardiovascular syphilis, the wall of the aorta behind the sinuses of Valsalva is spared, and the process begins immediately at the sinotubular junction. Distal to the sinotubular junction, every square millimeter of the aorta was affected until just past the origin of the celiac axis, and from that point distally, the aorta was normal.

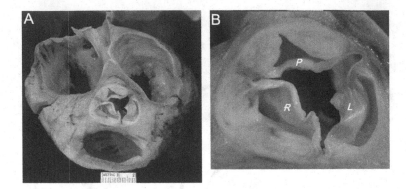

Figure 5 Heart of the patient described. (*A*) View from the cephalad direction of the right atrium, left atrium, aortic valve, and right ventricular outflow tract. (*B*) Close-up view of the aortic valve from above. The incision in the aorta is in the tubular portion just above the right (R) and posterior (P) cusps but in the sinus portion in the left (L) cusp. The sinus wall of the aorta was of normal thickness. The right coronary artery arose from the right cusp, and the wall of this aorta was of normal thickness because it was within the sinus. There was mild thickening of the margins of 2 cusps.

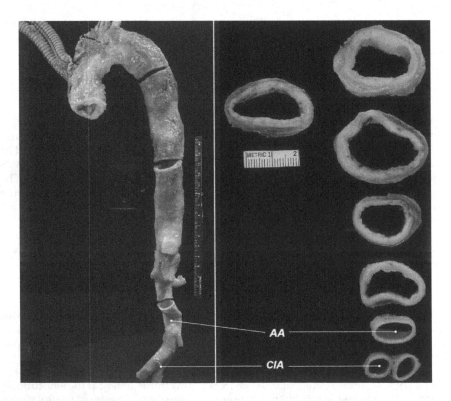

Figure 6 Tubular portion of the ascending aorta and the entire descending thoracic and abdominal aorta. The wall of the thoracic aorta was very thick, and the wall of the abdominal aorta (AA) was entirely normal. Likewise, the walls of the common iliac arteries (CIA) were entirely normal.

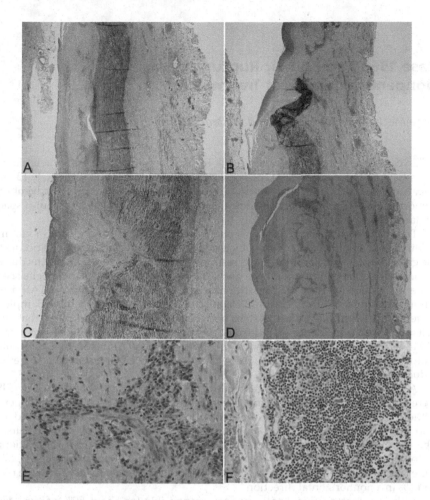

Figure 7 Histologic sections of the wall of the innominate artery aneurysm. The wall in all sections (*A to D*) was extremely thick. (*A to C*) Movat tissue stains showing marked disruption of the elastic fibers of the media, indeed a total disruption of the media in (*B*), and marked thickening of the intima and adventitia. (*D*) Collections of inflammatory cells in both adventitia and media. (*E,F*) Close-up of the inflammatory cells, consisting of plasmacytes and lymphocytes. (*A to C*) Movat stains at 20× and hematoxylin-eosin stains at (*D*) 20× and (*E,F*) 400×.

REFERENCES

1. Warfield CH. Roentgen diagnosis of aneurysms of the innominate artery. *AJR Am J Roentgenol* 1935;33:350–358.
2. Gay BB Jr, Walker FJ. Aneurysm of the innominate artery: review of clinical and radiologic findings in 18 cases. *Radiology* 1953;60:804–813.
3. Tadavarthy SM, Castaneda-Zuniga WR, Klugman J, Shachar JB, Amplatz K. Syphilitic aneurysms of the innominate artery. *Radiology* 1981;139:31–34.
4. Goei R, Tjwa MK, Snoep G. Luetic aneurysm of the innominate artery mimicking a mass in the right side of the anterior mediastinum: MR appearance. *AJR Am J Roentgenol* 1992;159:1343.

Case 1568 Fatal Aortic Rupture from Nonpenetrating Chest Trauma

Mina Mecheal Benjamin, MD, and William Clifford Roberts, MD

A 22-year-old man died following a side impact blow in an automobile accident. Necropsy showed a large tear in the posterior wall of the aorta approximately 12 mm distal to the insertion of ligamentum arteriosum (*Figures 1 and 2*). Subadventitial hemorrhage was prominent in the descending thoracic aorta. The left pleural space contained large quantities of blood.

Traumatic aortic rupture is the second most common cause of death in victims of blunt chest trauma from motor vehicle accidents.[1-3] Death usually (85%) occurs at the crash scene.[2-4] Aortic rupture was responsible for about 15% of the deaths due to automobile accidents until seat belts and air bags were introduced. Seat belts seem to be more effective than air bags in reducing traumatic aortic injury (TAI) after blunt frontal motor vehicle crashes.[5] Data from the National Automotive Sampling System Crashworthiness Data System between 1993 and 1998 indicated that seat belts reduced the incidence of TAI from 2.66% to 0.49% in crashes where an airbag did not deploy. Airbags alone do not significantly reduce TAI in survivors of frontal motor vehicle crashes. Airbags are more effective in those using seat belts, together reducing the incidence from 0.49% to 0.29%.[5]

According to Christopher and colleagues,[6] among patients with TAI, 71% were drivers, 23% were front-seat passengers, and 6% were back-seat passengers.[6] Although most reports focused on frontal impact crashes, side impact accidents also are a major cause of TAI, especially after the introduction of seat belts.[7, 8] The direction of the crash impact was known in 672 patients from the National Automotive Sampling System registry between 1998 and 2002; among those, 57% were frontal, 18% were at the driver's side, 16% at the passenger's side, 2% in the rear, and 6% in a nonhorizontal direction.[6]

Although motor vehicle accidents are responsible for about 80% of the cases of TAI,[9] other causes include, though much less frequently, falls from heights and crushes, penetrating (gunshot/stab) wounds, and iatrogenic causes (during interventional catheterization). If the rupture is not transmural, a partial tear may lead to an aneurysm (Figure 3).

In about 80% of reported cases of TAI, the site of the aortic tear is at the aortic isthmus between the ostium of the left subclavian artery and the ostium of the third pair of intercostal arteries.[10-15] The isthmus segment of the proximal descending aorta is the least mobile portion of the thoracic aorta, being "held down" by its attachment to the pulmonary trunk via the ligamentum arteriosum. A much less common site of rupture is the ascending aorta.[12]

Several mechanisms have been postulated as to why the isthmus portion is the most common site of aortic rupture. The most widely accepted theory suggests that in nonpenetrating chest traumas, sudden high-velocity deceleration is accompanied

From the Department of Internal Medicine (Benjamin) and the Baylor Heart and Vascular Institute (Roberts), Baylor University Medical Center at Dallas.

Corresponding author: William Clifford Roberts, MD, Baylor Heart and Vascular Institute, 3500 Gaston Avenue, Suite H-030, Dallas, Texas 75226 (e-mail: wc.roberts@baylorhealth.edu).

DOI: 10.1201/9781003408321-39

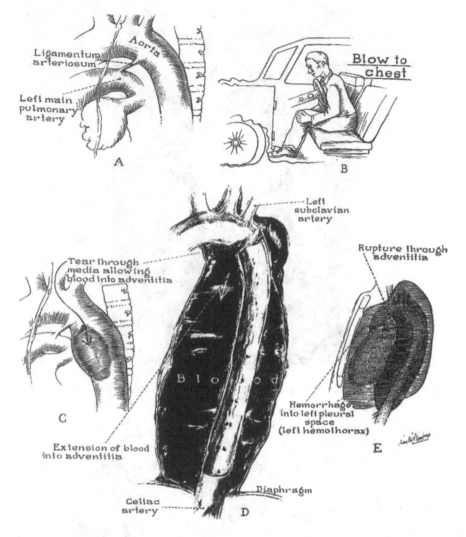

Figure 1 Most common pattern of full-thickness aortic rupture in motor vehicle accidents.

by hyperflexion of the spine leading to sudden chest compression and traction on the aortic isthmus, the point at which the mobile aortic arch meets the fixed proximal descending thoracic aorta.[16–22] Another theory suggests a "shoveling effect," as a lower thoracic impact results in cranial displacement of the mediastinum and torsion of the isthmus.[22] The "osseous pinch" theory suggests that the proximal descending aorta is pinched between the sternum, upper ribs, and clavicles anteriorly and the vertebral column posteriorly.[23] A less favorable theory suggests a "water-hammer" effect, where an acute rise in aortic pressure exerts maximum stress on the aortic isthmus.[20]

Rupture of the aorta is of course not the only type of cardiovascular injury from blunt chest trauma: rupture of the right or left ventricular free wall or ventricular septum,[24] left ventricular aneurysm,[25] and cardiac valve regurgitation[26] are some other cardiac consequences of blunt chest trauma.

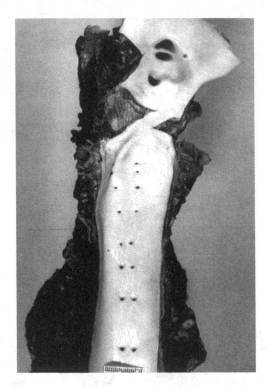

Figure 2 The site of the aortic tear in the patient described.

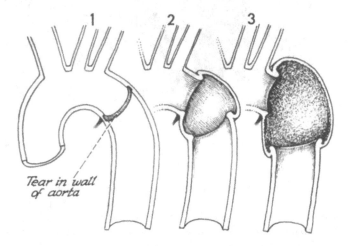

Figure 3 The mechanism of aortic aneurysm formation in the isthmic area after partial tear of the aorta.

Fatal cardiac arrest has been reported in a number of drivers of motorized vehicles. Usually, the driver becomes aware of the cardiac arrhythmia, pulls to the side of the road, and is then found pulseless slumped over the steering wheel without a crash into another vehicle or into a stationary structure on the side of the road.[27]

204

REFERENCES

1. Parmley LF, Marion WC, Mattingly TW. Nonpenetrating traumatic injury of the heart. *Circulation* 1958;18(3):371–396.
2. Greendyke RM. Traumatic rupture of aorta; special reference to automobile accidents. *JAM* 1966;195(7):527–530.
3. Symbas PN, Tyras DH, Ware RE, DiOrio DA. Traumatic rupture of the aorta. *Ann Surg* 1973;178(1):6–12.
4. Fabian TC, Richardson JD, Croce MA, Smith JS Jr, Rodman G Jr, Kearney PA, Flynn W, Ney AL, Cone JB, Luchette FA, Wisner DH, Scholten DJ, Beaver BL, Conn AK, Coscia R, Hoyt DB, Morris JA Jr, Harviel JD, Peitzman AB, Bynoe RP, Diamond DL, Wall M, Gates JD, Asensio JA, Enderson BL. Prospective study of blunt aortic injury: multicenter trial of the American Association for the Surgery of Trauma. *J Trauma* 1997;42(3):374–380.
5. Brasel KJ, Quickel R, Yoganandan N, Weigelt JA. Seat belts are more effective than airbags in reducing thoracic aortic injury in frontal motor vehicle crashes. *J Trauma* 2002;53(2):309–312.
6. Michetti CP, Hanna R, Crandall JR, Fakhry SM. Contemporary analysis of thoracic aortic injury: importance of screening based on crash characteristics. *J Trauma* 2007;63(1):18–24.
7. Ben-Menachem Y. Rupture of the thoracic aorta by broadside impacts in road traffic and other collisions: further angiographic observations and preliminary autopsy findings. *J Trauma* 1993;35(3):363–367.
8. Katyal D, McLellan BA, Brenneman FD, Boulanger BR, Sharkey PW, Waddell JP. Lateral impact motor vehicle collisions: significant cause of blunt traumatic rupture of the thoracic aorta. *J Trauma* 1997;42(5):769–772.
9. Keen G, Bradbrook RA, McGinn F. Traumatic rupture of the thoracic aorta. *Thorax* 1969;24(1):25–31.
10. Osborn GR. Findings in 262 fatal accidents. *Lancet* 1943;2:277–284.
11. Strassman G. Traumatic rupture of the aorta. *Am Heart J* 1947;33(4):508–515.
12. Parmley LF, Mattingly TW, Manion WC, Jahnke EJ Jr. Nonpenetrating traumatic injury of the aorta. *Circulation* 1958;17(6):1086–1101.
13. Zehnder MA. Delayed post-traumatic traumatic rupture of the aorta in a young healthy individual after closed injury: mechanical-etiological considerations. *Angiology* 1956;7(3):252–267.
14. Spencer FC, Guerin PF, Blake HA, Bahnson HT. A report of fifteen patients with traumatic rupture of the thoracic aorta. *J Thorac Cardiovasc Surg* 1961;41:1.
15. Conroy C, Hoyt DB, Eastman AB, Holbrook TL, Pacyna S, Erwin S, Vaughan T, Sise M, Kennedy F, Velky T. Motor vehicle-related cardiac and aortic injuries differ from other thoracic injuries. *J Trauma* 2007;62(6):1462–1467.
16. Sutorius DJ, Schreiber JT, Helmsworth JA. Traumatic disruption of the thoracic aorta. *J Trauma* 1973;13(7):583–590.
17. Lundevall J. The mechanism of traumatic rupture of the aorta. *Acta Pathol Microbiol Scand* 1964;62:34–46.
18. Feczko JD, Lynch L, Pless JE, Clark MA, McClain J, Hawley DA. An autopsy case review of 142 nonpenetrating (blunt) injuries of the aorta. *J Trauma* 1992;33(6):846–849.
19. Shkrum MJ, McClafferty KJ, Green RN, Nowak ES, Young JG. Mechanisms of aortic injury in fatalities occurring in motor vehicle collisions. *J Forensic Sci* 1999;44(1):44–56.
20. Giulini SM, Bonardelli S. Post-traumatic lesions of the aortic isthmus. *Ann Ital Chir* 2009;80(2):89–100.

21. Siegel JH, Belwadi A, Smith JA, Shah C, Yang K. Analysis of the mechanism of lateral impact aortic isthmus disruption in real-life motor vehicle crashes using a computer-based finite element numeric model: with simulation of prevention strategies. *J Trauma* 2010;68(6):1375–1395.
22. Siegel JH, Yang KH, Smith JA, Siddiqi SQ, Shah C, Maddali M, Hardy W. Computer simulation and validation of the Archimedes lever hypothesis as a mechanism for aortic isthmus disruption in a case of lateral impact motor vehicle crash: a Crash Injury Research Engineering Network (CIREN) study. *J Trauma* 2006;60(5):1072–1082.
23. Crass JR, Cohen AM, Motta AO, Tomashefski JF Jr, Wiesen EJ. A proposed new mechanism of traumatic aortic rupture: the osseous pinch. *Radiology* 1990;176(3):645–649.
24. Mason DT, Roberts WC. Isolated ventricular septal defect caused by nonpenetrating trauma to the chest. *Proc (Bayl Univ Med Cent)* 2002;15(4):388–390.
25. Glancy DL, Yarnell P, Roberts WC. Traumatic left ventricular aneurysm. Cardiac thrombosis following aneurysmectomy. *Am J Cardiol* 1967;20(3):428–433.
26. Chang JP, Chu JJ, Chang CH. Aortic regurgitation due to aortic root intimal tear as a result of blunt chest trauma. *J Formos Med Assoc* 1990;89(1):41–43.
27. Antecol DH, Roberts WC. Sudden death behind the wheel from natural disease in drivers of four-wheeled motorized vehicles. *Am J Cardiol* 1990;66(19):1329–1335.

Case 1667 Massive Diffuse Calcification of the Ascending Aorta and Minimal Focal Calcification of the Abdominal Aorta in Heterozygous Familial Hypercholesterolemia

William C. Roberts, MD[a,b,]*, Vera S. Won, BS[a], Matthew R. Weissenborn, MD[c], Adnan Khalid, MD[d], and Brian Lima, MD[e]

A 41-year-old woman, the mother of 3 offspring, with likely heterozygous familial hypercholesterolemia, had been asymptomatic until age 38 when angina pectoris and exertional dyspnea appeared leading to the discovery of severe multivessel coronary artery disease and a massively calcified ascending aorta. Coronary bypass grafting using the right and left internal mammary arteries did not alleviate the symptoms. Evidence of overt heart failure subsequently appeared and that led to heart transplantation at age 41. She died 22 days later. The occurrence of massive diffuse calcification of the ascending aorta and minimal focal calcification of the abdominal aorta is rare and in the patient described it appears to be the consequence of heterozygous familial hypercholesterolemia. © 2016 Elsevier Inc. All rights reserved. (Am J Cardiol 2016;117:1381–1385)

Heavy calcific deposits in the ascending aorta are infrequent. Patients with huge abdominal aortic aneurysms or huge calcific deposits in the wall of the abdominal aorta infrequently, for example, have significant calcific deposits in the ascending aorta. Patients with familial hypercholesterolemia, particularly the homozygous variety, typically have heavy calcific deposits in ascending aorta and few if any calcific deposits in abdominal aorta,[1] the reverse of the usual situation. Patients with non-familial hypercholesterolemia typically have heavy calcific deposits in their abdominal aorta and few, if any, in the ascending aorta. We recently studied a 41-year-old woman who had huge diffuse calcific deposits in the ascending aorta and minimal focal deposits in the abdominal aorta, and evidence of familial hypercholesterolemia of the heterozygous variety. Patients with a "porcelain" aorta are infrequently considered to have familial hypercholesterolemia.[2] A description of this occurrence in this setting is the purpose of this report.

DESCRIPTION OF PATIENT

This 41-year-old white woman was born in January 1973 and died in December 2014. Her family tree is shown in Figure 1. She underwent heart transplantation 22

[a]Department of Baylor Heart and Vascular Institute, [b]Department of Pathology, [c]Department of Radiology, [d]Division of Cardiology, Department of Internal Medicine, and [e]Department of Cardiothoracic Surgery, Baylor University Medical Center, Dallas, Texas. Manuscript received December 18, 2015; revised manuscript received and accepted January 22, 2016.

This study was funded by the Baylor Health Care System Foundation through the Cardiovascular Research Review Committee and in cooperation with the Baylor Heart and Vascular Institute.

* Corresponding author: Tel: +(214) 820–7911; fax: +(214) 820–7533.

E-mail address: wc.roberts@baylorhealth.edu (W.C. Roberts).

DOI: 10.1201/9781003408321-40

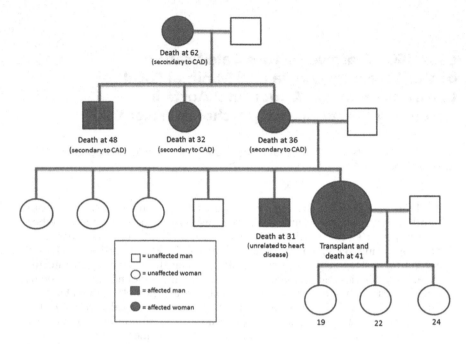

Figure 1 Diagram of patient's genetic pedigree. The large circle represents the patient described in this report. CAD = coronary artery disease.

days before death. (An autopsy was not performed.) A coronary artery bypass grafting procedure had been done in April 2012 because of angina pectoris and exertional dyspnea. Before that operation, coronary angiography had shown severe multivessel coronary disease (Table 1). A stent had been inserted in the proximal right coronary artery. Heavy calcific deposits had been noted in the left main, left anterior descending, and left circumflex coronary arteries and in the ascending aorta. In November 2014, the patient was referred to Baylor University Medical Center. Computed tomography confirmed the massive calcific deposits in the ascending aorta and only a few focal deposits in the abdominal aorta (Figure 2). Serum cholesterol and other values are shown in the table. She was on simvastatin 40 mg daily before these cholesterol values were evaluated. She had evidence of severe heart failure, a very low ejection fraction, and, global left ventricular hypokinesis.

The radiograph of the excised native heart (weight 495 g) is shown in Figure 3. All major epicardial coronary arteries were severely narrowed by atherosclerotic plaque. Scars were present in the left ventricular wall anteriorly, laterally, and posteriorly, and also in the ventricular septum (Figure 4). The left ventricular cavity was dilated (up to 4.5 cm). Heavy calcific deposits were present on the ventricular aspect of anterior mitral leaflet and on the aortic aspect of each of the 3 aortic valve cusps (Figure 3). Photomicrographs of sections of the left ventricular wall are shown in Figure 5. The entire ascending aorta was diffusely and heavily calcified, and the abdominal aorta was focally and minimally calcified (Figure 6).

DISCUSSION

The causes of "porcelain" aorta (*diffuse* calcific deposits in the tubular portion of ascending aorta) have recently been listed in a published review by Abramowitz and colleagues.[2] The list included diabetes mellitus, chronic kidney diseases, and

Table 1: Finding in our 41-year-old woman

Angina pectoris	+
Dyspnea on exertion	+
Precordial murmur	+ (grade3/6)
Diabetes mellitus (type II)	+
Systemic hypertension (by history)	+
Body mass index (Kg/m²)	26
Mitral regurgitation	2+/4+
Aortic valve stenosis	0
Hematocrit (%)	29
Total cholesterol (mg/dl)	135
Low-density lipoprotein cholesterol (mg/dl)	87
High-density lipoprotein cholesterol (mg/dl)	40
Triglycerides (mg/dl)	88
Blood urea nitrogen (mg/dl)	25
Creatinine (mg/dl)	1.2
B-type natriuretic peptide (pg/ml)	1970
Magnesium (mg/dl)	1.9
Thyroid stimulating hormone (uIU/ml)	0.95
Creatinine clearance (ml/min)	48
Coronary artery narrowing (% diameter reduction):	
Right	90%(ostial)
Left main	10%
Left anterior decending	99%
Left circumflex	10%
Coronary bypass	+
Intracardiac defibrillator	+
Ejection fraction (%)	25
Pulmonary artery (mmHg) (s/d)	35/26
Pulmonary arterial wedge (mmHg)	a17 b17 m16
Left ventricle (mmHg) (s/d)	113/10
Left ventricular angiogram	Global hypokinesis (severe)

s/d = peak systole; end diastole.

mediastinal irradiation, but not hyperlipidemia, whether familial or nonfamilial. Diabetes mellitus and chronic kidney disease of course affect millions of people, but diffuse calcification of the ascending aorta is extremely rare (depending on how "porcelain" is defined), and we were not able to find any reports demonstrating a diffusely calcified ascending aorta in either of these conditions. In contrast, most patients with homozygous familial hypercholesterolemia have diffuse calcification of the ascending aorta.[1,3] This condition, however, is rare (1/1,000,000). The heterozygous variety of familial hypercholesterolemia (occurrence 1/500) also is associated with calcific deposits in the ascending aorta but usually they are not as heavy as in the homozygous variety. Our patient appears to be the exception. Although we were unable to obtain serum lipid values in our patient before statin therapy (40 mg simvastatin) was began, the lipid values obtained were not those seen after statin therapy in patients with the homozygous variety of hyperlipidemia. The latter group of patients before lipid-lowering therapy generally have total cholesterol values >800 mg/dl and low-density lipoprotein (LDL) cholesterol levels >500 mg/dl. It would be impossible to reach the total and LDL-cholesterol levels that our patient had with simvastatin 40 mg dose if she had had the homozygous variety of familial hypercholesterolemia. The patients with the heterozygous variety of familial

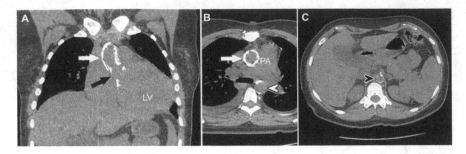

Figure 2 Noncontrast computed tomographic images from the patient before surgical intervention. (A) Coronal reformatted image of the left ventricular outflow tract, and (B) axial image through the level of the pulmonary trunk showing calcific deposits in the aortic sinuses (*black arrow*), heavy diffuse deposits in the ascending thoracic aorta (*white arrow*), and smaller focal deposits in the descending thoracic aorta (*white arrowhead*). Each is of normal caliber. (C) Axial image through the abdomen showing focal calcific deposits in the abdominal aorta (*black arrowhead*), which is also normal in caliber. LV = left ventricle; PA = main pulmonary artery.

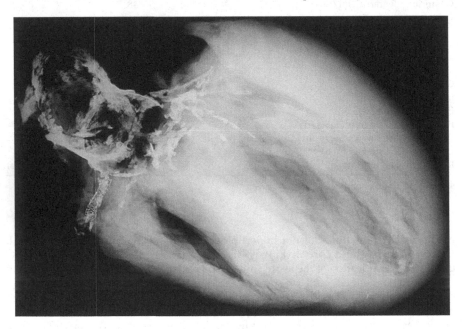

Figure 3 Radiograph of the patient's explanted heart showing massive diffuse calcific deposits in the ascending aorta, proximal epicardial coronary arteries, aortic valve cusps, and anterior mitral leaflet.

hypercholesterolemia generally have total cholesterol levels about 300 mg/dl and LDL-cholesterol levels about 200 mg/dl. Also, our patient's age (namely 38 years) when she was first discovered to have heart disease is obviously characteristic of the heterozygous variety and not of the homozygous variety. The latter group without lipid-lowering therapy usually dies in the teens, not in the fourth or fifth decade, as did our patient. Thus, although our patient did have diabetes mellitus

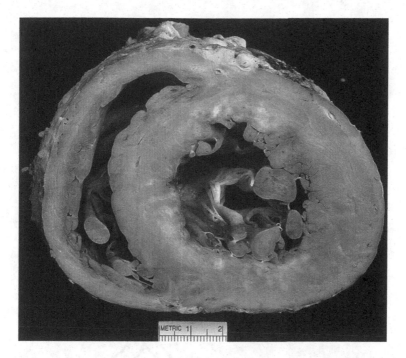

Figure 4 Photograph of the basal aspect of the heart showing both ventricular cavities to be dilated and the left ventricular free wall and ventricular septum to be focally scarred.

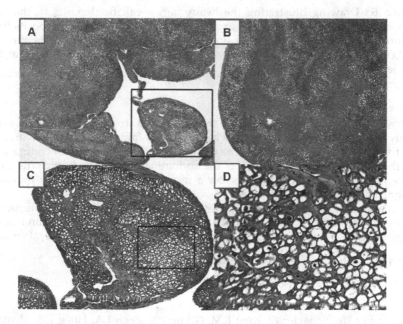

Figure 5 Photomicrographs of left ventricular subendocardial region, mainly papillary muscle, showing focal but extensive scarring and extensive vacuolization of myofibers. Trichrome stains: ×100 (A); ×40 (B); ×40 (C), and ×400 (D).

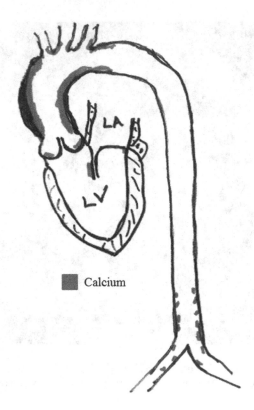

Figure 6 Drawing illustrating the heavy *diffuse* calcific deposits in the tubular portion of ascending aorta and arch and minimal focal calcific deposits in the abdominal aorta. Focal calcific deposits are present on the aortic aspects of each of the 3 cusps and on the ventricular aspect of anterior mitral leaflet. LA = left atrium; LV = left ventricle.

(discovered at age 38 years), we believe the evidence is strong—including the strong family history—that our patient had heterozygous familial hypercholesterolemia and that the latter is the cause of the diffuse calcification of the ascending aorta, and the minimal focal calcification of the abdominal aorta, a finding characteristic of the homozygous variety but possibly a more common finding they previously recognized in the heterozygous variety.

Although patients with diabetes mellitus or chronic renal disease for long periods of time may have calcific deposits in the ascending aorta, they are focal and smaller and not diffuse and large as in the patients with familial hypercholesterolemia.

DISCLOSURES

The authors have no conflicts of interest to disclose.

REFERENCES

1. Sprecher DL, Schaefer EJ, Kent KM, Gregg RE, Zech LA, Hoeg JM, Mcmanus B, Roberts WC, Brewer HB. Cardiovascular features of homozygous familial hypercholesterolemia: analysis of 16 patients. *Am J Cardiol* 1984;54:20–30.

2. Abramowitz Y, Jilaihawi H, Chakravarty T, Mack MJ, Makkar RR. Porcelain aorta. A comprehensive review. *Circulation* 2015;131:827–836.
3. Grenon SM, Lachapelle K, Marcil M, Omerogulu A, Genest J, Varennes BD. Surgical strategies for severe calcifications of the aorta (porcelain aorta) in two patients with homozygous familial hypercholesterolemia. *Am J Cardiol* 2007;23:1159–1161.

Case 1674 Origin of the Left Subclavian Artery as the First Branch and Origin of the Right Subclavian Artery as the Fourth Branch of the Aortic Arch with Crisscrossing Posterior to the Common Carotid Arteries

Junlin Zhang, MD, PhD, Joseph M. Guileyardo, MD, and William C. Roberts, MD

We describe an aortic arch anomaly consisting of the origin of the left subclavian artery as the fourth branch and the right subclavian artery as the first branch off the aortic arch with crisscrossing of these two arteries anterior to the trachea without clinical consequences. This anomaly, to our knowledge, has not been reported previously.

Anomalous origin of one or more arteries from the aortic arch (AA) is frequent. Liechty and associates[1] studied 1000 adult cadavers and found "departures from the anatomic norm" in 350 cases (35%). Karacan and colleagues[2] studied 1000 adults by computed tomographic angiography and found "variations from the norm in aortic arch branching patterns" in 208 cases (21%). Origin of the right subclavian artery (RSA) from the fourth branch of the AA with coursing to the right arm posterior to the AA is a relatively common AA anomaly. Origin of the RSA as the fourth AA branch, however, combined with origin of the left subclavian artery (LSA) as the first branch of the AA with crisscrossing posterior to the AA must be an extremely rare anomaly.

CASE DESCRIPTION

A 69-year-old hypertensive, diabetic, and obese (body mass index 39 kg/m²) woman had cardiac arrest outside the hospital the day of death. Forty days earlier, she had a debilitating stroke. Necropsy disclosed no grossly visible myocardial lesions and minimally narrowed coronary arteries. Examination of the AA disclosed the LSA to be the first branch and the RSA to be the fourth branch of the AA, and both coursed posterior to the AA and anterior to the trachea. The RSA coursed posterior to the LSA, and both coursed posterior to the common carotid arteries. The lumen of all four arteries arising from the AA were wide open (*Figure*).

DISCUSSION

We have found no example of the anomaly described herein in any previously published report.

From the Baylor Heart and Vascular Institute (Zhang, Roberts) and the Departments of Pathology (Guileyardo, Roberts) and Internal Medicine, Division of Cardiology (Roberts), Baylor University Medical Center at Dallas, Texas. Dr. Zhang is now with the Department of Physical Therapy, Arkansas State University.

Corresponding author: William C. Roberts, MD, Baylor Heart and Vascular Institute, Baylor University Medical Center, 3500 Gaston Avenue, Dallas, TX 75246 (e-mail: william.roberts1@bswhealth.org).

DOI: 10.1201/9781003408321-41

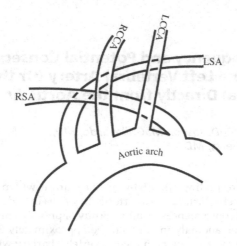

Figure 1   The origin of the arteries from the aortic arch. LCCA indicates left common carotid artery; LSA, left subclavian artery; RCCA, right common carotid artery; RSA, right subclavian artery.

REFERENCES

1. Liechty JD, Shields TW, Anson BJ. Variations pertaining to the aortic arches and their branches; with comments on surgically important types. *Q Bull Northwest Univ Med Sch* 1957;31(2):136–143.
2. Karacan A, Türkvatan A, Karacan K. Anatomical variations of aortic arch branching: evaluation with computed tomographic angiography. *Cardiol Young* 2014;24(3): 485–493.

Case 1675 Frequency and Potential Consequences of Origin of the Left Vertebral Artery (Or the Arteria Thryoidea Ima) Directly from the Aortic Arch

Junlin Zhang, MD, PhD, Joseph M. Guileyardo, MD, and William C. Roberts, MD

Described herein are findings in a 58-year-old man in whom necropsy disclosed origin of the left vertebral artery (or the arteria thryoidea ima) directly from the aortic arch. No functional consequences resulted. Study of previous publications disclosed the frequency of this anomaly in adults to be approximately 3.5%. Dissection has been reported to be more frequent in the left vertebral artery when it arises directly from the aorta than when it arises from the left subclavian artery.

We recently encountered, as an incidental autopsy finding, origin of the left vertebral artery (LVA) (or possibly the arteria thryoidea ima [ATI]) directly from the aortic arch (AA). Being unfamiliar with this variation, we studied previously published reports of its frequency and potential consequences. The results of that search and a brief description of the anomaly encountered in our patient is the purpose of this report.

CASE DESCRIPTION

A 58-year-old man died 10 years after bilateral lung transplantation for chronic obstructive lung disease. Figure 1 shows the AA with the anomalously arising artery between the left common carotid and the left subclavian arteries. The anomalous artery produced no apparent detrimental consequences.

DISCUSSION

The reported frequency of origin of the LVA from the AA among large numbers of patients studied at necropsy or by angiography/computed tomography is summarized in Table 1. Of 1000 subjects studied at *necropsy* by Liechty et al,[1] the LVA arose anomalously in 25 (2.5%). Of 6439 patients studied by *angiography/computed tomography* and reported by Komiyama et al,[2] Uchino et al,[3] Karacan et al,[4] Lale et al,[5] Huapaya et al,[6] and Tapia et al,[7] the LVA arose anomalously from the AA in 240 (3.7%). Additionally, four small necropsy studies (each <75 patients) found an anomalous LVA from the AA in 17 (8%) of 214 cases.[8–11]

Only one reported study of origin of the LVA from the AA has reported any hazardous consequences, and that was by Komiyama and colleagues,[2] who described by angiograms acute dissection in 4 of 21 patients (19%) having origin of the LVA from the AA. In contrast, these same authors described dissection by angiogram in 9 of 837 patients (1.1%) with LVA arising normally from the left subclavian artery.

From the Baylor Heart and Vascular Institute (Zhang, Roberts) and the Departments of Pathology (Guileyardo, Roberts) and Internal Medicine, Division of Cardiology (Roberts), Baylor University Medical Center at Dallas, Texas. Dr. Zhang is now with the Department of Physical Therapy, Arkansas State University.

Corresponding author: William C. Roberts, MD, Baylor Heart and Vascular Institute, Baylor University Medical Center, 3500 Gaston Avenue, Dallas, TX 75246 (e-mail: william.roberts1@bswhealth.org).

 DOI: 10.1201/9781003408321-42

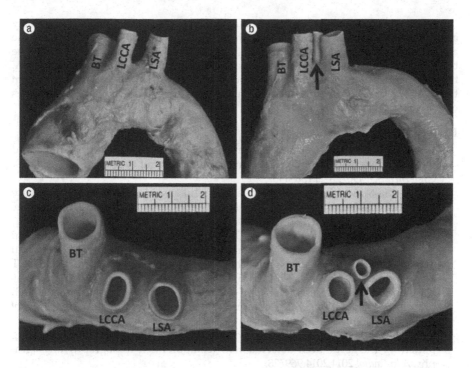

Figure 1 Photographs of the aortic arch showing the **(a)** (anterior view) and **(a′)** (superior view) *normal origin* of the three arteries (brachiocephalic trunk [BT]; left common carotid artery [LCCA], and left subclavian artery [LSA]) and **(b, b′)** origin of the left vertebral artery (LVA) directly from the aortic arch. The black arrow points to the anomalously arising LVA. (Photographs by Saba Ilyas.)

Table 1: Summary of the frequency of the left vertebral artery arising from the aortic arch

First author (year)	Number of patients	Age range (yrs)	Method of diagnosis	Frequency of the LVA arising from the AA
Liechty (1957)	1000	Adults	Autopsy	25 (2.5%)
Komiyama (2001)	860	—	Angio	21 (2.4%)
Uchino (2013)	2287	—	CT Angio	94 (4.1%)
Karacan (2014)	1000	17–94	CT Angio	41 (4.1%)
Lale (2014)	881	19–93	CT Angio	25 (2.8%)
Huapaya (2015)	361	—	CT Angio	8 (2.2%)
Tapia (2015)	1050	18–89	CT	51 (4.8%)
Total	7439	17–94		265 (3.5%)

Angio indicates angiography; AA, aortic arch; CT, computed tomography; LVA, left vertical artery; —, no information available.

This report has a major limitation. We were not able to follow the anomalously arising artery from the AA to its destination. Therefore, it is possible that the anomalously arising artery, rather than being the LVA, is the ATI. Both have been reported to arise directly from the AA, as in the present report. The LVA, however, appears to be the more common of the two to arise anomalously from the AA. No functional consequences have been reported when the ATI arises directly from the AA.

REFERENCES

1. Liechty JD, Shields TW, Anson BJ. Variations pertaining to the aortic arches and their branches; with comments on surgically important types. *Q Bull Northwest Univ Med Sch* 1957;31(2):136–143.
2. Komiyama M, Morikawa T, Nakajima H, Nishikawa M, Yasui T. High incidence of arterial dissection associated with left vertebral artery of aortic origin. *Neurol Med Chir (Tokyo)* 2001;41(1):8–11.
3. Uchino A, Saito N, Takahashi M, Okada Y, Kozawa E, Nishi N, Mizukoshi W, Nakajima R, Watanabe Y. Variations in the origin of the vertebral artery and its level of entry into the transverse foramen diagnosed by CT angiography. *Neuroradiology* 2013;55(5):585–594.
4. Karacan A, Türkvatan A, Karacan K. Anatomical variations of aortic arch branching: evaluation with computed tomographic angiography. *Cardiol Young* 2014;24(3):485–493.
5. Lale P, Toprak U, Yagiz G, Kaya T, Uyanik SA. Variations in the branching pattern of the aortic arch detected with computerized tomography angiography. *Adv Radiol* 2014;2014:969728.
6. Huapaya JA, Chávez-Trujillo K, Trelles M, Dueñas Carbajal R, Ferrandiz Espadin R. Anatomic variations of the branches of the aortic arch in a Peruvian population. *Medwave* 2015;15(6):e6194.
7. Tapia GP, Zhu X, Xu J, Liang P, Su G, Liu H, Liu Y, Shu L, Liu S, Huang C. Incidence of branching patterns variations of the arch in aortic dissection in Chinese patients. *Medicine (Baltimore)* 2015;94(17):e795.
8. Nayak SR, Pai MM, Prabhu LV, D'Costa S, Shetty P. Anatomical organization of aortic arch variations in the India: embryological basis and review. *J Vasc Bras* 2006;5(2):95–100.
9. Shin IY, Chung Y-G, Shin W-H, Im SB, Hwang SC, Kim BT. A morphometric study on cadaveric aortic arch and its major branches in 25 Korean adults: the perspective of endovascular surgery. *J Korean Neurosurg Soc* 2008;44(2):78–83.
10. Patil ST, Meshram MM, Kamdi NY, Kasote AP, Parchand MP. Study on branching pattern of aortic arch in Indian. *Anat Cell Biol* 2012;45(3):203–206.
11. Budhiraja V, Rastogi R, Jain V, Bankwar V, Raghuwanshi S. Anatomical variations in the branching pattern of human aortic arch: a cadaveric study from central India. *ISRN Anatomy* 2013;2013:828969.

Case 1705 Asymptomatic Ascending Aorta Aneurysm with Severe Aortic Regurgitation Caused by Multiple Intimal-Medial Tears Unassociated with Aortic Dissection

Carlos E. Velasco, MD[a,b,c],*, Helen Hashemi, MD[a], Christina P. Roullard, OMS[a], Juan Machannaford, MD[d], and William C. Roberts, MD[a,b,c,e]

A 62-year-old man was found to have an asymptomatic ascending aortic aneurysm (6.6 cm) associated with severe aortic regurgitation. Operative resection of the wall of the aneurysm disclosed its cause to be multiple healed intimal-medial tears without dissection involving a previously normal aorta. The concept of an intimal-medial tear unassociated with aortic dissection is a poorly recognized entity and these tears appear to be asymptomatic and after the aortic tearing lead to aneurysmal formation. © 2017 Elsevier Inc. All rights reserved. (Am J Cardiol 2018;121:668–669)

Aneurysms involving the ascending aorta have multiple causes.[1] When aneurysms involve both the sinus and the tubular portions, the etiology is usually the Marfan syndrome or forme fruste varieties of it and, histologically, there is severe loss of medial elastic fibers.[2] When aneurysms involve only the tubular portion of aorta, syphilis, systemic hypertension, and aortic dissection are the most common causes.[3-6] The occurrence of a large aneurysm involving both the sinus and the tubular portions of ascending aorta unassociated with dissection or with loss of medial elastic fibers is most unusual. Such was the case, however, in the patient to be described herein.

CASE REPORT

A 62-year-old white man with known systemic hypertension, dyslipidemia, and prostate cancer was referred to one of us (CEV) because of an asymptomatic ascending aortic aneurysm found on a routine chest x-ray. His indirect blood pressure was 155/50 mm Hg. He had no features of the Marfan syndrome. A grade 3/6 precordial diastolic blowing murmur was audible. Echocardiogram, computed tomogram (Figure 1), and aortogram (Figure 1) disclosed a large (6.6 cm) aneurysm involving both the sinus and the tubular portions of ascending aorta associated with severe aortic regurgitation (Figure 1). The left ventricular cavity was quite dilated.

[a]Division of Cardiology, Department of Internal Medicine, Baylor University Medical Center at Dallas, Dallas, Texas; [b]Baylor Jack and Jane Hamilton Heart and Vascular Hospital, Dallas, Texas; [c]Department of Internal Medicine, Texas A&M College of Medicine, Dallas Campus, Dallas, Texas; [d]Department of Cardiothoracic Surgery, Baylor University Medical Center at Dallas, Dallas, Texas; and [e]Department of Pathology, Baylor University Medical Center at Dallas, Dallas, Texas. Manuscript received November 29, 2017; revised manuscript received and accepted December 3, 2017.
* Corresponding author: Tel: (214) 826–6044; fax: (214) 370–3022.
E-mail address: carlos.velasco@bswhealth.org (C.E. Velasco).

DOI: 10.1201/9781003408321-43

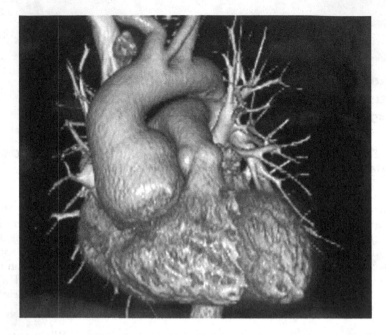

Figure 1 Spiral computed tomogram of the chest shows aneurysmal dilatation of the ascending aorta measuring up to 6.6 cm in diameter at the level of the takeoff of the left main coronary artery. There is no evidence of a dissection flap.

The direct left ventricular pressure was 120/18 mm Hg. The epicardial coronary arteries were free of significant narrowing.

The ascending aortic aneurysm was resected and the 3-cuspid nearly normal aortic valve was suture supported but not replaced.[7] Postbypass transesophageal echocardiogram demonstrated only trace aortic regurgitation and a less dilated left ventricular cavity. Four months after the operation, the patient was asymptomatic, and no precordial murmur was present.

The operatively excised wall of the ascending aorta is illustrated in Figure 2. On its intimal surface, several stretched out tears covered by fibrous tissue produced large gaps in the intima. The tears extended down to the outer media which was now covered by uniform fibrous tissue, allowing the thickness of stretched tears to be almost as thick as the nontorn portion of media. The adventitia was thickened by dense fibrous tissue, produced presumably by its contact with the adjacent structures (right atrium, pulmonary trunk, superior vena cava).

DISCUSSION

The concept of intimal-medial tears in the ascending aorta without accompanying aortic dissection has received little attention. Such tears without associated dissection are most common in patients with the Marfan syndrome and in the forme fruste varieties of the syndrome.[2] Such patients have associated severe loss of medial elastic fibers both in the stretched out tears and in the nontorn portions of the media, which often is quite thin. The present patient had multiple intimal-medial tears in the ascending aorta without accompanying aortic dissection and also without loss of medial elastic fibers or thinning of the nontorn aortic media. The appearance of the aneurysm, that is, involving both the sinus and the tubular portions, and of the aorta, however, is similar to that occurring in the Marfan patients. Despite our

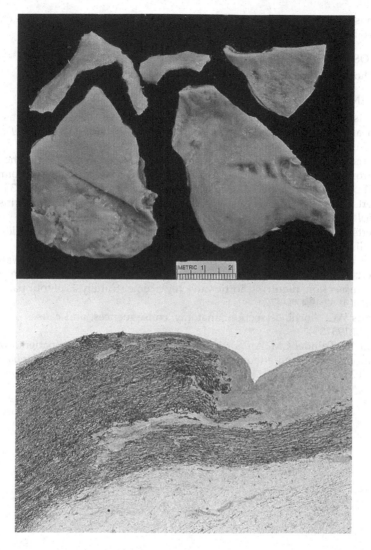

Figure 2 Shown in the upper panel are 5 fragments of ascending aorta excised at operation. The 2 larger portions show intimal-medial tears without dissection. The tears in some areas are "stretched out" and the surfaces of the resulting gaps are irregular and gray in color in contrast with the slightly yellow-colored surfaces of the normal portions of aorta. Shown in the lower panel is a photomicrograph at the site of 1 tear. The black-staining elastic fibers are torn and the resulting stretched portion at the site of the tear is now covered by fibromuscular connective tissue (Movat stain, x40).

patient's having multiple intimal-medial tears in the ascending aorta unassociated with dissection, at no time did he experience chest pain. Thus, these intimal-medial tears unaccompanied by dissection appear to be asymptomatic at the time of the tear and subsequently. It appears that the greater the number of intimal-medial tears, the greater the dilatation of the aorta irrespective of whether or not the nontorn portion of aorta is thinned. Also, the greater the aortic dilatation, the greater the chance of considerable aortic regurgitation.

DISCLOSURES

The authors have no conflicts of interests to disclose.

REFERENCES

1. Roberts WC. The aorta: its acquired diseases and their consequences as viewed from a morphologic perspective. In: Lindsay J Jr, Hurst JW, eds. *The Aorta.* New York: Grune & Stratton, Inc.; 1979:51–117.
2. Roberts WC, Honig HS. The spectrum of cardiovascular disease in the Marfan syndrome: a clinico-morphologic study of 18 necropsy patients and comparison to 151 previously reported necropsy patients. *Am Heart J* 1982;104:115–135.
3. Roberts WC, Ko JM, Vowels TJ. Natural history of syphilitic aortitis. *Am J Cardiol* 2009;104:1578–1587.
4. Roberts WC, Bose R, Ko JM, Henry AC, Hamman BL. Identifying cardiovascular syphilis at operation. *Am J Cardiol* 2009;104:1588–1594.
5. Waller BF, Zoltick JM, Rosen JH, Katz NM, Gomes MN, Fletcher RD, Wallace RB, Roberts WC. Severe aortic regurgitation from systemic hypertension (without aortic dissection) requiring aortic valve replacement: analysis of four patients. *Am J Cardiol* 1982;49:473–477.
6. Roberts WC. Aortic dissection: anatomy, consequences, and causes. *Am Heart J* 1981;101:195–214.
7. David TE, Feindel CM. An aortic valve-sparing operation for patients with aortic incompetence and aneurysm of the ascending aorta. *J Thorac Cardiovasc Surg* 1992;103:617–621.

Case 1739 Pseudoaneurysm of the Ascending Aorta at the Cannulation Site Diagnosed More Than Four Decades After Repair of Ventricular Septal Defect

Charles S. Roberts, MD[a,b,]*, Yusuf M. Salam, BS[c], Alastair J. Moore, MD[b,d], and William C. Roberts, MD[b,c,e]

Described herein is a 69-year-old woman who developed a large saccular aortic aneurysm at a previous cannulation site for repair of a ventricular septal defect at age 25 years. The aneurysm was resected and proved histologically to be a false one. The long interval between operations (44 years) exceeds those reported previously. © 2019 Published by Elsevier Inc. (Am J Cardiol 2019;124:1962–1965)

Although a pseudoaneurysm of the ascending aorta has many causes, the main one is a consequence of a previous penetration of the aortic wall during a cardiac or ascending aortic operation[1-6] (Figure 1). A number of publications have described results of reoperation to remove or repair the false aneurysm. None have provided gross or histologic descriptions of the pseudoaneurysm or emphasized the interval between the first operation and the reoperation. Such is the purpose of this report.

CASE DESCRIPTION

A 69-year-old white woman, who was born in December 1949, had a ventricular septal defect closed when she was 25 years of age. She thereafter was well until the age of 65 when she noted some transient nonspecific symptoms that prompted a chest radiograph which disclosed a right "suprahilar opacity" of uncertain etiology. A computed tomographic study then disclosed a saccular outpouching on the right side of the ascending aorta measuring up to 3.5 cm in maximal diameter (Figure 2). The aneurysm corresponded to the "suprahilar opacity" seen on chest radiograph.

The patient declined operative intervention on the aorta at that time and thereafter remained well until about a week before hospitalization at Baylor University Medical Center in May 2019, for transient nonspecific symptoms including nausea. Her body mass index was now 32 kg/m^2, up from 25 kg/m^2 4 years earlier. Repeat thoracic computed tomography now showed the saccular aneurysm to have a maximal diameter of 5.2 cm, a 33% increase during the previous 4 years. Coronary angiography showed a 70% diameter narrowing of the left anterior descending

[a]Department of Cardiac Surgery, Baylor University Medical Center, Baylor Scott & White Health, Dallas, Texas; [b]Department of Internal Medicine, Baylor University Medical Center, Baylor Scott & White Health, Dallas, Texas; [c]Baylor Scott & White Heart and Vascular Institute, Baylor University Medical Center, Baylor Scott & White Health, Dallas, Texas; [d]Department of Radiology, Baylor University Medical Center, Baylor Scott & White Health, Dallas, Texas; and [e]Department of Pathology, Baylor University Medical Center, Baylor Scott & White Health, Dallas, Texas. Manuscript received August 17, 2019; revised manuscript received and accepted September 10, 2019.
* Corresponding author: Tel: (469) 800–7760; fax: (469) 800–7770.
E-mail address: charles.roberts@bswhealth.org (C.S. Roberts).

0002-9149/© 2019 Published by Elsevier Inc.
https://doi.org/10.1016/j.amjcard.2019.09.023

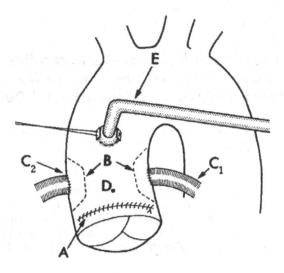

Figure 1 Drawing of the ascending aorta showing potential sites for development of pseudoaneurysm after a previous cardiac or ascending aortic operation. A = valvulotomy site; B = clamping site; C_1 and C_2 = anastomosis site; D = needle site; and E = cannulation site. Reproduced from Sullivan et al[1] with permission from publisher.

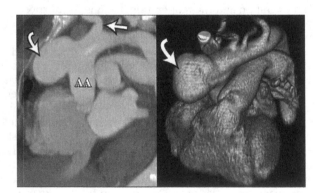

Figure 2 A computed tomography view (*left*) of the aneurysm in the ascending aorta (AA) aneurysm (*left arrow*) and a 3-dimensional volume rendering (*right*) derived from computed tomographic angiography. The off-axis oblique sagittal maximal intensity projection demonstrates the focal, saccular pouching-out (*curved arrow*) with a narrowed neck originating from the anteriolateral aspect of the mid tubular ascending aorta proximal to the origin of the innominate artery (*straight arrow*).

coronary artery and "irregularities" in the other major epicardial coronary arteries. Her blood hemoglobin was 7.4 g/L and the hematocrit was 25 mm/hour. The anemia proved to be an iron deficiency. One day before the operation, she was in atrial flutter; 1 day postoperatively she was in sinus rhythm (Figure 3).

At operation, the redo-sternotomy was uneventful, and aortic and atrial cannulation sites were prepared. After cardiopulmonary bypass was established, a high aortic crossclamp was applied and antegrade cardiologia delivered. A full

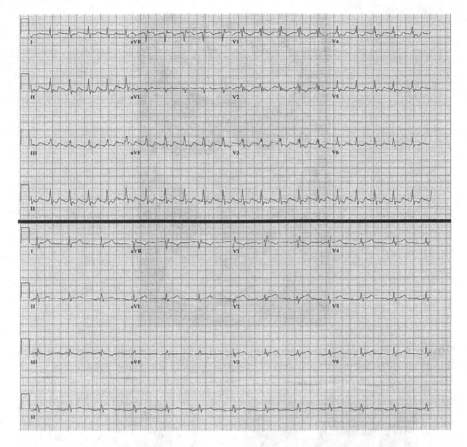

Figure 3 Electrocardiograms recorded just before (*upper*) and 1 day after resection of the aortic pseudoaneurysm (*lower*). Preoperatively, rapid atrial flutter is present and immediately postoperatively, sinus rhythm is present.

segment of aorta, including the mouth of the saccular aneurysm and the aneurysm itself, was resected, and replaced with a short, interposition 24 mm Dacron graft. No intraoperative or postoperative complication occurred.

Sutures partially covered by fibrous tissue were present at the junction of the normal-appearing aorta and the wall of the aneurysm. The wall of the aneurysm was much thinner than the wall of the adjacent aorta. The resected aneurysm weighed 9.6 g (Figure 4). Histologically, the wall of the adjacent aorta was normal. The wall of the aneurysm consisted of fibrous tissue, in most areas devoid of elastic fibers. No thrombus was present in the interior of the aneurysm (Figure 5).

DISCUSSION

The unique features of the present case are (1) the extremely long interval (44 years) between the aortic cannulation (used for cardiopulmonary bypass to close a ventricular septal defect) and the subsequent diagnosis of a saccular aneurysm in the ascending aorta, and (2) the presentation of the morphologic features (gross and histologic) of the saccular aneurysm, something not reported previously. Sullivan et al[1] summarized in 1988, thirty-one[1] previously reported

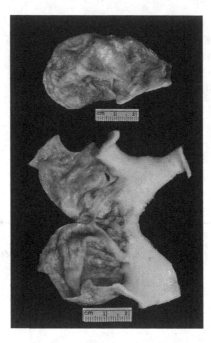

Figure 4 The intact false aneurysm (*upper*) and opened adjacent aorta and the aneurysm (*lower*). Sutures utilized 44 years earlier are shown by the arrows.

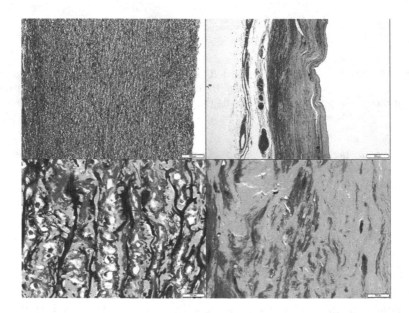

Figure 5 Photomicrographs of the aorta (*top left* and *bottom left*) and of the wall of the aneurysm (*top right* and *bottom right*). The aneurysmal wall is much thinner than the wall of the aorta. Movat stains: ×100 (*top left* and *top right*) and ×400 (*bottom left* and *bottom right*). Elastic fibers (black staining in the aortic media—*top left* and *bottom left*) and no elastic fibers in the wall of the aneurysm (*top right* and *bottom right*).

false aneurysms of the ascending aorta after previous operative penetration of the aortic wall: the mouth of the saccular aneurysm was at a previous aortic cannulation site in 11; at a saphenous venous insertion site for coronary artery bypass grafting in 8, and at the aortic incision done for an aortic valve operation in 12. The interval from the earlier operation to diagnosis of the pseudoaneurysm ranged from 1 to 108 months, with the interval in 13 being <6 months, mainly with superimposed infection and >30 months in only 9 patients, the longest being 108 months (9 years). Katsumata et al[2] described 10 patients with ascending aorta pseudoaneurysms and the longest interval between the 2 operations was 70 months (<12 months in 6, infection appearing to be the major culprit). Atik et al[3] described results in 42 patients who underwent ascending aortic pseudoaneurysm resection but the interval between the 2 operations is unclear. Malvindi et al[4] reviewed their experience with 43 patients who underwent a reoperation for postoperative development of an ascending aortic false aneurysm. The interval between the 2 operations ranged from 0.2 to 37 years (mean 8). Eusanio et al[5] encountered 22 ascending aortic false aneurysms after a previous operation but without information on the interval between operations. The stated interval in none of these reports was nearly as long as in the present patient.

Little data is available on the sizes of these false aneurysms. In none of the above reports was the size of the pseudoaneurysm described. Doria et al[7] reported an 8-cm-sized ascending aortic pseudoaneurysm and Parihas et al[8] described a 35-year-old man who had undergone aortic valve replacement and developed an ascending aortic pseudoaneurysm 5 months later. The aneurysm eroded through the sternum and reached a diameter of 10 cm.

The largest diameter of the pseudoaneurysm in the patient described herein was 5.2 cm. The inside of the aneurysm was devoid of thrombus. The wall of the adjacent aorta was histologically normal. In contrast, the wall of the aneurysm was much thinner than the wall of the adjacent aorta and it contained no elastic fibers, confirming that its wall was composed of structures different from the 3 layers of the aortic wall, the definition of a false one.

DISCLOSURES

The Authors have no commercial conflict of interest.

REFERENCES

1. Sullivan KL, Steiner RM, Smullens SN, Griska L, Meister SG. Pseudoaneurysm of the ascending aorta following cardiac surgery. *Chest* 1988;93:138–143.
2. Katsumata T, Moorjani N, Vaccari G, Westaby S. Mediastinal false aneurysm after thoracic aortic surgery. *Ann Thorac Surg* 2000;70:547–552.
3. Atik FA, Navia JL, Svensson LG, Vega PR, Feng J, Brizzo ME, Lytle BW. Surgical treatment of pseudoaneurysm of the thoracic aorta. *J Thorac Cardiovasc Surg* 2006;132:379–385.
4. Malvindi PG, Van Putte BP, Heijmen RH, Schepens MA, Morshuis WJ. Reoperation for aortic false aneurysms after cardiac surgery. *Ann Thorac Surg* 2010;90:1437–1443.
5. Eusanio MD, Berretta P, Bissoni L, Petridis FD, Marco LD, Bartolomeo RD. Re-operations on the proximal thoracic aorta: results and predictors of short- and long-term mortality in a series of 174 patients. *Eur J Cardiothorac Surg* 2011,40:1072 1076.
6. Malvindi PG, Cappai A, Raffa GM, Barbone A, Basciu A, Citterio E, Settepani E. Analysis of postsurgical aortic false aneurysm in 27 patients. *Tex Heart Inst J* 2013;40:274–280.

7. Doria E, Ballerini G, Pepi M. Giant anastomotic pseudoaneurysm after Bentall operation causing late postoperative cardiogenic shock. *Ital Heart J* 2001;2:627–630.
8. Parihar B, Choudhary LS, Madhu AP, Alpha MK, Thankachen R, Shukla V. Pseudoaneurysm of ascending aorta after aortic valve replacement. *Ann Thorac Surg* 2005;79:705–707.

Case 1773 Combined Cardiovascular Syphilis and Type A Acute Aortic Dissection

William C. Roberts, MD[a,b,c],*, and Charles S. Roberts, MD[a,d]

The occurrence of acute aortic dissection with the initiating tear in the ascending aorta superimposed on cardiovascular syphilis is an exceedingly rare occurrence. Such was the case, however, in a recently seen patient who presented with typical features of acute dissection (type A). Operative repair yielded the entire ascending aorta to examine both grossly and histologically and classic features of both conditions were observed. @2021 Elsevier Inc. All rights reserved. (Am J Cardiol 2022;168:159–162)

INTRODUCTION

A number of authors for many decades have listed cardiovascular syphilis as a potential predisposing factor for aortic dissection. We have been hesitant to accept this relationship because cardiovascular syphilis begins in the adventitia, causes severe focal loss of medial elastic fibers, replacing them with scar tissue, and considerable thickening of the intima. Aortic dissection, in contrast, is a medial disease associated with none or only minimal loss of its elastic fibers and is unassociated with thickening of either the adventitia or intima. Recently, we encountered for the first time a patient who underwent resection of the ascending aorta because of a large intimal-medial tear leading to dissection of the ascending aorta and beyond and associated with classic morphologic features of cardiovascular syphilis.

CASE STUDY

A 78-year-old man with known cerebral aneurysm and infarction was in his usual state of health until about one hour before admission to Baylor University Medical Center (BUMC) when while sitting watching television he suddenly passed out and when awakening noted severe right arm and chest pain and nausea. Emergency medical service brought him to the hospital. At examination, his blood pressure was 115 / 70 mm Hg. A precordial murmur was absent. The left-sided radial pulses were absent. His heart rate was 65 beats/minute. Not long after arriving to BUMC he had cardiac arrest. Cardiac resuscitation was initiated. Orotracheal intubation was carried out. Circulation was restored. A nasogastric tube was inserted. An electrocardiogram was negative for myocardial ischemia. Computed thoracic angiogram disclosed a type A acute aortic dissection (Figure 1). There was delayed

From the [a]Baylor Scott & White Heart and Vascular Institute, the Departments of [b]Internal Medicine, [c]Pathology, and [d]Cardiac and Thoracic Surgery, Baylor University Medical Center, Baylor Scott & White Health, Dallas, Texas. Manuscript received October 4, 2021; revised manuscript received and accepted October 29, 2021.
* Corresponding Author: William C. Roberts, MD, Baylor Scott & White Heart and Vascular Institute, 621 N. Hall Street, Suite H-030, Dallas, Texas 75226, (214) 820–7911 Office, (214) 820–7533 Fax
E-mail address: william.roberts1@bswhealth.org (W.C. Roberts).

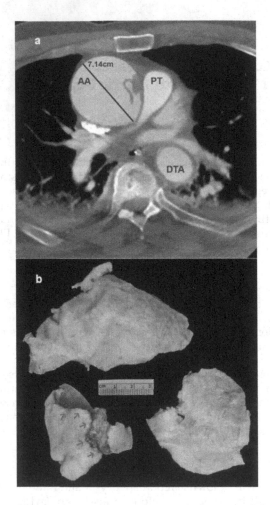

Figure 1 Shown here is the computer tomographic image of the heart and great arteries before the ascending aorta (AA) was resected. a The ascending aorta is hugely dilated, and it narrows a bit the adjacent pulmonary trunk (PT). The ascending aorta is much larger than the descending thoracic aorta (DTA). b Fragments of aorta resected by the surgeon (CSR). There is diffuse abnormality of the aortic intima -every square mm abnormal. The dissection tear is present in the lower left portion of this figure (arrows).

filling of the common carotid arteries and the right subclavian artery. At operation, a large tear was present just cephalad to the sino-tubular junction, the ascending aorta was resected, and the 3 aortic cusps were resuspended at their commissures (Figure 2.)

The ascending aorta was removed in 3 pieces, one of which contained a large intimal-medial tear that initiated the acute medial dissection (Figures 1 and 2). The intimal surface was diffusely abnormal. Histologically, (Figure 3) the adventitia was thickened by fibrosis tissue that contained numerous focal collections of plasmacytes and lymphocytes. Additionally, scattered in other areas of the adventitia were many eosinophils. The vasa vasora in the adventitia had thickened walls and narrowed

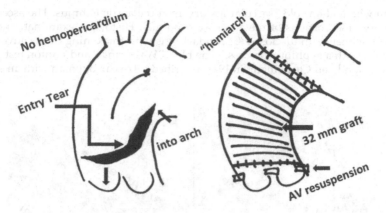

Figure 2 An illustration depicting the ascending aortic entry tear and the subsequent graft replacement.

lumens. The dissection was in the very outer media and often between the external elastic membrane and the outer media. There was massive loss of medial elastic fibers. The intima was thickened, mainly by fibrous tissue, and also by focal calcific deposits.

DISCUSSION

In the last 60 years we have studied about 200 patients with fatal acute aortic dissection at autopsy and also about 200 patients who had resection of the ascending aorta because of acute medial dissection (type A, zone 0).[1-16]

What are the classic morphologic features of cardiovascular syphilis? Exactly what are these features in the first 10 or so years after the occurrence of the presenting syphilitic lesion is unclear to us. The patients with cardiovascular syphilis we have studied at necropsy or after excision of the syphilitic aorta had their primary syphilitic lesion 15 to 40 years earlier. Thus, the aorta in them was thicker than normal due to fibrous thickening of the intima and fibrous thickening of adventitia. The fibrous tissue in the adventitia contained focal clumps of plasma cells and lymphocytes and thickened vasa vasora. The media was not thickened but there was extensive focal loss of its elastic fibers and occasionally inflammatory cells were present in this portion of the aorta. We have never seen *T. pallida* organisms in the aorta.

The classic morphologic lesion of acute aortic dissection is well known. A discrete intimal-medial tear is present (most commonly in the ascending portion and next most commonly in the descending thoracic aorta). The dissection is present in the media, usually in its outer portion, and neither the intima nor the adventitia is thickened. The media most commonly is normal before the onset of the dissection.[8]

Thus, aortic dissection is a medial disease and cardiovascular syphilis in a pan-aortic wall disease. Syphilis leads to medial scars which prevent propagation of the dissection and therefore make dissection an incredibly rare event in persons with cardiovascular syphilis. Indeed, cardiovascular syphilis might be viewed as a protective against the occurrence of aortic dissection.

As mentioned, the present case is the only one we have encountered in 60 years despite having a wide experience with both cardiovascular syphilis and aortic dissection.[1-16]

There have appeared, however, publications describing aortic dissection and cardiovascular syphilis in the same patient. Weiss[17] in 1938 described a 61-year-old woman who had an "old" saccular aneurysm at the aortic isthmus. The ascending and transverse portions of the aorta were normal. Histologic examination of the wall of the aneurysm disclosed ". . . endarteritis with thickening of the adventitia. consistent with a syphilitic process." The blood Wasserman and Hinton tests were positive. Bland and Castleman[18] in 1941 described a 47-year-old man with an earlier

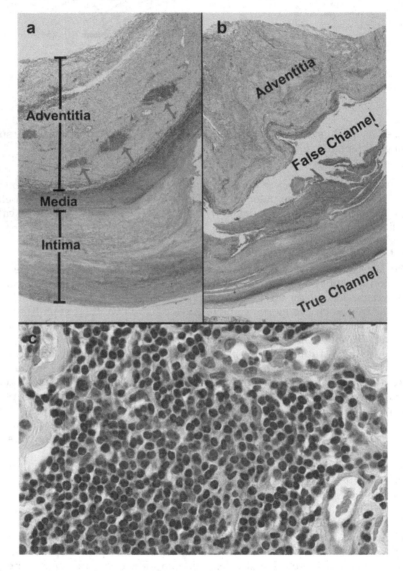

Figure 3 Shown here are photomicrographs of the ascending aorta in the patient described. a A section of the aorta showing the adventitia, the media, and the intima. The intima and adventitia are greatly thickened by fibrous tissue and the media, although not thickened, has lost most of its elastic fibers. Clumps of cells shown in c are designated by the arrows in the adventitia in a. b Section of aorta; the false channel is in the very outer media. The adventitia again is quite thick. c A close up of some of the cells designated by the arrow in a.

penile lesion, positive blood Hinton reaction, who had ". . . stellate scarring and linear tree barking . . ." in the tubular portion of aorta and its arch and a transverse intimal-medial tear about 2 cm cephalad to the sino-tubular junction. "The dissection had not ascended above the point of intimal tear, stopping short at the point where the syphilitic aortitis became evident." The authors indicated ". . . that the syphilitic scarring prevented the distal extension of the dissection." These were insightful comments. Other cases of both cardiovascular syphilis and aortic dissection have been described but the descriptions of the cardiovascular syphilis were inadequate to confirm its presence.[19]

DECLARATION OF INTERESTS

The authors declare that they have no known competing financial interests or personal relationships that could have appeared to influence the work reported in this paper.

REFERENCES

1. Roberts WC. Aortic dissection: Anatomy, consequences, and causes. *Am Heart J* 1981;101:195–214.
2. Warnes CA, Kirkmen PM, Roberts WC. Aortic dissection in more than one family member. *Am J Cardiol* 1985;55:236–238.
3. Roberts WC, Statler LF, Wallace RB. Hemodynamic confirmation of peripheral pulmonary stenosis caused by aortic dissection. *Am J Cardiol* 1989;63:1418–1420.
4. Roberts CS, Roberts WC. Aortic dissection with the entrance tear in transverse aorta: Analysis of 12 autopsy patients. *Ann Thor Surg* 1990;50:762–766.
5. Roberts CS, Roberts WC. Dissection of the aorta associated with congenital malformation of the aortic valve. *J Am Coll Cardiol* 1991;17:712–716.
6. Roberts CS, Roberts WC. Aortic dissection with the entrance tear in the descending thoracic aorta: Analysis of 40 necropsy patients. *Ann Surg* 1991;213:356–358.
7. Roberts CS, Roberts WC. Combined thoracic aortic dissection and abdominal aortic fusiform aneurysm. *Ann Thor Surg* 1991;52:537–540.
8. Roberts WC, Vowels TJ, Ko JM, Guileyardo JM. Acute aortic dissection with tear in ascending aorta not diagnosed until necropsy or operation (for another condition) and comparison to similar cases receiving proper operative therapy. *Am J Cardiol* 2012;110:728–735.
9. Roberts WC, Kapoor P, Main ML, Guileyardo JM. Acute aortic dissection with intussusception of the partition between the true and false channels leading to near total aortic occlusion (true aortic stenosis). *Am J Cardiol* 2017;119:340–344.
10. Roberts WC, Ko JM, Vowels TJ. Natural history of syphilitic aortitis. *Am J Cardiol* 2009;104:1578–1587.
11. Roberts WC, Bose R, Ko JM, Henry AC, Hamman BL. Identifying cardiovascular syphilis at operation. *Am J Cardiol* 2009;104:1588–1594.
12. Roberts WC, Lensing FD, Kourlis H Jr, Ko JM, Newberry JW, Smerud MJ, Burton EC, Hebeler RF Jr. Full blown cardiovascular syphilis with aneurysm of the innominate artery. *Am J Cardiol* 2009;104:1595–1600.
13. Roberts WC, Vowels TJ, Kitchens BL, Ko JM, Filardo G, Henry AC, Hamman BL, Matter GJ, Hebeler RF Jr. Aortic medial elastic fiber loss in acute ascending aortic dissection. *Am J Cardiol* 2011;108:1639–1644.
14. Barbin CM, Weissenborn MR, Ko JM, Guileyardo JE, Roberts WC. Computed tomographic and morphologic features of syphilis of the aorta. *Am J Cardiol* 2015;116:1311–1314.
15. Roberts WC, Kondapalli N. Operative recognition of syphilis of the aorta. *Am J Cardiol* 2018;122:898–904.

16. Roberts WC, Moore AJ, Roberts CS. Syphilitic aortitis: Still a current common cause of aneurysm of the tubular portion of ascending aorta. *Cardiovasc Pathol* 2020;46:107175.
17. Weiss S. Dissecting aneurysm of the aorta. *N Eng J Med* 2009;218:512–517.
18. Mallory TB. Cabot case 27302—(Bland EF and Castleman B). Dissecting aneurysm of the aorta with rupture into pericardium. *N Eng J Med* 1941;225:155–159.
19. Flaxman N. Dissecting aneurysm of the aorta. *Am Heart J* 1942:654–664.

Index

Note: Page numbers in *italics* indicate a figure and page numbers in **bold** indicate a table on the corresponding page.

A

abdominal aortic aneurysm, 189–191, *190*
acetaminophen overdose, massive
    cardiac consequences, 75–78
    laboratory test after ingestion, **78**
    left ventricular myocardium, *78*
    myocardium, histologic sections of, 75, *77*
    patient history, 75
    ventricular septum, *76*
adrenalin, 35
alveolar septum, 42, *44*
alveolitis, 46
amitriptyline, 96
annular subvalvular left ventricular
    aneurysms, 133
anticoagulation, 17
aortic aneurysm, 166
    massive perigraft, 177–181, *178–180*
    mechanism of, *204*
aortic arch anomaly, 214, *215*
aortic arch syndrome, 127, 140
aortic dissection, 173, 185, *186–188*,
    187–188, 231
    multiple intimal-medial tears with,
        219–221, *220, 221*
aortico-left ventricular tunnel (ALVT), in
    adulthood, *79*
aortic regurgitation, 151, 177
aortic rupture, fatal, 202–204, *203, 204*
aortic stenosis, 192
aortic valve cusps, 86
aortic valve replacement, 192–194, *193*
aortitis, and myocarditis, 133
aortitis, idiopathic, 129
ascending aorta, 183–184, *184*
    calcific deposits, 207
    and minimal focal calcification, 207–210,
        208, **209**, *210, 211*, 212
Aspergillus fumigatus thrombi, 63–65, *64, 65*
atherosclerosis, risk factors, 169
atherosclerotic plaque, 66, 91
atrioventricular nodes, 52
atypical bacteria, significance of, 151
autopsy
    rubella syndrome, 156, *157, 158*
    traumatic left ventricular aneurysm,
        13–14

B

Bentall procedure, 181
bilateral interstitial nephritis, 20, *21*
birefringent particles, 46
blood cultures, 148
blood urea nitrogen, 19
blunt chest trauma, 15, 202, *203*
bone marrow aspiration, 4
butyl nitrite, 170

C

calcific deposits, 26, 29, *32*, 34, 35, 86; *see also*
    massive calcific deposits
    in ascending aorta, 207
    atherosclerotic, 33
cardiac arrest, fatal, 204
cardiac aspergillosis, 63
cardiac tamponade, 21–22
    and cholesterol pericarditis with congenital
        hypothyroidism, 80–83, *81–83*
cardiac transplantation, 93–95, *95*
cardiopulmonary bypass, 16
cardiopulmonary resuscitation, 96
cardiovascular disease, radiation-induced,
    85–89
cardiovascular syphilis, 199
    examination, 233
    morphologic features of, 231
    patient history, 229, 230
chloramphenicol, 144
cholesterol pericarditis, 80–83, *81–83*
chronic kidney disease, 209
chronic thromboembolic disease, 98
circulatory impairment, 30
Citrobacter freundii, 97
clicks, systolic, 55–57, *55–57*
cocaine intoxication, 171, *172*
computed tomography
    ascending aorta, 230, *230*
    heterozygous familial
        hypercholesterolemia, 208
    massive calcific deposits, 115, *116*
    pseudoaneurysm, 223, *224*
congenital hypothyroidism
    cholesterol pericarditis and cardiac
        tamponade with, 80–83, *81–83*

foam cells, 81, *82*
heart at necropsy, 81
lipid deposits on epicardium, 81, *82*, 83
L-triiodothyronine, 80
patient history, 80–81
coronary angiography, 89, 114, 208, 223
coronary artery bypass graft, 208, 227
coronary cinearteriography, 12
coronary panarteritis, *147*
corticosteroids, 121

D

death in disco, 168–170, *169*
diabetes mellitus, 209
and chronic kidney disease, 209
Mönckeberg's calcinosis and, 35
diastolic murmur, 58–62, *59*, *60*
diuretic therapy, 70–74
dual-chamber transvenous pacemaker, 93
dyspnea, with hemoglobin SC disease
diagnosis, 96–101
imaging studies, 97–98
laboratory tests, 96–97, **97**
microscopic examination, 97
muscular pulmonary artery, *102*, *103*
pathology report, 101–104
patient history, 96–97

E

echocardiogram
massive calcific deposits, 114, 115, *116*
pericardial effusion, massive bloody,
111, *112*
perigraft aortic aneurysm, 177, *179*
electrocardiogram
acetaminophen overdose, massive, 75, *76*
acute dissecting aortic aneurysm,
complications of, 163
congenital hypothyroidism, 80
Gaucher's disease, 4, 5
idiopathic panaortitis, 127, *128*
massive calcific deposits, *117*
Mönckeberg's calcinosis, 27, *28*
pericardial effusion, massive bloody,
111, *112*
pseudoaneurysm, 224, *225*
pulmonary arterial and venous
hypertension, 66, *67*
pulseless disease, 142
rubella syndrome, 154, *155*
schizophrenia, 72, *72*, *73*
traumatic left ventricular aneurysm, 11,
12, *13*
ventricular septal defect, isolated, 107,
108, 109

endocarditis, infective, 149
eosinophilic nodular lesions, of glomerular
lobules, 29, *33*
erythromycin, 144
Escherichia coli, 97

F

familial hypercholesterolemia, 168
calcific deposits, 208–209
patient history, 207–208
foam cells, 81, *82*

G

ganglionitis, 52
Gaucher cells, 3, 5–6, 8, 9
Gaucher's disease
diagnosis, 4–5, 5, *6*, 9
heart, 5, *6*
muscular pulmonary arteries, 6, *7*
neurological signs, 3
patient history, 4–8
pulmonary alveolar capillaries, 5, *7*
giant cell chronic arteritis, 132
glomerulosclerosis, intercapillary, 29
glycolipid, 8
granulomatous myocarditis, 130, 132, 133
Graves' disease, 121–123, *122*, **123**

H

hemoglobin SC disease
diagnosis, 96–101
imaging studies, 97–98
laboratory tests, 96–97, **97**
microscopic examination, 97
muscular pulmonary artery, *102*, *103*
pathology report, 101–104
patient history, 96–97
hemosiderin-laden macrophages, 46–47, *47*
hepatosplenomegaly, 4
heroin, 42
hyperbetalipoproteinemia, 168
hypercholesterolemia, 169
hypokalemia, 73
hypoxemia, 100

I

idiopathic aortitis, 129
idiopathic panaortitis
diagnosis, 127, *128*
examination, 127, 129–135
patient history, 127, 129
idiopathic pulseless disease, 127, 129
immunoelectrophoresis, 142

inflammatory infiltrate, 150–151
innominate artery aneurysm, 195–199, *196–197, 199–201*

L

laparotomy, 49
left atrial appendage, 37–39, *39*
left main coronary artery (LMCA), 91
left ventricular calcification, 66–69, *67–69*
left ventricular cavity, massive calcific
    deposits in
    clinical findings, 114
    examination, 118–119, **119**
    patient history, 114–117
left vertebral artery (LVA), 216, *217*, **217**, 218
leukocytosis, 107, 150
lipid deposits, 81, *82*, 83
liquid protein-modified-fast (LPMF) diet, 52
low density lipoprotein (LDL), 168
L-triiodothyronine, 80

M

malignant hypertension
    bilateral interstitial nephritis, 20, *21*
    cardiac tamponade, 21–22
    necropsy findings, 20–21
    patient history, 19–20
    renal cortical hemorrhages, 20, *21*
    renal pelvis, 20, *23*
    renal tubular changes, 20, *22*
Marfan syndrome, 177
massive acetaminophen overdose
    cardiac consequences, 75–78
    laboratory test after ingestion, **78**
    left ventricular myocardium, *78*
    myocardium, histologic sections of, 75, *77*
    patient history, 75
    ventricular septum, *76*
massive calcific deposits
    of ascending aorta and minimal focal
        calcification, 207–210, *208*, **209**, *210*, *211*, 212
    clinical findings, 114
    examination, 118–119, **119**
    patient history, 114–117
massive hemoptysis, 9
methylphenidate, 42
microvascular infarction, 100
microvascular occlusion, 100
miliary tubercules, 133
Mönckeberg's calcinosis
    abdominal arteries, 29, *31*, *32*
    calcific deposits, 29, *32*, 34, 35
    circulatory impairment, 30
    coronary arteries, 29, *30*

and diabetes mellitus, 35
diagnosis, 27, *27*, *28*
eosinophilic nodular lesions of
    glomerular lobules, 29, *33*
examination, 26–27
in heart, 27–28
histologic examination, 29
intercapillary glomerulosclerosis, 29
patient history, 26–31
postmortem roentgenograms, 29, *30*, *32*
transmural myocardial scar, 29, *29*
monoclonal gammopathy, 150
multiple myeloma, 149–150
mural thrombosis, 15–16
muscular pulmonary arteries, 6, 7
myocardial contusion, 15–16
myocardial infarction, 58
myocardial scar, transmural, 29, *29*
myocarditis, aortitis and, 133
myocarditis, focal granulomatous, 132

N

necropsy
    acetaminophen overdose, massive, 75
    cardiovascular and pulmonary diseases
        (CPC), 168
    idiopathic panaortitis, 129, *130*
    innominate artery, 197
    massive calcific deposits, 116
    perigraft aortic aneurysm, 177, *180*
    pulseless disease, 144–145, *145*
    radiation-induced cardiovascular
        disease, 85
    sudden death, 183
nephritis, interstitial, 20, *21*, 22–24
neuritis, 52
nonpenetrating chest trauma, 15
nonpenetrating trauma, 106–109

O

"osseous pinch" theory, 203

P

panaortitis, idiopathic
    diagnosis, 127, *128*
    examination, 127, 129–135
    patient history, 127, 129
penicillin, 140, 141, 143, 144
pericardial effusion, massive bloody
    diagnosis, 111–113
    laboratory test, **113**
    patient history, 111
pericardial friction rub, 20
pericardiocentesis, 111, 112

pericardium, *138*
peri-composite graft aneurysm, 179
perigraft aortic aneurysm, *180*
peripheral pulmonary stenosis, 173, *174,*
    175, 176
peritoneal dialysis, 27
phonocardiogram
    pulseless disease, 144
    systolic clicks, 55, *55*
pleural tuberculosis, 96
"porcelain" aorta, 208
portopulmonary hypertension, 98
precordial murmur, 108–109
prednisone, 49
prolonged QT interval-ventricular
    tachycardia syndrome, 52–54, *53, 54*
pseudoaneurysm
    examination, 225, 227
    features of, 225
    operation, 224–225
    patient history, 223–224
pulmonary alveolar capillaries, 5, *7*
pulmonary arterial and venous
    hypertension, 66–69, *67–69*
pulmonary artery, right
    severe obstruction of, 166
    stenosis of, 163, *164–166,* 167
pulmonary embolism, 99
pulmonary granulomatosis, self-induced,
    42–47
    alveolar septum, 42, *44*
    birefringent particles, 46
    diagnosis, 44–47
    hemosiderin-laden macrophages, 46–47, *47*
    necropsy findings, 42–44, **45**
    patient history, 42
    pulmonary and cardiac findings, 42
    pulmonary function, alterations in, 46
    pulmonary hypertension, 42, *44*
    talc granulomas in pulmonary
        interstitium, 42, *43*
pulmonary hypertension, 42, 44, 66, 69, 98
pulmonic valve, acute rupture of
    balloon-tipped catheter withdrawal, 58–62
    cusp, 62
    diastolic murmur, 58–62, *59, 60*
    nitroprusside infusion, 58
    patient history, 58–59
    regurgitation, 59
pulmonic valve cusp, *50,* 58, 59, 62
pulmonic valve regurgitation, 59
pulseless disease, 127
    diagnosis, 127, *128*
    examination, 148–152
    example of, 129–130
    histologic study, 151
    idiopathic form, 127

pathologic findings, 135
patient history, 127, 129, 140–142
prepulseless phase of, 140–152, *142, 143,*
    145–149
serum electrophoresis, 142, *142*

R

radiation-induced cardiovascular disease
    clinical and necropsy findings, 85
    examination, 86
    morphologic findings, 86–87
    patient history, 85–86
    treatment, 88
radiography
    congenital hypothyroidism, 80
    massive calcific deposits, 115, *116*
    pericardial effusion, massive bloody,
        111, *111*
    schizophrenia, 72, *72*
    systolic clicks, 55, *56*
    ventricular septal defect, isolated, 106, *107*
radiotherapy, 85
redo-sternotomy, 224
renal cortical hemorrhage, 20, *21*
renal insufficiency, 24
renal pelvis, 20, *23*
renal sonogram, pericardial effusion, 112
right pulmonary artery
    severe obstruction of, 166
    stenosis of, 163, *164–166,* 167
right subclavian artery, 214
right ventricular outflow obstruction, 49–51
rituximab, 121
roentgenogram
    Gaucher's disease, 4, *6, 9*
    idiopathic panaortitis, 127, *128*
    Mönckeberg's calcinosis, 27, *27, 28*
    pulmonic valve, acute rupture of, 58
    pulseless disease, 142, *143*
    traumatic left ventricular aneurysm,
        11, *12*
roentgenologic interpretation, 152
rofecoxib, 96
rubella syndrome
    characteristic vascular lesion in, 159
    clinical manifestations, 160–161
    diagnosis, 154
    features of, 154
    histology, 158, *159*
    patient history, 154–158

S

schizophrenia
    chest radiography, 72, *72*
    diagnosis, *72,* 72–73, *73*

diuretic therapy, 70–74
  fatal water intoxication, 70–74
  patient history, 70–72
  treatment, 73–74
sickle cell chronic lung disease, 101
sickle cell disease, 100
sputum culture, 97, 98
stenosis
  of coronary ostium, 85–89, *87, 88*
  of right pulmonary artery, 163,
    164–166, 167
streptomycin, 143, 144
sucking action
  left atrial appendage, 37–39, *39*
  negative pressures within ventricles, 40
  patient history, 37
  role of hemorrhage from right ventricle,
    40–41
sudden coronary death, 169–170
sudden death, 183–184, *184*
sulfamethoxazole, 96
supra-aortic arteries, 127–138, *136*
suprahilar opacity, 223
symptomatic coronary heart disease, 169
syphilis *see* cardiovascular syphilis
systemic hypertension, 26
  diuretic therapy for, 70–74
systolic clicks, 55–57, *55–57*

T

Takayasu's arteriopathy, 150
talc granulomas, 42, *43*
thoracic aorta, *134, 135,* 144, 156
thrombocytopenia, in pregnancy, 122–123
thrombotic thrombocytopenic purpura
    (TTP), 121–123, *122,* **123**
thrombus
  in pulmonic valve cusps, 49, *50*
  right ventricular outflow obstruction
    from, 49–51
  in right ventricular outflow tract, 49, *50*
traumatic aortic rupture, 202

traumatic left ventricular aneurysm
  autopsy, 13–14
  coronary cinearteriography, 12
  coronary thrombosis, 15
  diagnosis, 11–13, *12–14*
  left cineventriculograms, 13, *14*
  left ventricular thrombus, 13, *14*
  mural thrombosis, 15–16
  operative findings, 11–12
  patient history, 11–14
  postoperative embolization, 16
  treatment, 11–12
tricuspid regurgitation, 151
trimethoprim, 96
TTP *see* thrombotic thrombocytopenic
    purpura (TTP)
type II hyperlipoproteinemia, 168

U

urinalysis, 19, 24, 97, 141

V

Valsalva maneuver, 144
vascular cell adhesion molecule 1
    (VCAM-1), 100
ventricular diastolic pressure, 40
ventricular septal defect, 94
  nonpenetrating trauma, 106–109
  patient history, 106
  precordial examination, 106
  precordial murmur, 108–109
  spectral phonocardiogram, *107*
ventricular septum, *76*
very low density lipoprotein, 168
vitamin D, 35

W

warfarin sodium, 11
"water-hammer" effect, 203
water intoxication, fatal, 70–74

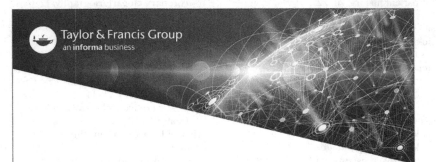

Printed in the United States
by Baker & Taylor Publisher Services